Regional Therapeutics for Advanced Malignancies

WITHDRAWN FROM STOCK

Regional Therapeutics for Advanced Malignancies

Editor

Martin D. Goodman
MD FACS
Assistant Professor of Surgery
Tufts Medical Center
Director of the Peritoneal Surface Malignancy Program
Boston, Massachusetts, USA

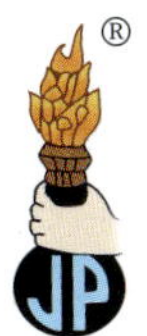

JAYPEE BROTHERS MEDICAL PUBLISHERS (P) LTD

New Delhi • Panama City • London

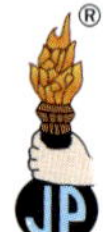
Jaypee Brothers Medical Publishers (P) Ltd

Headquarter
Jaypee Brothers Medical Publishers (P) Ltd
4838/24, Ansari Road, Daryaganj
New Delhi 110 002, India
Phone: +91-11-43574357
Fax: +91-11-43574314
Email: jaypee@jaypeebrothers.com

Overseas Offices

JP Medical Ltd
83 Victoria Street London
SW1H 0HW (UK)
Phone: +44-2031708910
Fax: +02-03-0086180
Email: info@jpmedpub.com

Jaypee-Highlights Medical Publishers Inc
City of Knowledge, Bld 237, Clayton
Panama City, Panama
Phone: +507-301-0496
Fax: +507-301-0499
Email: cservice@jphmedical.com

Website: www.jaypeebrothers.com
Website: www.jaypeedigital.com

Inquiries for bulk sales may be solicited at: jaypee@jaypeebrothers.com

Regional Therapeutics for Advanced Malignancies

First Edition: **2012**

ISBN 978-93-5025-887-3

Printed at: Ajanta Offset & Packagings Ltd., New Delhi

Dedicated to

My kids Rachel, Max and Simon
Who make me proud to be called their Dad.

All patients with cancer, their families and
caregivers who face this disease head on.

Contributors

Abby Crume DO
Surgical Resident
Maine Medical Center
Portland, Maine, USA

Andrea Cercek MD
Assistant Attending
Gastrointestinal Oncology Service
Memorial Sloan-Kettering Cancer
Center, New York, NY, USA

Andrew Hayes MA PhD FRCS
Consultant Surgeon
Sarcoma and Melanoma Unit
Royal Marsden Hospital
London, United Kingdom

Anne Garrison MD
Assistant Professor
Division of Gynecologic Oncology
University of Massachusetts
Medical Center
Worcester, Massachusetts, USA

Benedict D.T. Daly MD
Professor and Chairman
Department of Cardiothoracic Surgery
Boston Medical Center
Boston, Massachusetts, USA

C. William Helm MA MB.BChir
Professor, Gynecologic Oncology
Gynecology and Women's Health
Saint Louis University
School of Medicine
St Louis, Missouri, USA

Chaitan K. Narsule MD
Fellow, Department of
Cardiothoracic Surgery
Boston Medical Center
Boston, Massachusetts, USA

Daniel C. Wiener MD
Assistant Professor of Surgery
Division of Thoracic Surgery
Tufts Medical Center
Boston, Massachusetts, USA

David L. Bartlett MD FACS
Bernard Fisher Professor of Surgery
Vice Chairman Surgical Oncology
Director of the David D. Koch
Regional Perfusion Cancer
Therapy Center
Director of the Multidisciplinary
Disease Site Clinical and Research
Programs
University of Pittsburgh Medical
Center and Research Institute
Pittsburgh, Pennsylvania, USA

Douglas L. Fraker MD FACS
Jonathan E. Rhoads Professor of
Surgical Science
Chief Division of Endocrine and
Oncologic Surgery
Hospital of the University of
Pennsylvania
Philadelphia, Pennsylvania, USA

Giorgos C. Karakousis MD
Assistant Professor of Surgery
Hospital of the University of
Pennsylvania
Philadelphia, Pennsylvania, USA

H. Richard Alexander Jr MD FACS
Professor of Surgery
Associate Chairman for Clinical
Research, Surgery
Division of Surgical Oncology
University of Maryland School of
Medicine, Baltimore, Maryland, USA

Haroon A. Choudry MD FACS
Assistant Professor of Surgery
University of Pittsburgh Medical
Center and Research Institute
Pittsburgh, Pennsylvania, USA

Hebat Allah Mohamed Saad El-Din Fouad
Assistant Lecturer at the
Department of Radiology
Faculty of Medicine
Cairo University Hospitals
(Kasr Al-Ainiteaching Hospital)
Cairo, Egypt

Hiran C. Fernando MBBS FRCS FACS
Associate Professor
Department of Cardiothoracic Surgery
Director
Minimally Invasive Thoracic Surgery
Boston Medical Center
Boston, Massachusetts, USA

Jesus Esquivel MD FACS
Director
Peritoneal Surface Malignancy Program
St Agnes Hospital
Baltimore, Maryland, USA

Lisa Rutstein MD FACS
Associate Professor of Surgery
Department of Surgical Oncology
Maine Medical Center
Portland, Maine, USA

Martin D. Goodman MD FACS
Assistant Professor of Surgery
Director of the Peritoneal Surface
Malignancy Program
Tufts Medical Center
Boston, Massachusetts, USA

Nancy E. Kemeny MD
Attending Physician
Memorial Sloan-Kettering
Cancer Center
Professor of Medicine
Weill Medical College at Cornell
University, New York, NY, USA

Neil A. Christie MD FRCS(C) FACS
Assistant Professor of Surgery
Department of Cardiothoracic Surgery
University of Pittsburgh Medical
Center, Pittsburgh, Pennsylvania, USA

Paul H. Sugarbaker MD FACS FRCS
Director, Program in Peritoneal
Surface Malignancy
Washington Hospital
Washington DC, USA

Robert C.G. Martin II MD PhD FACS
Sam and Lolita Weakley Endowed
Chair in Surgical Oncology
Professor of Surgery
Director, Division of Surgical Oncology
University of Louisville
School of Medicine
Louisville, Kentucky, USA

Sarah H. Hughes MD
Assistant Professor
Division of Gynecologic Oncology
University of Massachusetts
Medical Center
Worcester, Massachusetts, USA

Sarah McPartland MD
Surgical Resident
Tufts Medical Center
Boston, Massachusetts, USA

Susan B. Kesmodel MD FACS
Assistant Professor
Division of Surgical Oncology
University of Maryland
School of Medicine
Baltimore, Maryland, USA

Terence C. Chua BMedSc (Hons) MBBS MRCS (Ed)
Hepatobiliary and Surgical
Oncology Unit, St George Hospital
Sydney, Australia

Tim Pencavel MB BS MRCS
Surgical Research Fellow
Sarcoma/Melanoma Unit
The Royal Marsden Hospital
London, United Kingdom

Preface

As I started my career, I never thought I would be a surgical oncologist treating patients with advanced and metastatic malignancies. As treatment modalities improve, more and more patients are living longer. Palliation for patients has been shown to improve not only quality of life but improve survival. At times, when there appeared to be no hope, advanced treatments can turn a hopeless situation into a chronic problem. Over the past 25 years, the use of multimodality treatments has been proven time and time again to be the approach to treat cancer. Regional therapies have been developed and proven in the literature to not only palliate symptoms, but to prolong survival, improve quality of life, and sometimes even cure in what seems a hopeless situation.

In-transit metastasis of a limb from melanoma or peritoneal disease only from colon cancer can be looked at not as a systemic disease but a regional disease. This book *Regional Therapeutics for Advanced Malignancies* is the most comprehensive collaboration of some of the world's experts on this topic. More and more centers across the world are changing their approach to regional disease and treatments. This book will help educate and guide medical professionals who treat patients with these difficult scenarios.

I would like to thank the authors for their time and knowledge in creating and contributing to *Regional Therapeutics for Advanced Malignancies*. I would also like to acknowledge Payal Bharti of Jaypee Brothers Medical Publishers, New Delhi, India for her expertise and guidance in the preparation of this project.

Martin D. Goodman

If children have the ability to ignore all odds and percentages, then may be we can all learn from them. When you think about it, what other choice is there but to hope? We have two options, medically and emotionally: give up, or fight like hell.

—Lance Armstrong

Contents

Section 3: Melanoma, Sarcoma and Lung

Section 4: Liver

Section I

Peritoneal Disease

1 Pathophysiology of Peritoneal Malignancies and Modalities of Treatment

Sarah McPartland, Martin D. Goodman

INTRODUCTION

Cancers of the peritoneal cavity are a unique subset of malignancies. They can behave different from other malignancies, particularly in regards to propagation and systemic spread. Once considered universally fatal with few treatment options, multimodality therapies have been shown to palliate symptoms which improve quality of life as well as achieve significant lengths of survival. An understanding of the anatomic, physiologic and distinctive malignant properties is important to properly evaluate and treat patients with peritoneal-based cancers.

THE PERITONEAL CAVITY

Embryologic Origins

The primitive origin of the peritoneal cavity originates in the third week of gestation. During this time the intraembryonic mesoderm differentiates into two layers: (1) the somatic and (2) the splanchnic mesoderm layers. The somatic mesoderm layer forms the parietal peritoneum, which lines the abdominal and pelvic walls. The splanchnic mesodermal lining forms the visceral peritoneum. Early in development, these two layers of the peritoneum are connected to each other via the dorsal mesentery, which suspends the entire primordial gut from the midline of the posterior abdominal wall[1,2] (Fig. 1).

The primitive mesentery of the foregut, midgut and hindgut has both ventral and dorsal divisions; initially has a broad attachment to the posterior abdominal wall. Early in development, the liver grows into the ventral mesentery; essentially dividing it into two peritoneal attachments: the falciform ligament and the lesser omentum. The dorsal mesentery is identified as the greater omentum in the adult. Initially formed as an omental bursa or sac in front of the transverse mesocolon, a portion of its anterior and posterior layers eventually join to form a single plane. This omental layer then fuses with the transverse colon and its mesentery to form the gastrocolic ligament.[1,3]

Anatomy

Although no true compartmentalization of the peritoneal cavity exists, it is helpful to divide the space into compartments, particularly to emphasize technical considerations of operating in each area. The greater peritoneal sac encompasses the main anterior portion of the peritoneal cavity. The lesser sac (omental bursa) lies posterior to the stomach. Its superior recess extends up to the diaphragm and its inferior recess is a sac-like structure that extends caudally between the two layers of the greater omentum. The greater and lesser sacs communicate via the foramen of Winslow, located on the posterior edge of the hepatoduodenal ligament.[2]

The transverse mesocolon effectively divides the peritoneal cavity into supracolic and infracolic compartments. The supracolic compartment contains the stomach, liver and spleen, and can further be divided between the infrahepatic and the suprahepatic spaces. The infracolic compartment contains the small and large bowel, and is lateralized to left and right subdivisions by the small

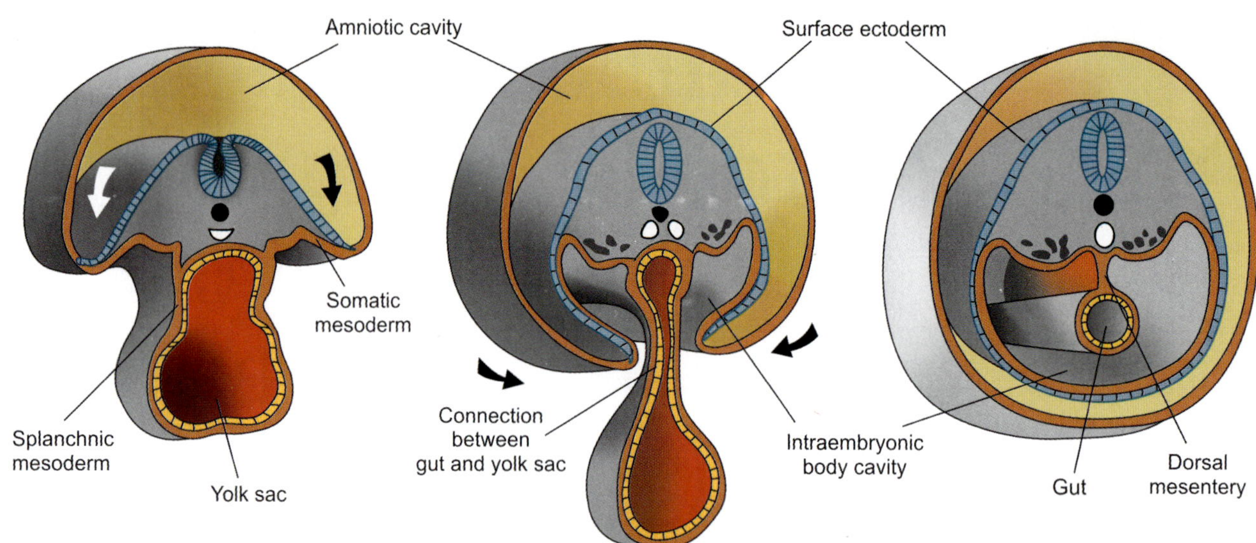

Figure 1 Embryologic origin of the peritoneal cavity
[*Source*: Reprinted with permission from Sadler TW. Langman's Medical Embryology, 9th edition. 2004[1]]

bowel mesentery. The left paracolic gutter is completely contained within the left infracolic compartment by the phrenocolic ligament. This ligament does not exist on the right, thereby allowing free communication between the right paracolic gutter and the supracolic compartment. Inferiorly, fluid, infection or malignant cells can find a pathway into the pelvis along the paracolic gutters.[2,3]

Of additional clinical importance is the fact that, in males, the peritoneal cavity is a closed system. The peritoneum protrudes into the rectovesical pouch in males, creating a separation between the rectum and bladder. In females, however, the peritoneal cavity is contiguous with the pelvic organs (fimbria, ovaries, fallopian tubes, uterus and vagina), creating yet another pathway for the spread of malignancy. Additionally, the pelvic peritoneum creates two pouches in women: (1) the rectouterine pouch (separates bladder from rectum) and (2) the vesicouterine pouch (separates bladder from uterus).

The arterial supply and venous drainage of parietal peritoneum occur via branches of the abdominal wall vessels. These include the superior and the inferior epigastric arteries, lumbar vessels, musculophrenic artery and deep circumflex arteries. The visceral peritoneum derives its blood supply from branches of the viscera it covers. Nerve supply to the parietal and visceral peritoneum follows a similar pattern, with adjacent visceral nerves supplying the visceral peritoneum, and those of the abdominal wall (and diaphragm) supplying the parietal peritoneum.

The majority of lymphatic drainage from the peritoneal cavity occurs via the subdiaphragmatic lymphatic system. Intercommunicating plexuses on either side of the diaphragm are found in variable distribution within the muscular portion of the diaphragm. Lymphatic fluid is absorbed at specific sites on the diaphragm (lymphatic lacuna) and then travels through large substernal collecting ducts associated with the internal mammary vessels, eventually reaching the anterior mediastinal lymph nodes. A small portion of the lymphatic drainage from the diaphragm may go to the bronchial lymph nodes or proceed caudally into the retroperitoneal fat lymph nodes and eventually, the cisterna chyli. The main thoracic duct plays a very small role in lymphatic drainage of the peritoneal cavity.[4]

Physiologic and Immune Function

The mesothelial cell lining of the peritoneal cavity has an active role in the physiologic functioning of the peritoneal cavity and forms the "plasma peritoneal barrier". One role of these cells is the secretion of surfactant that works as a lubricant to decrease friction between the abdominal organs.[5] Mesothelial cells are actively involved in the initiation and regulation of peritoneal cavity's immune functions. These cells secrete inflammatory mediators and play a gatekeeper role for leukocyte extravasation into the peritoneal cavity at times of infection. This is part of the peritoneal cavity's complex system to resist microbial proliferation, which consists of both physical barriers and immune-mediated functions. First-line defenses against infectious insults include lymphatic uptake of particulate matter at the diaphragm and opsonization of microorganisms with subsequent macrophage-associated phagocytosis.[6,7]

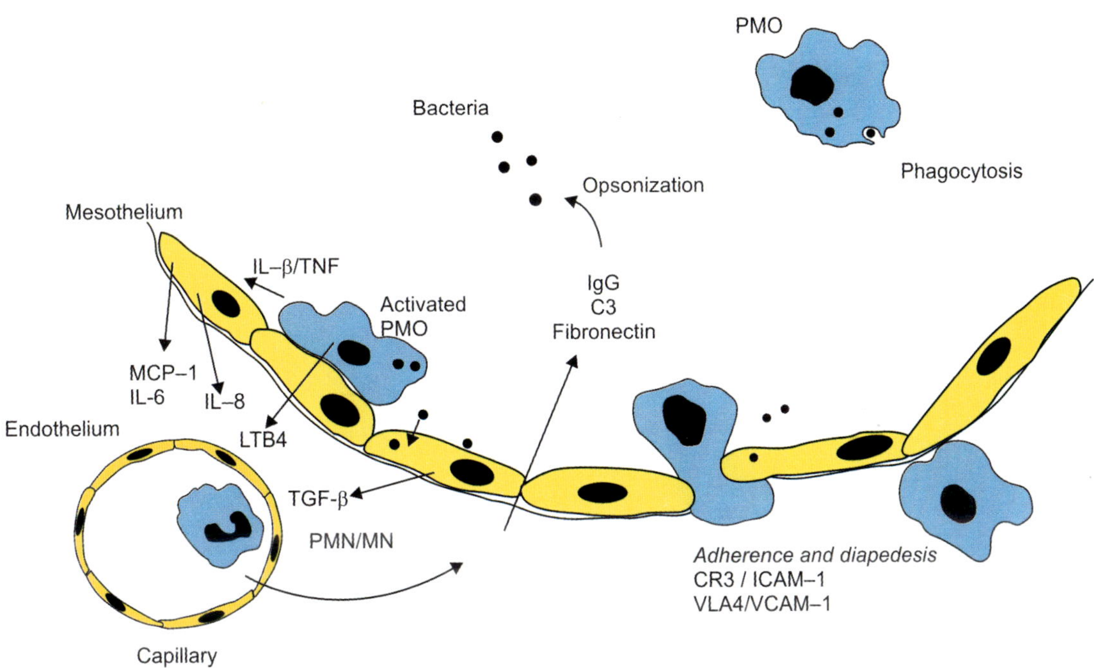

Figure 2 Activation of peritoneal macrophages following bacterial contamination, and role of mesothelium in local host defenses [*Source*: Reprinted with permission from Brulez HF, Verbrugh HA. Perit Dial Int. 1995;15(7 Suppl):S24-33][7]

The peritoneal fluid contains a variety of resident and migratory immunogenic cells, factors and peptides, even in the uninfected patient. Of the leukocytes, monocytes/macrophages are the most dominant. However, the fraction of any individual cell type on peritoneal fluid cell differential is highly variable. The percentage of leukocytes that are macrophages may range 20–95%, with lymphocytes having similar variability.[7,8] Neutrophils are present in only small amounts in the normal state of health; however, their concentration and activity dramatically increases during times of active infection.[8]

Macrophages are also found in perivascular and submesothelial areas of the peritoneum.[7] They secrete a variety of inflammatory factors including cytokines, prostaglandins, chemoattractants and leukotrienes[6] (Fig. 2). Additionally, perivascular lymphoid aggregates have been identified in various tissues including the omentum and pouch of Douglas. These aggregates termed "milky spots", harbor macrophages as well as lymphocytes, which can be released into the peritoneal cavity following inflammatory stimuli.[9]

Malignancies of the Peritoneal Cavity

Primary Peritoneal Malignancies

Primary *de novo* malignancy of the peritoneal cavity is exceedingly rare. A study examining 24 population-based registries in the United States from 1995 to 2004 found the incidence of primary peritoneal cancer to be 6.78 per million.[10] White women accounted for the largest cohort of patients, with the disease least likely to affect black women. Mean age at diagnosis was 67 years. Subtypes of primary peritoneal malignancies and their important features are outlined in Table 1.

Secondary Peritoneal Malignancies

The majority of peritoneal malignancies are due to secondary spread of cancer cells. Appendiceal, ovarian and colorectal cancers are common sources of intraperitoneal disease. Gastric, endometrial, small bowel, pancreatic, breast cancers, sarcomas and pulmonary mesothelioma can also demonstrate peritoneal spread.

Appendiceal: Appendiceal cancers are exceedingly rare, and can encompass varying histopathologic subtypes including adenocarcinoma (with or without mucin production), signet ring cell adenocarcinoma, carcinoid, and adenocarcinoid. One study that evaluated 15 years of patient data from the National Cancer Institute's Surveillance, Epidemiology and End-Results (SEER) database found the annual incidence of all types of appendiceal cancer to be 0.12 per million people.[23] Mucinous adenocarcinoma was the most common subtype reported in this study. Epithelial appendiceal cancers which are associated with peritoneal disease, are

Table 1 Types and key features of primary peritoneal malignancies

Types	*Features*
Peritoneal serous papillary carcinoma (PSPC)	• Similar clinical and histopathologic features to ovarian serous papillary carcinoma (OSPC), however, has been diagnosed in women following oophorectomy[11,12] • Ovarian mass must be excluded to ensure peritoneal disease is not metastatic lesion • One study examining 199 patients with presumed epithelial ovarian cancer found PSPC in 15% of the patients at the time of laparotomy[13] • Omental caking with extensive calcifications is a common CT scan finding, and can help to differentiate between PSPC and mesothelioma[14]
Malignant peritoneal mesothelioma	• Male>>Female • Typical age at diagnosis 40–60 years • Only a small minority of patients have history of significant asbestos exposure • Late diagnosis with advanced peritoneal disease at presentation is common • Useful tumor markers are CA 125 and CA 15-3 • Three histopathologic subtypes: epithelioid (most common), sarcomatoid, biphasic[15]
Cystic mesothelioma	• Female>>Male • Benign/no malignant potential • Recurrence rate 25–50% • Lesions typically grapelike clusters of mesothelium-lined cysts, separated by fibrous tissue • Pelvic region often involved • Does not typically cause mass effect or calcifications[15]
Benign papillary mesothelioma	• Affects both males and females, although seen more commonly in women[16] • Most are inactive/indolent and, therefore, considered benign[17] • Grossly appears similar to metastatic implants which may result in intraoperative diagnostic dilemma[17] • Typically recommended adjuvant therapy only, in cases of disease progression[17] • Very rarely, can also occur in the tunica vaginalis[18]
Desmoplastic small round cell tumor	• 4:1 male:female incidence (typically found in young adult males) • Very aggressive tumor with poor long-term survival • Multiphenotypic differentiation—coexpression of epithelial, mesenchymal and neural cell markers[19] • Reported occurrences in pleura and central nervous system[20,22] • Can metastasize to lymph nodes, pleura, liver and pericardium[21]
Lymphoproliferative malignancies • Granulocytic sarcoma • Lymphomatosis • Plasmacytoma • Leukemias	
Mesenchymal tumors (benign) peritoneal hemangiomatosis	• Reported in infants • Often associated with diffuse disease that also involves the gastrointestinal tract[22]
Leiomyomatosis peritonealis disseminata (LPD)	• Found most commonly in pregnant women
Lymphangioma	• Typically appears as large, thin-walled, multiloculated cysts at CT[15] • Significant mesenteric infiltration, requiring bowel resection for complete removal, is common[15]
Lipoma	• Often an incidental finding on imaging without clinical implications
Gastrointestinal stromal tumors (GIST)	• Malignant potential
Mesenchymal tumors (malignant) • Peritoneal angiosarcoma • Peritoneal histiocytoma • Liposarcoma • Fibrosarcoma • Synovial sarcoma • Malignant fibrous histiocytoma • Leiomyosarcoma	

very difficult to diagnose preoperatively; the majority of these cancers are diagnosed during postoperative histopathological review.[24]

Ovarian: Ovarian epithelial cancer is an aggressive disease that often demonstrates intraperitoneal spread. The current standard for therapy includes cytoreductive surgery and adjuvant chemotherapy (platinum-based agent plus taxane). Only half of all patients obtain a complete clinical response with this regimen, a state which is maintained at the 5-year mark in less than 50% of the patients.[25,26] These cancers commonly become chemotherapy-resistant following an initial response, further complicating the treatment algorithm. Long-term survival is poor.

Colorectal: Colorectal cancers spread to the peritoneal cavity with relative frequency, second only to the liver. This will often lead to peritoneal carcinomatosis. At the time of primary surgery, peritoneal disease is already detectable in approximately 7% of patients with colon cancer.[27] Historically, peritoneal carcinomatosis was regarded as distant metastatic disease (M1/stage IV), and offered a grave prognosis. Patients were typically offered only palliative chemotherapy. When offered, surgery too was usually palliative in nature (e.g. intestinal bypass for obstruction).

In population-based studies, the improved application of palliative chemotherapy regimens over the past 15 years appears to have increased the overall survival of patients with colorectal carcinomatosis from approximately 35 weeks to 66 weeks.[28] Within this cohort, patients with isolated peritoneal disease who were treated with systemic chemotherapy had the longest median survival. This "peritoneal-only" group of patients with colorectal carcinoma is thought to make up approximately 25% of all the patients with colorectal carcinomatosis. Recently, it has been suggested that these patients may be better served by treating their disease as locoregional extension as opposed to systemic metastases.

Pseudomyxoma peritonei: Pseudomyxoma peritonei (PMP) is a clinical syndrome of gelatinous mucinous ascites with a characteristic pattern of peritoneal and omental implants, resulting from peritoneal contamination from a mucinous tumor, commonly of appendiceal or ovarian etiology. Interestingly, these tumor cells lack the adhesion molecules necessary to arbitrarily bind to any tissue and are, therefore, often just "redistributed" around the peritoneal cavity until they reach specific areas of the peritoneum rich in lymphatic stomata. It is at these sites that tumor adherence is most likely to occur in the early stages of disease.[29,30]

The mucin produced by these tumors is a glycoprotein encoded for by the MUC family of genes, which MUC gene a cell expresses is dependent on location (e.g. MUC-2 is expressed by small intestine and colonic goblet cells; MUC-5AC is expressed by the stomach and respiratory tract). Mucin is produced by epithelial cells and has both a membrane-associated and secreted form.[30]

The exact origin of PMP in women has been debated in the literature. The question has been raised as to whether an ovarian malignancy is responsible for PMP, with secondary spread to the peritoneal cavity and appendix. The possibility of multifocal neoplasia or multiple primary tumors coexisting has also been raised.[31,32] Studies examining the clinical and immunohistochemical properties of these tumors, however, have demonstrated convincing evidence that ovarian tumors seen in PMP are from a primary appendiceal malignancy; therefore, representing regional solid organ metastases.[33,34]

Tumor Biology of Peritoneal Malignancies

Biology of a Cancer Cell in the Peritoneal Cavity

Kusumara et al. described three mechanisms for development of peritoneal carcinomatosis. First, as previously discussed, primary peritoneal malignancies can arise spontaneously or following carcinogenic exposure, e.g. asbestos (Fig. 2).[30]

Second, peritoneal carcinomatosis can occur independently in the setting of another primary tumor. This phenomenon of individual tumors with polyclonal multifocal origin is seen with peritoneal disease in the setting of ovarian tumors of low malignant potential (OTLMP) or peritoneal serous papillary carcinoma (PSPC). In this scenario the tumors appear histopathologically similar but behave differently from a pathophysiological standpoint. The independent origin of these tumors can be demonstrated by analyzing their patterns of X-chromosome inactivation. Early in development, normal somatic cells in women randomly undergo inactivation of one of their X chromosomes, resulting in mosaicism amongst the somatic cells. This pattern of inactivation remains constant throughout the life of the cell. Tumors of monoclonal origin would be expected to have identical patterns of X chromosome inactivation. In cases of peritoneal disease and OTLMP (or PSPC), polyclonicity (i.e. different patterns of X chromosome inactivation) has been demonstrated.[30,35,36]

Finally, tumor cells of a gastrointestinal or gynecological primary tumor can gain entry into the peritoneal cavity via a number of routes. A serosal invading malignancy may "shed" tumor cells directly into the peritoneal cavity. These cells can also gain entry into the peritoneal cavity following tumor rupture, as is commonly the case in appendiceal-derived mucinous malignancies. Intraoperatively, contamination of the peritoneal cavity can occur by disruption of vessels or lymphatics, with subsequent dispersal of tumor cells within the blood or lymphatic fluid. Additionally, manipulation of the tumor itself during the course of resection can introduce tumor cells into the peritoneal cavity.

Once in the peritoneal cavity, these rogue cells are then spread throughout with relative ease, aided by gravity and intra-abdominal movement as a consequence of intestinal peristalsis and respiration-generated changes in intra-abdominal pressure.[30] Attachment and proliferation of these cells is outlined in Figure 3.

Following tumor detachment and dissemination within the peritoneal cavity, tumor cells may follow the transmesothelial pathway, translymphatic pathyway (e.g. PMP), or utilize both mechanisms for metastasis (e.g. colon cancer).[30]

Treatment of Peritoneal Malignancies

In general, carcinomatosis portends a shortened survival and poor quality of life. There are many treatment options available but not one alone has been shown to have any or minimal affect on survival. Most of these patients have a survival of 6–12 months depending on the disease and therapy provided. This has been a major problem in treating cancer patients for hundreds of years. The past 50 years has shown great promise in this field with improved chemotherapy, palliative treatments and novel multimodality therapy.

Systemic Chemotherapy

Systemic chemotherapeutic agents employ their cytotoxic effects through a variety of mechanisms, from generalized inhibition of DNA/RNA synthesis to more targeted pathways for specific proteins and enzymes. Systemic therapy, as compared to locoregional application of chemotherapy, is advantageous in that it can potentially reach undetectable distant malignant cells. However, because these therapies reach both malignant and healthy tissues, they are accompanied by the potential cytotoxic damage to healthy tissue leading to a variety of often undesirable, sometimes dose-limiting and, occasionally, life-threatening side effects.

In addition to potential side effects, the benefits of systemic chemotherapy for peritoneal-based malignancies have thus far had a very limited role. In fact, for appendiceal malignancies, currently available regimens of neoadjuvant systemic chemotherapy may have deleterious effects on outcomes.[37] The reason why systemic chemotherapy is so ineffective for peritoneal-based disease is its multifactorial nature.

The "kinetic model" for drug resistance proposes that slow growing cancers are more likely to be drug resistant because the "window" during which time the cell is in a mitotic state, and is susceptible to cytotoxicity from chemotherapy occurs less frequently (longer intervals between cell division) as compared to a fast-growing malignancy. This theory is limited by a considerable number of exceptions (e.g. the blast cell phase of chronic myelogenous leukemia, which is often extremely fast growing but refractory to chemotherapy) but its principles may be contributory in some cancers, such as peritoneal mucinous tumors, which are often slow growing.[38,39]

Another mechanism that may help to describe the inadequacy of systemic chemotherapy for peritoneal malignancies is the "multicellular spheroid model" or diffusion model. This proposes that high drug concentrations cannot be obtained throughout large tumors due to inadequate drug diffusion. That is, as tumor depth increases, concentration of drug and associated cytotoxic effects decrease. Given that peritoneal malignancies often develop into bulky disease by the time they are diagnosed, it would be plausible that this theory may indeed apply to the inherit drug resistance seen in these cancers. In practice, however, it is often the higher molecular weight agents that impart superior malignant degradation, somewhat discrediting this theory as one would expect lower diffusion capabilities of these drugs.[40,44]

The "Goldie-Coldman" model for drug resistance is a useful tool to explain the overall poor performance of systemic chemotherapy for the treatment of peritoneal cancers. This mathematical model takes into account the generally accepted theory that resistance to chemotherapy is, at least in part, due to the generation of phenotypic drug resistance. Studies which investigated single tumor cell suspensions found that those cells responded to cytotoxic agents in a manner consistent with the clinical response of the larger tumor from which they were harvested, suggesting that it is the individual cell characteristics that dictate drug resistance.[41,42,44]

The tumor cell can develop this drug resistance through random mutations in its genetic code ("genetic instability theory"), which alters the gene products, and thereby changes the phenotypic drug responsiveness.[44] A single mutation can result in significant drug resistance by changing cell membrane permeability to specific compounds ("pleiotropic drug resistance"). The "fluctuation test of Lunia and Delbruck" is a method of mathematically predicting the frequency of these

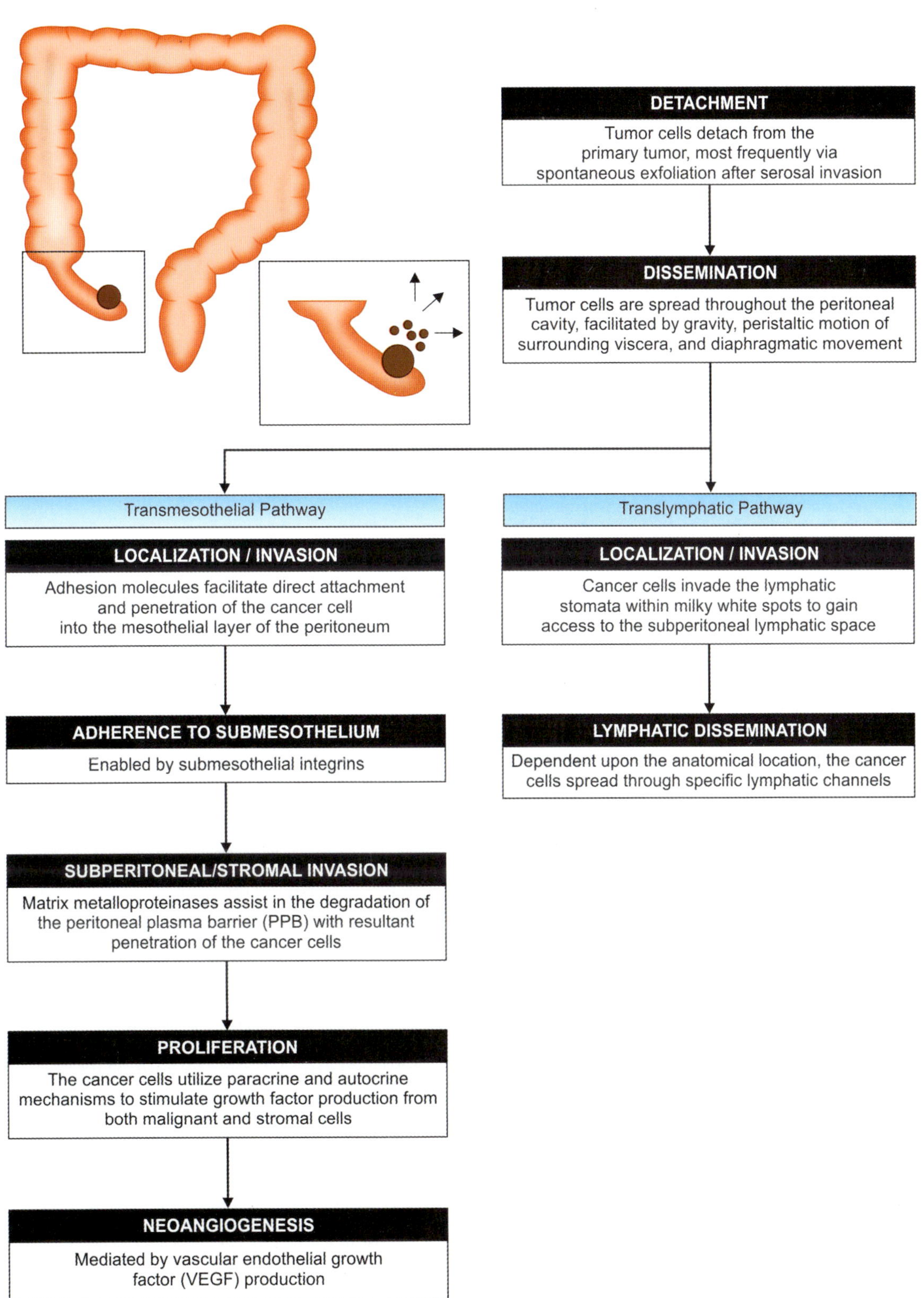

Figure 3 Attachment and dissemination of cancer cells within the peritoneal cavity

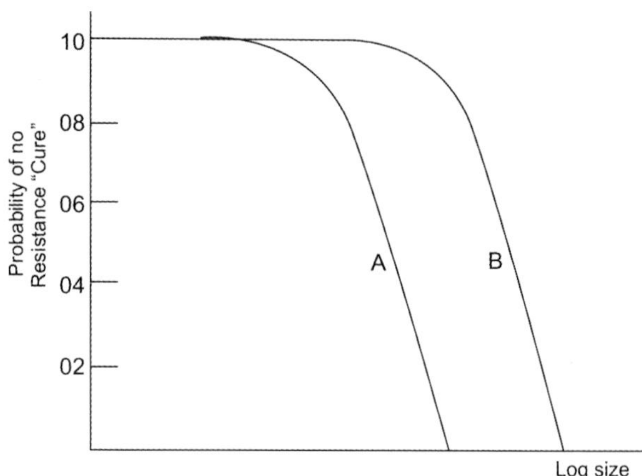

Figure 4 Goldie-Coldman mathematical model (probability of resistance for a given tumor size/mutation rate). Plot of the function $p = \theta^{-\alpha N}$ for two different mutation rates, A and B; where A > B. The function defines the probability of therebeing zero resistant cells present for any given value of the tumor size, and the mutation rate to resistance. Where treatment is capable of eradicating all nonresistant cells, then this probability approaches the value of potential cure. For tumor burdens distributed over the steep portion of the curve, relatively small increases in tumor mass will have a disproportionate effect on reducing curability. [*Source*: Reprinted with permission from Goldie JH, Coldman AJ. Cancer Res. 1984;44:3643-53][44]

random mutations.[43,44] Taking these principles of genetic variability into account, the Goldie-Coldman model demonstrates that the larger the tumor, the greater the likelihood of a mutant cell type arising.[44] That is, the likelihood of a cure (p) = $\theta^{-\alpha N}$, where "α" represents mutation rate per cell generation and "N" is the number of cells.[44]

This theory can be applied to most tumors with the exception of those that are highly curable or incurable as these lie on the flat part of the sigmoid curve (Fig. 4).[44] For peritoneal cancers, which are often large, bulky and at the time of diagnosis, the Goldie-Coldman model would predict a high likelihood of phenotypic drug resistance. Additionally, this theory essentially supports the role of cytoreductive surgery prior to chemotherapy, which decreases the concentration of tumor cells thereby shifting the curve to the left (decreased probability of drug resistance).

Surgery

Surgical resection is the mainstay of treatment for many types and stages of gastrointestinal and gynecological malignancy. Surgical cytoreduction to the point of no measurable malignant cells by postoperative peritoneal cytology can be achieved and is associated with improved outcomes as compared to incomplete debulking.[45]

Unfortunately, however, gastrointestinal malignancies have a high rate of local recurrence at anastomotic regions and within the peritoneal cavity, even when complete resection (negative surgical margins and no gross disease) were achieved.[46] The proposed mechanism for this recurrence is centered on the concept of "tumor cell entrapment", which begins when tumor microemboli are disseminated into the peritoneal cavity during surgical resection.[47] Intraoperative blood loss provides the opportunity for malignant cells in the venous blood to spread throughout the peritoneal cavity. Additionally, disruption of both lymphatic channels and tumor margins allow for tumor cell dispersal. These events can occur in even the most meticulously executed open and laparoscopic surgical procedures. Fibrin deposition, which occurs as part of the normal postsurgical inflammatory process, then entraps these cells, and essentially protects them as they propagate, while also providing a vascular framework further fostering tumor growth.

Intraperitoneal Chemotherapy

The peritoneal plasma barrier (PPB) allows for higher concentrations of cytotoxic agents to be administered intraperitoneally as compared to systemic administration. For many drugs, the PPB contributes to slower diffusion, thereby maintaining higher intraperitoneal concentrations over time. The regional exchange rate for pharmacologic agents introduced into the peritoneal cavity is 5–25 milliliters per minute, depending on the properties of the drug.[48]

Bioavailability refers to the extent to which a drug reaches the systemic circulation. The bioavailability of intraperitoneal chemotherapy is significantly lower than that of intravenous or oral chemotherapy due to first-pass hepatic metabolism. It has been suggested that the majority of intraperitoneally administered chemotherapy is absorbed by the visceral peritoneum.[49] As discussed previously, the vascular drainage of this portion of the peritoneum follows that of the viscera, and its mesentery (i.e. the mesenteric veins to the portal circulation), subject to hepatic metabolism. Conversely, the parietal peritoneum, which follows the venous drainage of the anterior abdominal wall via the epigastric vessels, bypasses the portal system. The predilection for portal venous drainage of the peritoneal cavity dramatically decreases the amount of drug that reaches the systemic circulation.

The substantial drug concentrations attainable via peritoneal-based chemotherapy can be demonstrated by measuring the area under the curve (AUC) following drug administration. The AUC is a measure of drug exposure, calculated by taking the integral of plasma concentration versus time—$\int([\text{drug, plasma}] \times Dt)$. Sugarbaker et al. calculated AUC for intraperitoneal delivery of Mitomycin C (MMC), and 5-fluorouracil (5FU) in patients undergoing early postoperative intraperitoneal chemotherapy (EPIC).[55] In this group of patients, it was found that the AUC for peritoneal fluid drug concentration versus plasma drug concentration was 117:1 for 5FU, and 21.6 for MMC. This allows for a dose intensive regimen of locoregional cytotoxic agents with a general avoidance of systemic toxicity. Additionally, this study demonstrated that intraperitoneal 5FU exhibited a high rate of first-pass hepatic metabolism (i.e. high portal venous drug concentration, and low systemic plasma drug concentration). The slow rate of peritoneal 5FU absorption and, therefore, the avoidance of hepatic over saturation contributed to the liver's capacity to metabolize the drug.

Unfortunately, in the absence of operative resection, intraperitoneal chemotherapy as a monotherapy or in conjunction with systemic chemotherapy has not been shown to impart significant disease-free or overall survival for peritoneal malignancies. Likely contributing to this failure is the observation that 90% of the concentration advantage that intraperitoneal chemotherapy provides (as compared to systemic therapy) is only maintained to a depth of up to one millimeter (100 cell layers).[50]

Hyperthermia

Hyperthermia—administered as tumor-directed therapy, locoregionally, or to the whole body—can be used as an adjunct to chemotherapy and radiation therapy, where it has been shown to have a synergistic effect in certain clinical situations. To some degree, elevated temperature can also independently induce tumor cell death or necrosis.

The scope of damage elicited by heat on cells was summarized by Hildebrandt et al. (Table 2). Malignant cells are more susceptible—as compared to normal tissues—to hyperthermic damage for a number of reasons. The microenvironment of tumor cells contributes to their temperature sensitivity. Tumor growth often occurs at a rate unsupported by their vascular supply, resulting in nutritional deprivation. This also generates acidic and hypoxic conditions, making these cells more susceptible to the cytotoxic effects of hyperthermia. The application of heat likely only further impairs blood flow to the tumor. Interestingly, tumor cells may indeed "get hotter" and "stay hotter" when compared to non-malignant cells due to their chaotic and insufficient vascular supply, which does not reliably cool the cells (and itself is more susceptible to heat-induced damage).[51,52]

Table 2 The range of hyperthermia's cellular effects

Effects of hyperthermia on tumor cells
Change in the fluidity and stability of the cell membrane
Changes in cell shape
Impaired transmembrane transport
Changes in membrane potential
Modulation of transmembrane efflux pumps
Induction of apoptosis
Impairment of protein synthesis
Protein denaturation
Aggregation of proteins at the nuclear matrix
Induction of heat sensitive protein synthesis
Impairment of DNA and RNA synthesis
Inhibition of enzyme repair
Altered DNA conformation
Alteration of intracellular metabolism of other substrates
Alteration of gene expression and signal transduction

(*Source*: Adapted from Hildebrandt B, et al. Critical Reviews in Oncology/Hematology. 2002;43:33–56)[57]

Cell death from hyperthermia is a function of both temperature and length of exposure. It occurs in two stages. First, at the start of the heat exposure, linear growth arrest occurs (reversible). This is followed by an exponential rate of cell death. While a selective tumor killing being effective is exhibited within a range of 40°C to 44°C, research has shown that the ability to progress to the exponential phase of cell death is decreased considerably if temperatures are less than 43°C. In clinical practice, 43°C is a target temperature for therapy. The "thermal isoeffect dose" (TID) allows for the conversion of other thermal therapies into "units" of equivalent heating time at 43°C.[53,57]

Sugarbaker et al. found that heat has synergistic properties with some chemotherapeutic agents including MMC, doxorubicin and Cisplatin.[54] These drugs have an increased "thermal enhancement ratio", a ratio of percentage of cell death from an agent at normothermia and hyperthermia. The exact etiology of this synergism is unclear, and it is not demonstrated universally among cytoxic drugs. It is likely that heat-induced chemosensitization is a multifactorial process, involving changes in the tumor vascular supply, membrane sensitivity or permeability to specific agents, and local changes in the tumors microenvironment. Interestingly, heat may have an additional advantage of helping to overcome drug resistance with MMC, cisplatin, doxorubicin and nitrosureas.[59]

In practice, hyperthermia has been found to be safe when applied to the peritoneal cavity. In a small prospective study examining 16 patients with gastric cancer who underwent open instillation of intraperitoneal chemotherapy (without peritonectomy), hyperthermia by itself was not found to induce any additional peritoneal injury or inflammation, as measured by postoperative ascitic amount and protein concentration.[55] Additionally, safe and effective methods for the intraoperative application of heated chemoperfusate have been developed. Spratt et al. studied intracavitary hyperthermia in an animal model, forming a basis for the development of a perfusion system.[56]

An important feature of hyperthermia in the treatment of malignancy is that prior cellular exposure to hyperthermia may have a deleterious effect on sensitivity—referred to as "thermal tolerance". This is at least partially due to the development of heat-shock proteins following initial exposure to elevated temperature.[57] These proteins are expressed on the surface of malignant cells following non-lethal application of heat, but are not produced by normal cells.[59] This is an important concept to consider when anticipating time to optimal temperature intraoperatively and also for situations of reoperative surgery.

Multimodality Treatment: The Role of Cytoreductive Surgery with Intraoperative Hyperthermic Chemotherapy

In summary, systemic chemotherapy, surgery, locoregional chemotherapy and hyperthermia have properties important in the treatment of peritoneal malignancy. Unfortunately, as monotherapy, each of these therapies fails in regards to long-term achievement of a disease-free state and overall lengths of survival.

A case series examining patient data from M.D. Anderson Hospital during the mid-1950s to late-1970s, revealed an actuarial survival rate of 54% and 18% at 5 and 10 years respectively, in a cohort of 38 patients with ovarian or appendiceal PMP treated with cytoreductive surgery and adjuvant chemotherapy.[58] Appendiceal origin was associated with significantly worse outcomes in this study. Data from 56 patients treated at the Mayo Clinic during a similar time period found 1-, 5- and 10-year survival rates at 98%, 53% and 32% respectively.[59] Thirteen percent of these patients underwent normothermic intraperitoneal chemotherapy. Interestingly, the only adverse predictor of outcome in this group was administration of systemic adjuvant chemotherapy, which 27% of the patients received. Recurrence rate was 50%, irrespective of degree of operative cytoreduction.

These results have been improved by combining surgical resection with intraoperative application of regional hyperthermia and intraperitoneal chemotherapy, with or without adjuvant chemotherapy. This has become the mainstay of treatment for certain peritoneal-based malignancies, and is becoming a more commonly accepted treatment for other locoregionally advanced gastrointestinal malignancies.

Cytoreductive surgery and intraoperative hyperthermic chemotherapy (CRS-HIPEC) have been employed in the treatment of some primary peritoneal malignancies with promising results. Median survival of patients with malignant mesothelioma is approximately one year when treated with systemic chemotherapy alone.[60,61] However, multiple studies investigating the use of CRS-HIPEC for this disease have demonstrated a median survival in the range of 28–35 months.[62,63] Yano et al. performed CRS-HIPEC with doxorubicin and cisplatin (followed by early postoperative chemotherapy in select patients), and achieved a median survival of 3.7 years (range 0.7–6.9 years) for eight patients who were optimally debulked.[64]

Many studies have investigated the use of CRS-HIPEC for PMP and appendiceal cancers. Often times, however, the data for various pathologic origins of peritoneal disease (e.g. colorectal, gastric, appendiceal) are pooled, making assessment of outcomes based on tumor type difficult. Table 3 presents findings from some larger studies that examined CRS-HIPEC for PMP and appendiceal cancers. Of the pathological subtypes of appendiceal carcinoma, disseminated peritoneal adenomucinosis (DPAM) imparts a more favorable prognosis when compared to peritoneal mucinous carcinomatosis (PMCA), and those mucinous tumors with intermediate or discordant features.[43] However, there is a benefit of treatment with CRS-HIPEC for even high-grade tumors.[65]

While historically the focus of treatment with CRS-HIPEC was appendiceal-related malignancies and PMP, its use for ovarian, colorectal and gastric malignancies has shown promising results. Glehen et al. performed a multi-institutional study of 1,290 patients with various peritoneal-based cancers including PMP, peritoneal mesothelioma, gastrointestinal

Table 3 Select investigations of CRS-HIPEC in the treatment of pseudomyxoma peritonei and appendiceal cancers[66,67]

Author, study date	Pathologic origin	N [# CC0-1]	Chemotherapy type, dose [temp, duration]	Survival
Cioppa et al., 2008[75]	PMP	53 [53]	CIS 100 mg/m² + MMC 16 mg/m² [41.5°C, 60 min] two patients with MMC only due to preoperative platinum toxicity	5-year OS, 94% 10-year OS, 84.6% 5-year DFS, 80% 10-year DFS, 70%
Deraco et al., 2004[76]	PMP	31 [31]	CIS 25 mg/m²/L + MMC 3.3 mg/m²/L [42.5°C, 60 min]	5-year OS, 97% 5-year PFS, 43% 5-year LR-PFS, 59%
Elias et al., 2010[77]	PMP	301 [206] HIPEC = 255	HIPEC MMC [41-42°C, 60-120 min] + oxaliplatin [43°C, 30 min] [N = 255]; EPIC MMC, day 1 + 5FU, day 2-5 {N = 46]	1-year OS, 89.4% 5-year OS, 72.6% 10-year OS, 54.8% 5-year DFS, 56% In CC-0 group: 5-year OS. 84%; 10-year OS, 61%
Loungnarath et al., 2005[78]	PMP	27 [11]	CIS 0.7 mg/kg + MMC 0.5 mg/kg [42–42.5°C, 90 min]	Median OS not reached (median follow-up 23 months; range 3–82) Actuarial 1-year survival, 100% Actuarial 5-year survival, 52%
Marcotte et al., 2008[79]	Appendiceal	38 [28] HIPEC = 23	Oxaliplatin 460 mg/m² [30°C, 30 min]	3-year OS [HIPEC], 86% 3-year DFS [HIPEC], 49%
Sugarbaker, Chang, 1999[80]	Appendiceal	385 [250]	HIPEC MMC 12.5 mg/m² (males), MMC 10 mg/m² (females) [N = 205]; EPIC 5FU/MMC + IP 5FU + IV MMC x 3 cycles [N = 156]; EPIC + IP 5FU/MMC x 3 cycles [N = 21]; EPIC 5FU x 12 cycles [N = 3]	5-year OS (adenomucinosis), 86% 5-year OS (hybrid pathology), 50% 5-year OS (CC > 2), 20%
Stewart et al., 2006[81]	Appendiceal	110 [R0 = 31]	MMC 30 mg + 10 mg added after 60 min [38.5–42°C, 60–120 min]	1-year OS, 79.9% 5-year OS, 53.4%
Smeenk et al., 2007[82]	PMP	103 [NR]	MMC 35 mg/m² [40–41°C, 90 min] Adjuvant IV 5FU/leucovorin x 6 months [N = 30]	Median DFS, 25.6 months 3-year DFSP, 43.6% 5-year DFSP, 37.4%
Witkamp et al., 2000[83]	PMP	46 [40]	MMC 15–40 mg/m² [40–41°C, 90 min] Adjuvant 5FU/leucovorin [N = 22]	2-year actuarial OS, 91% 3-year actuarial OS, 81%

(MMC = mitomycin C; CIS = cisplatin; CC-O = complete cytoreduction; CC>2 = incomplete cytoreduction; OS = overall survival; DFS = disease-free survival; LR-PFS = locoregional progression-free survival; PFS = progression-free survival; DFSP = disease-free survival probability; EPIC = early postoperative intraperitoneal chemotherapy)

adenocarcinomas (colorectal, gastric, appendiceal, small bowel), primary peritoneal serous carcinoma and peritoneal sarcomatosis.[68] About 91.8% of these patients underwent optimal surgical debulking (CC0-1) followed by either HIPEC (85.8%) and/or EPIC (16.6%). Median follow-up was 45.4 months (range 20.3–90.0 months), and overall median survival of 34 months was achieved for all patients. Further analysis demonstrated median survivals of 30 months, 9 months, 41 months and 77 months for peritoneal carcinomatosis from colorectal, gastric, peritoneal mesothelioma and appendiceal adenocarcinoma respectively. Median survival of PMP patients was not reached.

In a Phase III randomized trial by Verwaal et al., that compared CRS-HIPEC plus adjuvant chemotherapy with palliative surgery followed by systemic chemotherapy, a statistically significant survival advantage was observed in the CRS-HIPEC group with median survival of 22.3 months, compared with 12.6 months in the palliative arm.[69] Of additional interest are studies comparing patients with peritoneal disease from colorectal cancer with those who have isolated hepatic colorectal metastases.[70,71] Following optimal cytoreduction of the peritoneal disease or margin-negative hepatic metastasectomy, these patients had similar 1- and 5-year survival rates. This again makes a strong argument that isolated peritoneal metastases should be regarded as locoregional extension, and not systemic disease.

Additionally, there is some data to suggest that HIPEC may play a palliative role in patients who undergo suboptimal debulking, whereby it has reduced ascites and improved quality of life.[72]

What accounts for the significant survival and disease-free progression period when therapies are combined? First, effective cytoreductive surgery removes any pre-existing adhesive tissue, and allows exposure of all aspects of the peritoneal cavity. Surgical mobilization and peritonectomy "prime" the peritoneal tissues for responsiveness to cytotoxic agents by exposing the submesothelium. Additionally, with the abdomen already exposed, insertion of intraperitoneal catheters and application of chemoperfusate in the operating suite is relatively simple.

Second, the probability of chemotherapy resistance amongst the remaining tumor cells following cytoreduction is dramatically decreased, as demonstrated by Goldie-Coldman model, where the likelihood of chemotherapy resistance is proportionate to tumor cell concentration. Additionally, surgical resection stimulates the tumor cells to reenter the proliferative phase of the cell cycle, making them more susceptible to cytotoxic agents.[30] In practice, intraperitoneal chemotherapy has been shown to be significantly more effective when utilized in the intraoperative or early postoperative period. The reason for this is multifold. As previously discussed, adhesive tissues that develop in the postoperative period are nidus for implantation by the rogue remnant tumor cells that remain following surgery. They provide a skeletal framework for attachment and subsequent malignant proliferation. These same adhesive tissues also cause compartmentalization of the peritoneal cavity which can prevent complete distribution of cytotoxic agents introduced into the peritoneal space.

Interestingly, the pharmacokinetics of intraperitoneal drug absorption—physiology of the plasma peritoneal barrier—seem to change over time. Evidence suggests that when cytotoxic agents are administered on consecutive days in the postoperative period, their clearance increases over time; in that the plasma concentrations of a cytotoxic agent are significantly higher following repetitive exposure and duration following surgery.[73] This supports the argument for one-time intraoperative intraperitoneal chemotherapy. Additionally, a linear relationship between cell death and intraperitoneal exposure has been suggested, even with limited exposure time.[74]

The treatment of this dynamic group of intraperitoneal malignancies continues to evolve. Improvements in our understanding of the pathophysiology of these tumors will hopefully shed light on new and improved therapies. Operative cytoreduction and intraperitoneal chemotherapy will likely continue to be a staple in the treatment of peritoneal malignancies. There are challenges to overcome, however, which include the need for standardization of the operative procedure, improvements in the diagnostic and preoperative evaluation of disease, burden in this cohort of patients and increasing the availability of CRS-HIPEC to a larger number of patients. More effective systemic adjuvant therapies are also needed.

REFERENCES

1. Sadler TW. Langman's Medical Embryology, 9th edition. Philadelphia: Lippincott Williams & Wilkins; 2004.
2. Moore KL, Dalley AF. Clinically Oriented Anatomy, 4th edition. New York: Lippincott Williams & Wilkins; 1999.
3. Skandalakis JE. Anatomical Complication in General Surgery. Texas: McGraw-Hill; 1983.
4. Khanna R, Mactier R, Twardowski ZJ, et al. Peritoneal cavity lymphatics. Perit Dial Int. 1986;6:113-21.
5. Dobbie JW, Anderson JD. Ultrastructure, distribution, and density of lamellar bodies in human peritoneum. Perit Dial Int. 1996;16(5):482-7.
6. Faull RJ. Peritoneal defenses against infection: winning the battle but losing the war? Semin Dial. 2000;13(1):47-53.
7. Brulez HF, Verbrugh HA.First-line defense mechanisms in the peritoneal cavity during peritoneal dialysis. Perit Dial Int. 1995;15(7 Suppl.):S24-33.
8. Lewis S, Holmes C. Host defense mechanisms in the peritoneal cavity of continuous ambulatory peritoneal dialysis patients. Perit Dial Int. 1991;11(1):14-21.
9. Krist LF, Eestermans IL, Steenbergen JJ, et al. Cellular composition of milky spots in the human greater omentum: an immunochemical and ultrastructural study. Anat Rec. 1995;241(2):163-74.
10. Goodman MT, Shvetsov YB. Incidence of ovarian, peritoneal, and fallopian tube carcinomas in the United States, 1995-2004. Cancer Epidemiol Biomarkers Prev. 2009;18(1):132-9.
11. Bloss JD, Liao SY, Buller RE, et al. Extraovarian peritoneal serous papillary carcinoma: a case-control retrospective comparison to papillary adenocarcinoma of the ovary. Gynecol Oncol. 1993;50(3):347-51.
12. Tobacman JK, Greene MH, Tucker MA, et al. Intra-abdominal carcinomatosis after prophylactic oophorectomy in ovarian-cancer-prone families. Lancet. 1982;2(8302):795-7.
13. Halperin R, Zehavi S, Langer R, et al. Primary peritoneal serous papillary carcinoma: a new epidemiologic trend? A matched-case comparison with ovarian serous papillary cancer. Int J Gynecol Cancer. 2001;11(5):403-8.

14. Killackey MA, Davis DR. Papillary serous carcinoma of the peritoneal surface: matched-case comparison with papillary serous ovarian carcinoma. Gynecol Oncol. 1993;51(2):171-4.
15. Pickhardt PJ, Bhalla S. Primary neoplasms of peritoneal and sub-peritoneal origin: CT findings. Radiographics. 2005;25(4): 983-95.
16. Chua TC, Yan TD, Morris DL. Surgical biology for the clinician: peritoneal mesothelioma: current understanding and management. Can J Surg. 2009;52(1):59-64.
17. Daya D, McCaughey WT. Well-differentiated papillary mesothelioma of the peritoneum. A clinicopathologic study of 22 cases. Cancer. 1990;65(2):292-6.
18. Tzanakakis G, McCully KS, Vezeridis MP. Benign papillary mesothelioma of the peritoneum: a consideration in the differential diagnosis of peritoneal implants. South Med J. 1989;82(12):1579-80.
19. Chetty R. Well differentiated (benign) papillary mesothelioma of the tunica vaginalis. J ClinPathol. 1992;45(11):1029-30.
20. Ordóñez NG, el-Naggar AK, Ro JY, et al. Intra-abdominal desmoplastic small cell tumor: a light microscopic, immuno-cytochemical, ultrastructural, and flow cytometric study. Hum Pathol. 1993;24(8):850-65.
21. Tison V, Cerasoli S, Morigi F, et al. Intracranial desmoplastic small-cell tumor. Report of a case. Am J Surg Pathol. 1996; 20(1):112-7.
22. Gerald WL, Miller HK, Battifora H, et al. Intra-abdominal desmoplastic small round-cell tumor. Report of 19 cases of a distinctive type of high-grade polyphenotypic malignancy affecting young individuals. Am J Surg Pathol. 1991;15(6):499-513.
23. Ibarguen E, Sharp HL, Snyder CL, et al. Hemangiomatosis of the colon and peritoneum: case report and management discussion. Clin Pediatr (Phila). 1988;27(9):425-30.
24. McCusker ME, Cote TR, Clegg LX, et al. Primary malignant neoplasms of the appendix: a population-based study from the Surveillance, Epidemiology and End-Results program, 1973–1998. Cancer. 2002;94(12):3307-12.
25. Deans GT, Spence RA. Neoplastic lesions of the appendix. Br J Surg. 1995;82(3):299-306.
26. Conte PF, Gadducci A, Cianci C. Second-line treatment and consolidation therapies in advanced ovarian cancer. Int J Gynecol Cancer. 2001;11(Suppl. 1):52-6.
27. Diaz-Montes TP, Bristow RE. Secondary cytoreduction for patients with recurrent ovarian cancer. Curr Oncol Rep. 2005;7(6):451-8.
28. Koppe MJ, Boerman OC, Oyen WJ, et al. Peritoneal carcinomatosis of colorectal origin: incidence and current treatment strategies. Ann Surg. 2006;243(2):212-22.
29. Klaver YL, Lemmens VE, Creemers GJ, et al. Population-based survival of patients with peritoneal carcinomatosis from colorectal origin in the era of increasing use of palliative chemotherapy. Ann Oncol. 2011.
30. Kusamura S, Baratti D, Zaffaroni N, et al. Pathophysiology and biology of peritoneal carcinomatosis. World J Gastrointest Oncol. 2010;2(1):12-8.
31. Sugarbaker PH. Pseudomyxomaperitonei. A cancer whose biology is characterized by a redistribution phenomenon. Ann Surg. 1994;219(2):109-11.
32. Seidman JD, Elsayed AM, Sobin LH, et al. Association of mucinous tumors of the ovary and appendix. A clinicopathologic study of 25 cases. Am J Surg Pathol. 1993;17(1):22-34.
33. Kahn MA, Demopoulos RI. Mucinous ovarian tumors with pseudomyxoma peritonei: a clinicopathological study. Int J Gynecol Pathol. 1992;11(1):15-23.
34. Kaern J, Tropé CG, Abeler VM. A retrospective study of 370 borderline tumors of the ovary treated at the Norwegian Radium Hospital from 1970 to 1982. A review of clinicopathologic features and treatment modalities. Cancer. 1993;71(5):1810-20.
35. Chuaqui RF, Zhuang Z, Emmert-Buck MR, et al. Genetic analysis of synchronous mucinous tumors of the ovary and appendix. Hum Pathol. 1996;27(2):165-71.
36. Young RH, Gilks CB, Scully RE. Mucinous tumors of the appendix associated with mucinous tumors of the ovary and pseudomyxomaperitonei. A clinicopathological analysis of 22 cases supporting an origin in the appendix. Am J Surg Pathol. 1991;15(5):415-29.
37. Prayson RA, Hart WR, Petras RE. Pseudomyxoma peritonei. A clinicopathologic study of 19 cases with emphasis on site of origin and nature of associated ovarian tumors. Am J Surg Pathol. 1994;18(6):591-603.
38. Ronnett BM, Kurman RJ, Zahn CM, et al. Pseudomyxoma peritonei in women: a clinicopathologic analysis of 30 cases with emphasis on site of origin, prognosis, and relationship to ovarian mucinous tumors of low malignant potential. Hum Pathol. 1995;26(5):509-24.
39. Ronnett BM, Shmookler BM, Diener-West M, et al. Immunohistochemical evidence supporting the appendiceal origin of pseudomyxoma peritonei in women. Int J Gynecol Pathol. 1997;16(1):1-9.
40. Cuatrecasas M, Matias-Guiu X, Prat J. Synchronous-mucinous tumors of the appendix and the ovary associated with pseudomyxomaperitonei. A clinicopathologic study of six cases with comparative analysis of c-Ki-ras mutations. Am J Surg Pathol. 1996;20(6):739-46.
41. Gu J, Roth LM, Younger C, et al. Molecular evidence for the independent origin of extra-ovarian papillary serous tumors of low malignant potential. J Natl Cancer Inst. 2001;93(15): 1147-52.
42. Muto MG, Welch WR, Mok SC, et al. Evidence for a multi-focal origin of papillary serous carcinoma of the peritoneum. Cancer Res. 1995;55(3):490-2.
43. Baratti D, Kusamura S, Nonaka D, et al. Pseudomyxo-maperitonei: clinical pathological and biological prognostic factors in patients treated with cytoreductive surgery and hyperthermic intraperitoneal chemotherapy (HIPEC). Ann Surg Oncol. 2008;15(2):526-34.
44. Goldie JH, Coldman AJ. The genetic origin of drug resistance in neoplasms: implications for systemic therapy. Cancer Res. 1984;44(9):3643-53.
45. Shackney SE, McCormack GW, Cuchural GJ Jr. Growth rate patterns of solid tumors and their relation to responsiveness to therapy: an analytical review. Ann Intern Med. 1978;89(1): 107-21.
46. Sutherland RM, McCredie JA, Inch WR.Growth of multicell spheroids in tissue culture as a model of nodular carcinomas. J Natl Cancer Inst. 1971;46(1):113-20.

47. Buick RN, Mackillop WJ. Measurement of self-renewal in culture of clonogenic cells from human ovarian carcinoma. Br J Cancer. 1981;44(3):349-55.
48. Salmon SE, Alberts DS, Meyskens Jr. FL, et al. Clinical correlations of in vitro drug sensitivity. In: Salmon SE (Ed). Cloning of Human Tumor Stem Cells. New York: Alan R. Liss; 1980. pp. 223-46.
49. Siminovitch L. On the nature of hereditable variation in cultured somatic cells. Cell. 1976;7(1):1-11.
50. Law LW. Origin of the resistance of leukemic cells to folic acid antagonists. Nature. 1952;169(4302):628-9.
51. Loggie BW, Fleming RA, Geisinger KR. Cytologic assessment before and after intraperitoneal hyperthermic chemotherapy for peritoneal carcinomatosis. Acta Cytol. 1996;40(6):1154-8.
52. Minsky BD, Mies C, Rich TA, et al. Potentially curative surgery of colon cancer: patterns of failure and survival. J Clin Oncol. 1988;6(1):106-18.
53. Sugarbaker PH, Cunliffe WJ, Belliveau J, et al. Rationale for integrating early postoperative intraperitoneal chemotherapy into the surgical treatment of gastrointestinal cancer. Semin Oncol. 1989;16(4 Suppl. 6):83-97.
54. Collins JM. Pharmacologic rationale for regional drug delivery. J Clin Oncol. 1984;2(5):498-504.
55. Sugarbaker PH, Graves T, De Bruijn EA, et al. Early postoperative intraperitoneal chemotherapy as an adjuvant therapy to surgery for peritoneal carcinomatosis from gastrointestinal cancer: pharmacological studies. Cancer Res. 1990; 50(18):5790-4.
56. Gianni L, Jenkins JF, Greene RF, et al. Pharmacokinetics of the hypoxic radio sensitizers misonidazole and demethylmisonidazole after intraperitoneal administration in humans. Cancer Res. 1983;43(2):913-6.
57. Hildebrandt B, Wust P, Ahlers O, et al. The cellular and molecular basis of hyperthermia. Crit Rev Oncol Hematol. 2002;43(1):33-56.
58. Bleehen NM. Hyperthermia—a treatment method for cancer? J R Soc Med. 1981;74(12):865-7.
59. van der Zee J. Heating the patient: a promising approach? Ann Oncol. 2002;13(8):1173-84.
60. Sugarbaker PH. Intraperitoneal chemotherapy and cytoreductive surgery for the prevention and treatment of peritoneal carcinomatosis and sarcomatosis. Semin Surg Oncol. 1998;14(3):254-61.
61. Shido A, Ohmura S, Yamamoto K, et al. Does hyperthermia induce peritoneal damage in continuous hyperthermic peritoneal perfusion? World J Surg. 2000;24(5):507-11.
62. Spratt JS, Adcock RA, Sherrill W, et al. Hyperthermic peritoneal perfusion system in canines. Cancer Res. 1980;40(2): 253-5.
63. Issels RD. Hyperthermia adds to chemotherapy. Eur J Cancer. 2008;44(17):2546-54.
64. Fernandez RN, Daly JM. Pseudomyxomaperitonei. Arch Surg. 1980;115(4):409-14.
65. Gough DB, Donohue JH, Schutt AJ, et al. Pseudomyxomaperitonei. Long-term patient survival with an aggressive regional approach. Ann Surg. 1994;219(2):112-9.
66. Castagneto B, Botta M, Aitini E, et al. Phase II study of pemetrexed in combination with carboplatin in patients with malignant pleural mesothelioma (MPM). Ann Oncol. 2008; 19(2):370-3.
67. Vogelzang NJ, Rusthoven JJ, Symanowski J, et al. Phase III study of pemetrexed in combination with cisplatin versus cisplatin alone in patients with malignant pleural mesothelioma. J Clin Oncol. 2003;21(14):2636-44.
68. Sebbag G, Yan H, Shmookler BM, et al. Results of treatment of 33 patients with peritoneal mesothelioma. Br J Surg. 2000;87(11):1587-93.
69. Loggie BW, Fleming RA, McQuellon RP, et al. Prospective trial for the treatment of malignant peritoneal mesothelioma. Am Surg. 2001;67(10):999-1003.
70. Feldman AL, Libutti SK, Pingpank JF, et al. Analysis of factors associated with outcome in patients with malignant peritoneal mesothelioma undergoing surgical debulking and intraperitoneal chemotherapy. J Clin Oncol. 2003;21(24): 4560-7.
71. Deraco M, De Simone M, Rossi CR, et al. An Italian Multicentric Phase II study on peritonectomy and intraperitoneal hyperthermic perfusion (IPHP) to treat patients with peritoneal mesothelioma. J Exp Clin Cancer Res. 2003; 22(4 Suppl):41-5.
72. Brigand C, Monneuse O, Mohamed F, et al. Peritoneal mesothelioma treated by cytoreductive surgery and intraperitoneal hyperthermic chemotherapy: results of a prospective study. Ann Surg Oncol 2006;13(3):405-12.
73. Yano H, Moran BJ, Cecil TD, et al. Cytoreductive surgery and intraperitoneal chemotherapy for peritoneal mesothelioma. Eur J Surg Oncol. 2009;35(9):980-5.
74. Omohwo C, Nieroda CA, Studeman KD, et al. Complete cytoreduction offers long-term survival in patients with peritoneal carcinomatosis from appendiceal tumors of unfavorable histology. J Am Coll Surg. 2009;209(3):308-12.
75. Cioppa T, Vaira M, Bing C, et al. Cytoreduction and hyperthermic intraperitoneal chemotherapy in the treatment of peritoneal carcinomatosis from pseudomyxoma peritonei. World J Gastroenterol. 2008;14(44):6817-23.
76. Deraco M, Baratti D, Inglese MG, et al. Peritonectomy and intraperitoneal hyperthermic perfusion (IPHP): a strategy that has confirmed its efficacy in patients with pseudomyxoma peritonei. Ann Surg Oncol. 2004;11(4):393-8.
77. Elias D, Gilly F, Quenet F, et al. Pseudomyxoma peritonei: a French multicentric study of 301 patients treated with cytoreductive surgery and intraperitoneal chemotherapy. Eur J Surg Oncol. 2010;36(5):456-62.
78. Loungnarath R, Causeret S, Bossard N, et al. Cytoreductive surgery with intraperitoneal chemohyperthermia for the treatment of pseudomyxoma peritonei: a prospective study. Dis Colon Rectum. 2005;48(7):1372-9.
79. Marcotte E, Sideris L, Drolet P, et al. Hyperthermic intraperitoneal chemotherapy with oxaliplatin for peritoneal carcinomatosis arising from appendix: preliminary results of a survival analysis. Ann Surg Oncol. 2008;15(10):2701-8.

80. Sugarbaker PH, Chang D. Results of treatment of 385 patients with peritoneal surface spread of appendiceal malignancy. Ann Surg Oncol. 1999;6(8):727-31.
81. Stewart JH 4th, Shen P, Russell GB, et al. Appendiceal neoplasms with peritoneal dissemination: outcomes after cytoreductive surgery and intraperitoneal hyperthermic chemotherapy. Ann Surg Oncol. 2006;13(5):624-34.
82. Smeenk RM, Verwaal VJ, Antonini N, et al. Survival analysis of pseudomyxoma peritonei patients treated by cytoreductive surgery and hyperthermic intraperitoneal chemotherapy. Ann Surg. 2007;245(1):104-9.
83. Witkamp AJ, de Bree E, Kaag MM, et al. Extensive surgical cytoreduction and intraoperative hyperthermic intraperitoneal chemotherapy in patients with pseudomyxomaperitonei. Br J Surg. 2001;88(3):458-63.
84. Glehen O, Gilly FN, Boutitie F, et al. Toward curative treatment of peritoneal carcinomatosis from nonovarian origin by cytoreductive surgery combined with perioperative intraperitoneal chemotherapy: a multi-institutional study of 1,290 patients. Cancer. 2010;116(24):5608-18.
85. Verwaal VJ, van Ruth S, de Bree E, et al. Randomized trial of cytoreduction and hyperthermic intraperitoneal chemotherapy versus systemic chemotherapy and palliative surgery in patients with peritoneal carcinomatosis of colorectal cancer. J Clin Oncol. 2003;21(20):3737-43.
86. Shen P, Thai K, Stewart JH, et al. Peritoneal surface disease from colorectal cancer: comparison with the hepatic metastases surgical paradigm in optimally resected patients. Ann Surg Oncol. 2008;15(12):3422-32.
87. Cao CQ, Yan TD, Liauw W, et al. Comparison of optimally resected hepatectomy and peritonectomy patients with colorectal cancer metastasis. J Surg Oncol. 2009;100(7):529-33.
88. Deraco M, Rossi CR, Pennacchioli E, et al. Cytoreductive surgery followed by intraperitoneal hyperthermic perfusion in the treatment of recurrent epithelial ovarian cancer: a phase II clinical study. Tumori. 2001;87(3):120-6.
89. Sugarbaker PH, Klecker RW, Gianola FJ, et al. Prolonged treatment schedules with intraperitoneal 5-fluorouracil diminish the local-regional nature of drug distribution. Am J Clin Oncol. 1986;9(1):1-7.
90. Jol C, Kuppem P, Leeflang PA, et al. In vitro human ovarian cancer. In: Taguchi T, Andryse O (Eds). New Trends in Cancer Chemotherapy with Mitomycin C. Amsterdam: Excerpta Medica; 1987. pp. 181-91.

2

Pseudomyxoma Peritonei and Peritoneal Mucinous Carcinoma of Appendiceal Origin

Paul H. Sugarbaker

THE PRIMARY APPENDICEAL NEOPLASM

Mucocele of the Appendix

The appendix has no known contribution to gastrointestinal function. Therefore, it is removed as an incidental organ in many surgical procedures within the abdomen or pelvis. Upon study of the mucosa of the appendix, it is obvious that this structure contains many goblet cells and consequently its exocrine production of mucus is copious. The density of these goblet cells is far greater within the epithelium of the appendix than within the colon. If any important function for the appendix does exist, perhaps its role in mucus production and lubrication of the fecal contents within the right colon should be mentioned.

With this large proportion of mucus-producing epithelial cells, it is not surprising that a majority of the epithelial tumors of the appendix are mucinous. Also, it is not surprising that most appendiceal tumors begin as a mucocele (Fig. 1). The mucocele of the appendix may be symptomatic versus asymptomatic, small (less than 5 cm) versus large, neoplastic versus benign, unruptured versus ruptured. The precise incidence of a mucocele of the appendix over the lifespan of a human is not known. However, since a mucocele is so frequently encountered, it must be quite common. Fortunately, a great majority of mucoceles removed with appendectomy are benign.

When a mucocele of the appendix is first visualized, it is extremely important to determine if the wall is intact or is perforated. This gross assessment of the appendix either by open surgery or by laparoscopic surgery is essential. Also essential is the proper surgical management of the mucocele; rupture of a neoplastic mucocele by a traumatic appendectomy can be considered an iatrogenic surgical disaster.[1]

Important data regarding the management of appendiceal tumors was provided by Misdraji and colleagues at the Massachusetts General Hospital.[2] In 49 low-grade mucinous neoplasms, those with tumor confined within the appendix behaved as benign disease and no recurrence was seen with a six-year follow-up. In contrast, a low-grade tumor with extra-appendiceal spread had

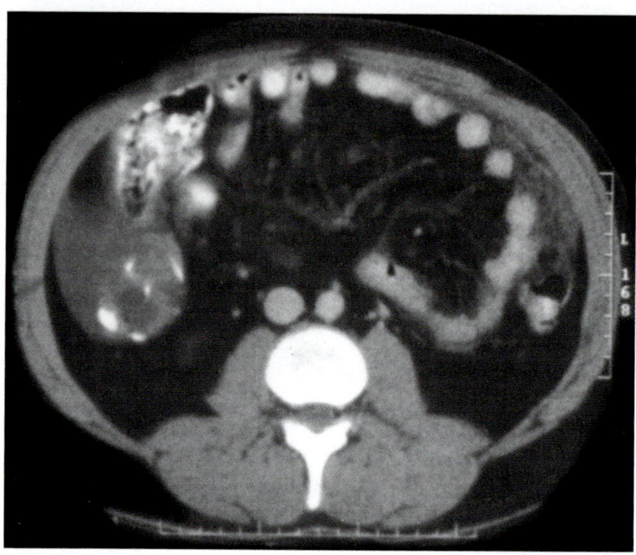

Figure 1 Mucocele of the appendix as seen on abdominal computed tomography
(*Source*: Sugarbaker PH. Epithelial appendiceal neoplasms. Cancer J. 2009; 15(3):225-35.)

only a 45% five-year survival. They concluded that an unruptured mucocele that contained low-grade cancer was a benign process and should be treated by simple appendectomy. In contrast, low-grade mucinous tumors (benign appearing histology), when there was access to the free peritoneal cavity, were often lethal.

Unfortunately, gross external examination of the appendix at the time of appendectomy and an assessment of the size of the mucocele cannot determine if it is benign or malignant.[2] The prudent surgical approach is to regard every mucocele of the appendix as malignant. This means that special care in the resection of an appendiceal mucocele must occur in order to avoid trauma and possible rupture of the appendix as it is removed. Often, this requires conversion of a laparoscopic appendectomy to an open laparotomy.

Not only the appendiceal mucocele must be removed intact by a gentle surgical technique but also the peritoneal spaces surrounding the appendix must be carefully studied. Fluid or mucus in the vicinity must not be suctioned away and discarded; it must be recovered and sent for cytologic examination. Recovery of fluid aspiration from beneath the right liver within the right retrohepatic space is indicated; also, aspiration of fluid from the pelvis is essential. Careful observation of both the right and left ovary looking for cystic tumors may establish the Krukenberg syndrome.[3] If these spaces and tissues are adequately sampled, the patient's subsequent treatment can be more knowledgeably planned.

Some patients with a neoplastic mucocele will have the wall of the appendix breached. Epithelial cells will escape and will be present in the mucus outside of the appendix. In this situation, the criteria for diagnosis of the pseudomyxoma peritonei syndrome have been established.[4] Of course, if tumor nodules outside of the appendix exist, these must be biopsied in order to confirm intracelomic disseminated disease.

Mucinous Appendiceal Neoplasms versus Intestinal Type

For colon cancer, approximately 10% of patients will have a mucinous histologic type of adenocarcinoma. In contrast, approximately 90% of appendiceal epithelial cancers are of a mucinous histologic type and the intestinal type of disease (nonmucinous) is unusual. When the intestinal type of disease occurs, the appendiceal malignancy is usually at the orifice of the appendix, and the cancer dissemination to lymph nodes was reported in 20% of patients.[5] Epithelial malignancies that exist along the lumen of the appendix or at its tip are of a mucinous histologic type; the initial cancer dissemination is through the wall of the appendix into the peritoneal space (Fig. 2). With high-grade mucinous tumors, the incidence of lymph node dissemination is approximately 5%. With low-grade tumors, lymph node dissemination is seldom if ever seen.[5]

Gross and Histologic Types of Mucinous Appendiceal Neoplasms

Essential to the proper management of mucinous appendiceal neoplasms is the recognition that a broad spectrum of aggressiveness exists. The histologic types were classified by Ronnett and coworkers from the extent of cellular atypia of the epithelial cells and the architecture of these cells within the peritoneal cancer deposits.[6] The least aggressive mucinous tumors present on peritoneal surfaces were classified as diffuse peritoneal adenomucinosis (DPAM) (Fig. 2). Misdraji et al. has referred to this type of tumor as low-grade mucinous appendiceal neoplasms.[2] Histologically, peritoneal adenomucinosis was characterized by multifocal mucinous tumors adherent to but not invading into visceral or parietal peritoneal surfaces. Microscopically, the peritoneal lesions contain scant histologically benign appearing mucinous epithelium within abundant extracellular mucus (Fig. 3). An intense hyalinizing fibrotic reaction that separates the pools of mucin was another important histologic feature. The need to distinguish secondary involvement of the ovaries by a

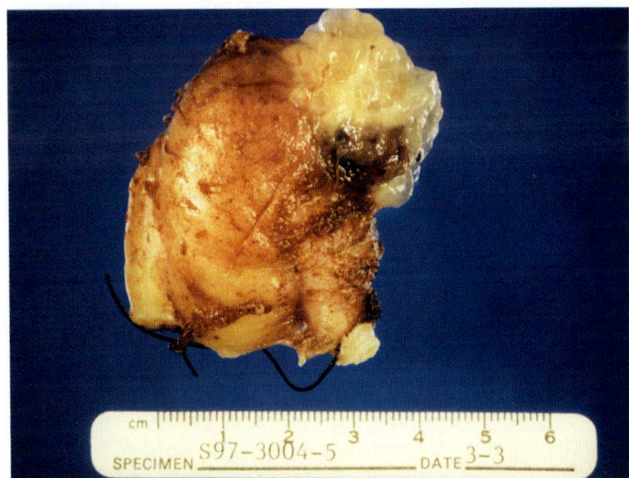

Figure 2 Ruptured appendiceal mucinous neoplasm with pathology of diffuse peritoneal adenomucinosis. Mucus containing malignant cells extruded into the free peritoneal cavity from the end of the appendix. The entire appendix and mesoappendix were removed in order to sample the appendiceal lymph nodes
(*Source*: Sugarbaker PH. Epithelial appendiceal neoplasms. Cancer J. 2009; 15(3):225-35.)

Chapter 2

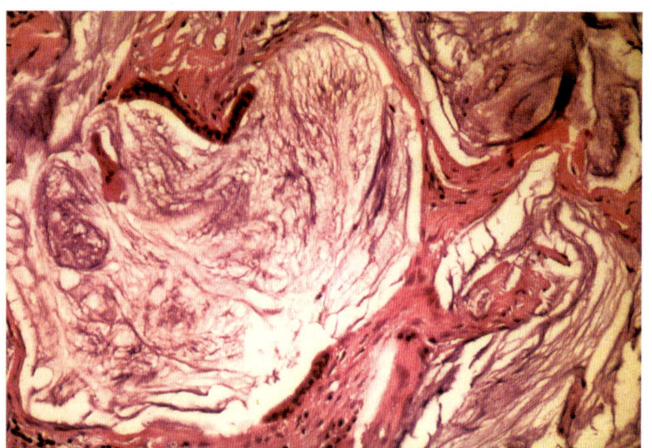

Figure 3 Peritoneal lesions of disseminated peritoneal adenomucinous showed simple mucinous epithelial strips with abundant extracellular mucin. Bland epithelium had no cytologic atypia or mitosis (hematoxylin and eosin, 400x)
(*Source*: Sugarbaker PH. Epithelial appendiceal neoplasms. Cancer J. 2009; 15(3):225-35.)

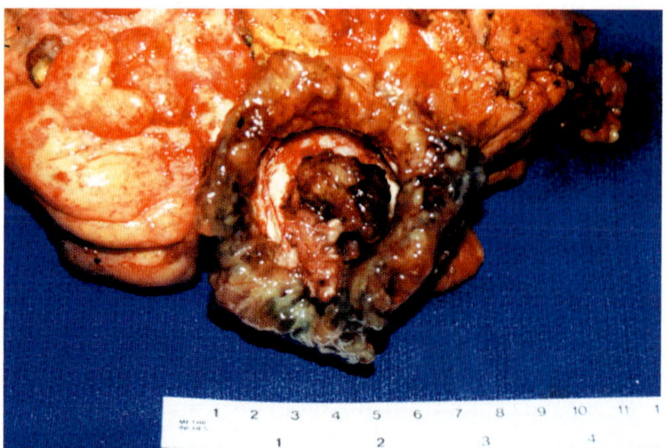

Figure 4 Ruptured appendiceal mucinous neoplasm with pathology of peritoneal mucinous carcinoma. The appendix has been destroyed by the progressive cancer
(*Source*: Sugarbaker PH. Epithelial appendiceal neoplasms. Cancer J. 2009; 15(3):225-35.)

perforated mucinous appendiceal tumor from mucinous borderline tumors of the ovary has been previously established.[7]

Peritoneal mucinous adenocarcinoma (PMCA) emanates from an invasive appendiceal primary tumor (Fig. 4). Misdraji et al. has referred to this type of tumor as high-grade mucinous appendiceal neoplasms.[2] The histology shows abundant epithelium with glandular or signet ring cell morphology with sufficient architectural complexity and cytological atypia to warrant a diagnosis of mucinous adenocarcinoma (Fig. 5). Mucinous adenocarcinomas could be further separated into three grades by evaluating the epithelial content of the tumor in order to more completely describe a histological progression of aggressive cancer behavior. Well-

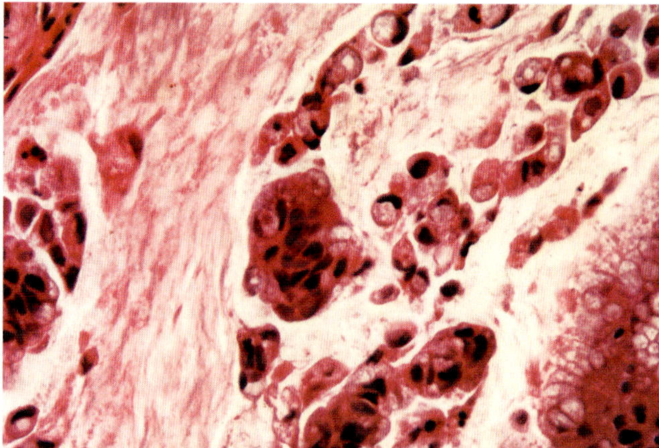

Figure 5 Peritoneal lesion of mucinous carcinomatosis showed the invasion of tumor cells with cytologic atypia. Signet ring cells are numerous (hematoxylin and eosin, 500x)
(*Source*: Sugarbaker PH. Epithelial appendiceal neoplasms. Cancer J. 2009; 15(3):225-35.)

differentiated mucinous adenocarcinoma was composed predominantly of single tubular glands. The tumor cells were well polarized similar to epithelium of an adenoma. Atypia of the tumor cells was evident and an invasive component was identified. Moderately differentiated mucinous adenocarcinoma showed characteristics between well-differentiated adenocarcinoma and poorly-differentiated adenocarcinoma. It was composed of solid sheets of malignant cells admixed with glandular formations. The polarity of the tumor cells was minimal or absent. Poorly-differentiated adenocarcinoma was composed of highly irregular glandular structures or lacked glandular differentiation. The polarity of the cancer cells had disappeared completely. Often, signet ring cells were present.[8]

An intermediate type, often referred to as hybrid type of appendiceal mucinous tumor, was also described by Ronnett.[6] In the intermediate or hybrid type of tumor the predominant histologic features were those of adenomucinosis; however, focal areas (lower than 5% of the field of view) were of mucinous adenocarcinoma (Fig. 6). Exhaustive study of the clinical material available from many different foci of peritoneal neoplasms may be necessary in order to establish an intermediate histologic type.

Adenocarcinoid Histologic Type

As the name implies, adenocarcinoid tumors of the appendix possess a dual morphology showing both carcinoid and mucinous adenocarcinoma components.[9] The carcinoid component is positive for

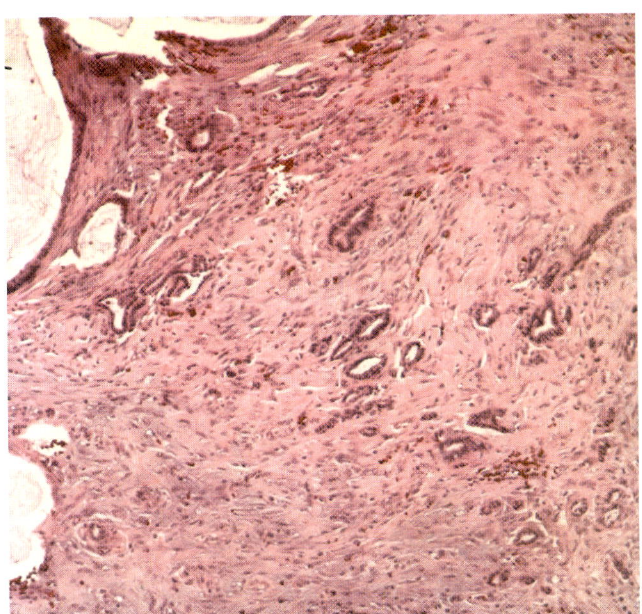

Figure 6 The hybrid type of appendiceal mucinous tumor predominantly demonstrated features of disseminated peritoneal adenomucinosis (right upper corner). However, as shown in the center of the photomicrograph, if sufficient tissue was examined, focal areas of well differentiated adenocarcinoma are identified (hematoxylin and eosin, 80x). In this patient, 15 slides showed disseminated peritoneal adenomucinosis, and in one of these, foci of mucinous adenocarcinoma were identified. The cystic foci seen in this figure adjacent to areas of adenocarcinoma are not likely to be dilated glands of carcinoma. They represent the predominant histologic pattern of diffuse peritoneal adenomucinosis seen in this patient
(*Source*: Sugarbaker PH. Epithelial appendiceal neoplasms. Cancer J. 2009; 15(3):225-35.)

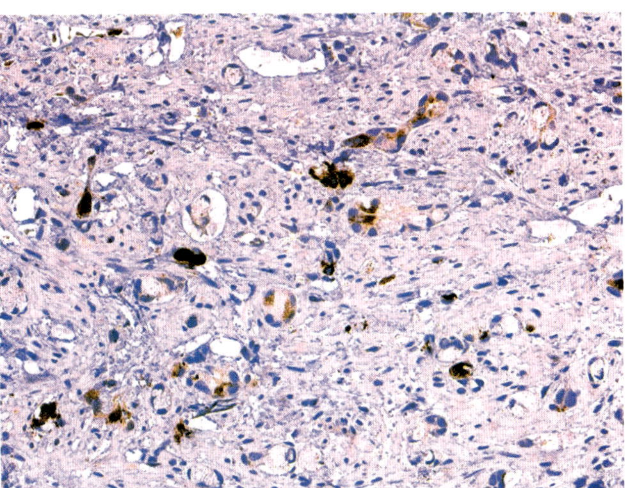

Figure 7 Adenocarcinoid shows an admixture of small uniform glands and single infiltrating tumor cells that resemble goblet cells. Some fields of view show copious mucus. Many cells stain by neuroendocrine immunostain, chromogranin (200x)
(*Source*: Sugarbaker PH. Epithelial appendiceal neoplasms. Cancer J. 2009; 15(3):225-35.)

neuroendocrine immunostains including synaptophysin, chromogranin and neurospecific enolase (Fig. 7). The biologic behavior of the adenocarcinoid tumors is similar to that of peritoneal mucinous carcinoma; signet ring morphology is common. Adenocarcinoids have a higher rate of spread to the ovaries. At the time of surgery it is sometimes recommended to remove the ovaries even if they are not involved with tumor.

Surgical Management of the Primary Appendiceal Neoplasm

Although solid evidence from the literature is lacking, epithelial neoplasms of the appendix over 2 cm in diameter have traditionally been managed by right colon resection. The rationale for prophylactic right colectomy was the resection of occult lymph nodal metastases within the ileocolic lymphatic system. Gonzalez and colleagues addressed this surgical tradition by analyzing clinical data on 501 patients with epithelial malignancy of the appendix.[10] All of these patients had peritoneal dissemination at the time of referral and were treated in a uniform manner by cytoreductive surgery and perioperative intraperitoneal chemotherapy. The surgical procedure was appendectomy in 198 patients and right colectomy in 280 patients and no colectomy in 23. Patients with a right colectomy did not have a survival advantage. Varisco and colleagues performed a retrospective chart review and meta-analysis for adenocarcinoid of the appendix.[11] Their data supported the use of appendectomy alone in localized cases of adenocarcinoid of the appendix, provided there was no cecal involvement and the tumor's histology was of low grade. Gonzalez, in his review, determined that the incidence of lymph node metastases was 4.2% with all the mucinous appendiceal malignancies including high-grade and low-grade primary tumors. It was statistically significantly higher with the intestinal type adenocarcinomas of the appendix (66.7%). The presence of lymph node metastases had no influence on prognosis ($p = 0.155$). These authors suggested that this new information on appendiceal mucinous neoplasms indicated a more selective approach to the use of right colectomy in the management of mucinous appendiceal tumors. Routine right colon resection can only be recommended with an intestinal type of appendiceal cancer. The conservation of colonic length is important because many patients with mucinous carcinomatosis require a left colon resection to clear the pelvis of tumor.

The current approach recommended by Sugarbaker and colleagues uses the sentinel node concept to help decide if right colectomy is necessary with an appendiceal tumor.[12] At the time of appendectomy or with a reoperation, the appendiceal lymph nodes are dissected away from the posterior aspect of the cecum. Four to seven nodes lie in and along the appendiceal artery. This en-bloc resection of the appendiceal lymph nodes is then submitted to the pathologist for cryostat section. If gross and microscopic examinations of these sentinel appendiceal lymph nodes are negative, prophylactic right colectomy is not required to remove occult appendiceal lymph nodes within the ileocolic system.

Also, a positive margin on the base of the appendix should not be used as an indication for a right colectomy. Cecectomy can be used to obtain a negative margin of excision and can save the right colon and ileocecal valve function for the patient.

Second Look Surgery in Patients with Appendiceal Mucinous Neoplasms

Recently, a new approach to the management of mucinous appendiceal neoplasms, a proactive approach, has evolved. Now, patients with a perforated mucocele of the appendix are knowledgeably evaluated and selectively brought back to the operating room for a second look surgery.

If the evaluation of the specimens obtained at the time of appendectomy shows the presence of mucinous peritoneal dissemination, the treatment recommended by this author is straightforward. This recommendation includes both DPAM and PMCA. The patient needs cytoreductive surgery and hyperthermic intraperitoneal chemotherapy for a long-term survival.[13] However, frequently a dilemma exists following the resection of a mucocele in which the wall of the appendix has been perforated but no diagnosis of peritoneal surface malignancy can be established. In this situation, my recommendation for management is as follows: If the appendiceal specimen with perforation shows adenomucinosis, follow-up with computed tomography (CT) scans on a six monthly basis for five years is recommended. With follow-up, if progressive pseudomyxoma peritonei is detected clinically, it should be sufficiently indolent to allow a curative approach to the disease process. In contrast, if the appendiceal tumor shows mucinous adenocarcinoma in the appendix specimen, a second look surgery should be recommended. This should be an open laparotomy with wide exposure of the abdomen and pelvis so that complete exploratory laparotomy can be performed. The undersurface of the diaphragms and the omental bursa must be exposed and clearly visualized. The ligament of Treitz and the left paracolic sulcus are important sites of disease. Of course, the rectovesical or rectouterine space must be inspected to its most inferior aspect. The small bowel should be visualized from the ligament of Treitz to the ileocecal valve.

In patients in whom progressive mucinous adenocarcinoma is documented, cytoreductive surgery to remove all evidence of mucinous adenocarcinoma is necessary. Also greater and lesser omentectomy, oophorectomy and sampling of the appendiceal lymph nodes must occur. If these lymph nodes are positive, right colectomy is indicated. The patient is treated with hyperthermic intraperitoneal chemotherapy in order to eradicate the nonvisible cellular component of the disease.

If recurrent mucinous adenocarcinoma cannot be established then the patient undergoes a sampling of the appendiceal lymph nodes, greater and lesser omentectomy, oophorectomy and treatment with hyperthermic intraperitoneal chemotherapy. This approach is seen as a prophylaxis against subclinical disease developing at a later time. The timing for the second look is recommended at approximately six months following removal of the primary tumor by appendectomy.

This selective second look is designed to prevent the rapid progression of a mucinous adenocarcinoma that may not be recognized by CT and tumor marker surveillance [carcinoembryonic antigen (CEA) and carbohydrate antigen (CA) 19–9]. The long-term results of treatment of mucinous adenocarcinoma are dependent on the extent of the disease. Large volume disease carries a reduced prognosis and a greater morbidity and mortality; in contrast, the treatment of small volume mucinous adenocarcinoma is associated with an improved prognosis.[14]

PERITONEAL DISSEMINATION OF MUCINOUS APPENDICEAL NEOPLASMS

Intracelomic Dissemination

The characteristic distribution of a mucinous appendiceal neoplasm throughout the abdomen and pelvis constitutes a characteristic feature of this disease process.[15,16] The unique pattern of dissemination with small bowel sparing was the original observation that led to the cytoreductive approach to this disease process.[17]

When the appendix bursts due to internal pressure from the mucus-producing neoplasm, mucus and mucinous tumor cells are released into the free peritoneal cavity. Because of the slippery fluid, these cells do not adhere only to the area proximal to the perforated appendix. Rather, by physical principles of fluid dynamics they follow the flow of peritoneal fluid. The fluid rises out of the pelvis along the right paracolic sulcus and moves around the abdomen in a clockwise direction. Large volumes of fluid are absorbed through the open lymphatic lacunae on the undersurface of the right hemidiaphragm and tumor cells are drawn to these sites of fluid resorption. The falciform ligament diverts nonabsorbed fluid down to the lower abdomen. Further fluid is removed by the open lymph pores on the greater omentum. Tumor becomes entrapped within the greater omentum and leads to the "omental cake" formation. This large accumulation of mucinous tumor within the greater and lesser omentum is the hallmark of the pseudomyxoma peritonei syndrome. Tumor cells also become entrapped in the left paracolic sulcus, especially where the sigmoid colon is attached, to the left lateral pelvic sidewall. Fluid and tumor cells cascade into the pelvis and by gravity are entrapped within the cul-de-sac. The ovaries, right or left on a monthly basis, present a "sticky surface" for tumor cell implantation.[3] Also, hormonal factors may cause more rapid progression of the disease once it becomes implanted within the ovarian stroma.

The small bowel, because of its continuous peristalsis, is relatively uninvolved with the mucinous tumor implants. The cul-de-sac created by the ligament of Treitz is a prominent site for accumulation of tumor cells. Also, the terminal ileum has a high density of lymph pores for peritoneal fluid resorption. Consequently, the volume of disease in and around the terminal ileum and ascending colon may be considerably greater than that which occurs along the course of the majority of the small bowel and small bowel mesentery.

This characteristic distribution of mucinous neoplasms of the appendix, both adenomucinosis and peritoneal mucinous carcinoma, creates the clinical picture called pseudomyxoma peritonei. If the clinical entity referred to as pseudomyxoma peritonei is caused by an appendiceal mucinous neoplasm, it is called the pseudomyxoma peritonei syndrome.[4]

The signs and symptoms of this disease are determined by the patterns of peritoneal dissemination of the mucinous tumor cells. Esquivel and Sugarbaker studied, in a retrospective review, the clinical characteristics of 217 patients with the diagnosis of pseudomyxoma peritonei syndrome.[18] The results of their study are shown in Table 1. The most common initial symptom in men and women combined was appendicitis. However, in none of these patients did the appendicitis occur as a first event in the dissemination of the disease and in the absence of mucinous tumor dissemination within the abdomen and pelvis. All patients presenting with appendicitis had moderate to large volume dissemination of the mucinous tumor within the peritoneal cavity. Apparently, the primary tumor had leaked mucin and mucinous tumor cells on many occasions prior to the episode of appendicitis.

Table 1 Clinical presentation of 217 patients with pseudomyxoma peritonei syndrome

	No. of patients	Men	Women
Appendicitis	58 (27)	36 (34)	22 (20)
Increased abdominal girth	49 (23)	28 (27)	21 (19)
Ovaraian mass	44 (20)	–	44 (39)
Hernia	30 (14)	26 (25)	4 (4)
Ascites	9 (4)	5 (5)	4 (4)
Abdominal pain	8 (4)	5 (5)	3 (3)
Other	19 (9)	5 (5)	14 (12)
Total	217 (100)	105 (48)	112 (52)

Values in parentheses are percentages

(*Source*: Esquivel J, Sugarbaker PH. Clinical presentation of the pseudomyxoma peritonei syndrome. Br J Surg. 2000;87(10):1414-8.)

The second most common symptom for men and third most common symptom for women were increasing abdominal girth as a result of progressive mucinous ascites. This "jelly belly" as it is often referred to, often progressed to enormous size before patients recognized the expanding abdomen (Fig. 8). For women, the most common symptom was an ovarian mass. This phenomenon is very similar in its pathobiology to the Krukenberg syndrome; in this syndrome gastric cancer cells move via the celomic space to the ovary. In pseudomyxoma peritonei, the mucinous tumor cells move from the appendix to the ovary. The fourth most common presentation in both men and women was a new onset hernia that was filled by a mucoid fluid. Approximately one-third of the hernias were right inguinal hernia, one-third left inguinal hernia and another one-third umbilical hernias.

Management of Appendiceal Mucinous Neoplasms with Peritoneal Dissemination

Current standard of care for patients with appendiceal mucinous neoplasms requires a "comprehensive

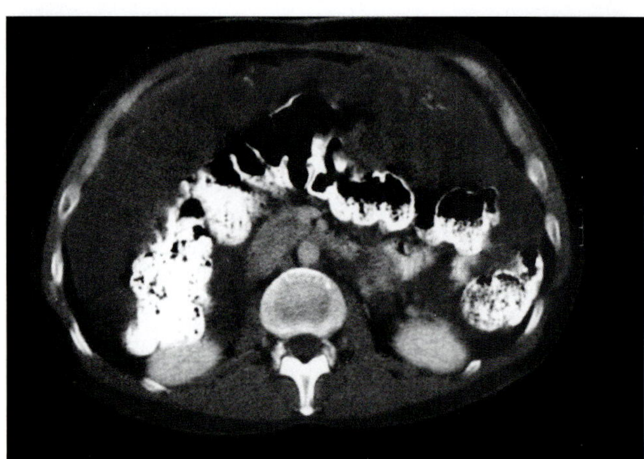

Figure 8 Computed tomography on a patient presenting with a large "omental cake" and a large volume of mucinous ascites
(*Source*: Sugarbaker PH. Epithelial appendiceal neoplasms. Cancer J. 2009; 15(3):225-35.)

management plan." For patients with peritoneal mucinous carcinoma, the first intervention we use at Washington Hospital Cancer Institute is a short course of systemic chemotherapy using 5-fluorouracil and oxaliplatin.[19] Then patients with DPAM and PMCA undergo cytoreductive surgery. This is a combination of visceral resections and peritonectomy procedures. After all visible evidence of tumor has been surgically removed, an attempt to eradicate microscopic disease and small tumor nodules occurs using a hyperthermic intraperitoneal chemotherapy treatment.

The cytoreductive surgery involves a series of visceral resections and peritonectomy procedures.[20] The various combinations of surgical procedures are listed in Table 2. It should be emphasized that no organ or peritoneal surfaces is resected unless there is visible tumor layered out on this structure. Oftentimes, with adenomucinosis, the mucinous tumor is noninvasive and can be wiped away from the involved visceral or parietal peritoneum; in this situation, the organ or peritoneal surface is not resected.

Very often, the visceral resections are performed in combination with peritonectomy procedures. For example, the old abdominal incision proceeds just prior to the complete anterior parietal peritonectomy. The left upper quadrant peritonectomy is performed prior to greater omentectomy and splenectomy so that these structures are elevated out of the left upper quadrant and can be removed under direct vision. The pelvic peritonectomy is begun as a first step in the resection of the rectosigmoid colon, the uterus and ovaries. The pelvic peritoneum, rectosigmoid colon and uterus are removed en bloc and submitted as a single specimen to the pathologist. The right upper quadrant peritonectomy proceeds the cholecystectomy. The cholecystectomy becomes the anatomic lead-in to the lesser omentectomy with stripping of the omental bursa.

These procedures have been diagrammed and described in several prior publications.[21]

There are multiple different chemotherapy regimens utilized to eradicate residual tumor nodules and free tumor cells within the peritoneal cavity. Over the past 23 years, an evolution of intraperitoneal treatments has occurred at the Washington Cancer Institute. The regimen currently in use is hyperthermic intraperitoneal doxorubicin and mitomycin C plus systemic 5-fluorouracil (HIPEC-plus). The standardized order for HIPEC-plus is given in Table 3. As shown in Figure 9 an open method for chemotherapy administration that allows for manual distribution of the heat and chemotherapy solution is used.[22]

Since the activity of all gastrointestinal chemotherapy regimens is dependent on a full dose of 5-fluorouracil, this drug is continued for four days after the HIPEC-plus treatments. Of course, the patient's tolerance for an adequate dose of 5-fluorouracil must be considered. Patients who have had extensive prior systemic chemotherapy will not tolerate full doses of postoperative chemotherapy. Chemotherapy given in the early postoperative period

Table 2 Visceral resections and peritonectomy procedures that may be required for complete cytoreduction

Cytoreduction	
Visceral Resections	*Peritonectomy Procedures*
• Resection of prior abdominal incisions	• Anterior parietal peritonectomy
• Greater omentectomy +/– splenectomy	• Left upper quadrant peritonectomy
• Rectosigmoid colon resection	• Pelvic peritonectomy
• Hysterectomy and oophorectomy	• Right upper quadrant peritonectomy
• Cholecystectomy	• Lesser omentectomy with stripping of the omental bursa

Table 3 Physicians orders for bidirectional intraoperative chemotherapy [Hyperthermic intraperitoneal chemotherapy (HIPEC) plus 5-fluorouracil]

1.	Add mitomycin C _______ mg to 2 liters of 1.5% dextrose peritoneal dialysis solution.
2.	Add doxorubicin _______ mg to the same 2 liters of 1.5% dextrose peritoneal dialysis solution.
3.	Dose of mitomycin C and for doxorubicin is 15 mg/m^2 for each chemotherapy agent.
4.	Add 1.5% dextrose peritoneal dialysis solution so that the total volume of chemotherapy solution to be instilled is 1.5 l/m^2.
5.	Add _______ mg 5-fluorouracil (400 mg/m^2) and leucovorin _______ mg (20 mg/m^2) to separate bags of 250 ml normal saline. Begin rapid IV infusion of both drugs simultaneous with intraperitoneal chemotherapy.
6.	Send all the above to operating room _______ at _______ O'Clock for 90-minute treatment.

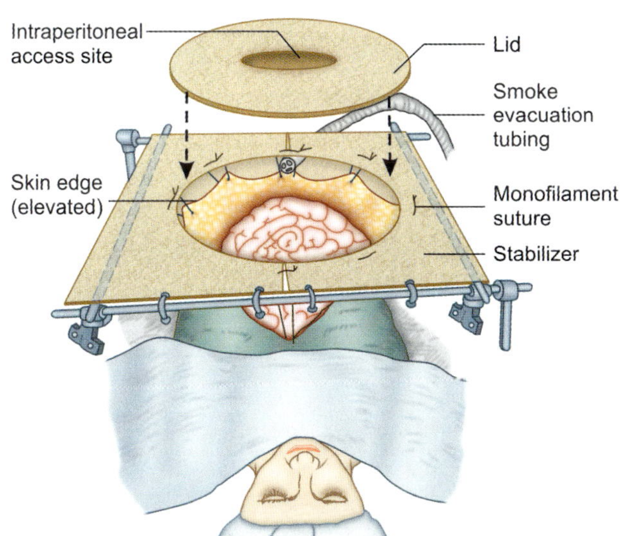

Figure 9 Apparatus for hyperthermic intraperitoneal chemotherapy administered by an open technique that attempts to achieve uniform distribution of heat and chemotherapy solution
(*Source*: Sugarbaker PH. Epithelial appendiceal neoplasms. Cancer J. 2009; 15(3):225-35.)

into the peritoneal cavity is referred to as early postoperative intraperitoneal chemotherapy (EPIC).[23]

OUTCOMES OF THE TREATMENT AT THE WASHINGTON CANCER INSTITUTE OF USING QUANTITATIVE PROGNOSTIC INDICATORS

Quantitative prognostic indicators by which to evaluate patients with appendiceal neoplasms may help understand the causes of success versus failure of treatment of this disease. Also, these quantitative prognostic indicators serve as guidelines in the selection of patients for treatments to maximize benefits of therapy and to exclude patients who have little or no likelihood for improvement.[24] They are of great utility in high risk and costly management protocols in order to prevent patients who are unlikely to benefit from entering into these treatments. Requirements of a useful quantitative prognostic indicator include reproducibility, prediction of morbidity and mortality, and prediction of survivorship. The goal is to establish management protocols and patient selection criteria that will standardize the decision-making process for multiple institutions. Collaborative studies between institutions are greatly facilitated when standardized clinical tools for patient management of peritoneal surface malignancy are available. The data presented in the following paragraphs are extracted from a database of 925 patients having surgery for peritoneal dissemination of an appendiceal epithelial neoplasm.[14]

Histopathology as a Quantitative Prognostic Indicator

Mucinous appendiceal neoplasms have a broad spectrum of biological aggressiveness and the histology of the neoplasm can estimate this factor. The survival of patients with mucinous appendiceal neoplasm, when treated in a uniform fashion using cytoreductive surgery and perioperative intraperitoneal chemotherapy, is profoundly affected by the patient's histologic type. Adenomucinosis describes a noninvasive peritoneal surface malignancy that may become widely disseminaed on peritoneal surfaces. In contrast, peritoneal mucinous adenocarcinoma may show the same propensity for widespread intraperitoneal dissemination that is facilitated by large quantities of mucus, but this histopathology shows invasion into surrounding structures. Also, an intermediate (often called hybrid) type of disease exists in which 95% or more of the fields of view show adenomucinosis, but areas of mucinous adenocarcinoma exist.[5] In the histologic assessment of prognosis presented below the intermediate type is included with the mucinous carcinoma group.

The survival of patients treated at the Washington Cancer Institute by histopathology is shown in Figures 10A and B. The top portion of Figures 10A and B includes all patients with a complete and an incomplete cytoreduction that are in the database. The bottom graph is limited to patients who have had a complete cytoreduction. The impact of histopathology on survival persists with complete cytoreduction.

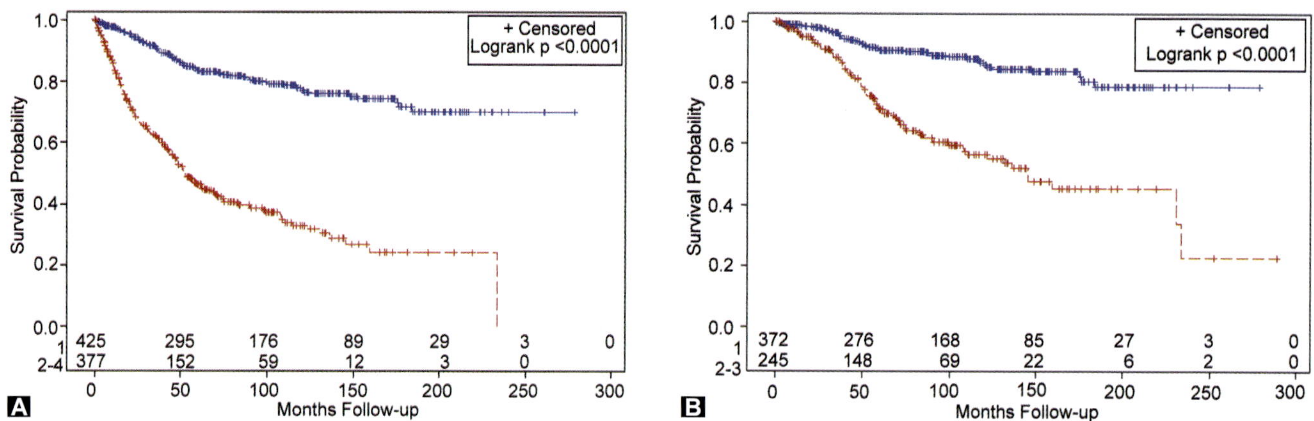

Figures 10A and B Peritoneal surface malignancy of appendiceal origin. Survival by histopathology of patients treated at Washington Cancer Institute. (A) The graph on the left includes all patients. The blue line (N = 425) indicates patients with adenomucinosis. The red line (N = 377) indicates patients with mucinous adenocarcinoma and includes patients with intermediate type histology; (B) The graph on the right is limited to patients with a complete cytoreduction. There were 372 adenomucinosis patients (blue line), and 245 patients (red line) with mucinous adenocarcinoma

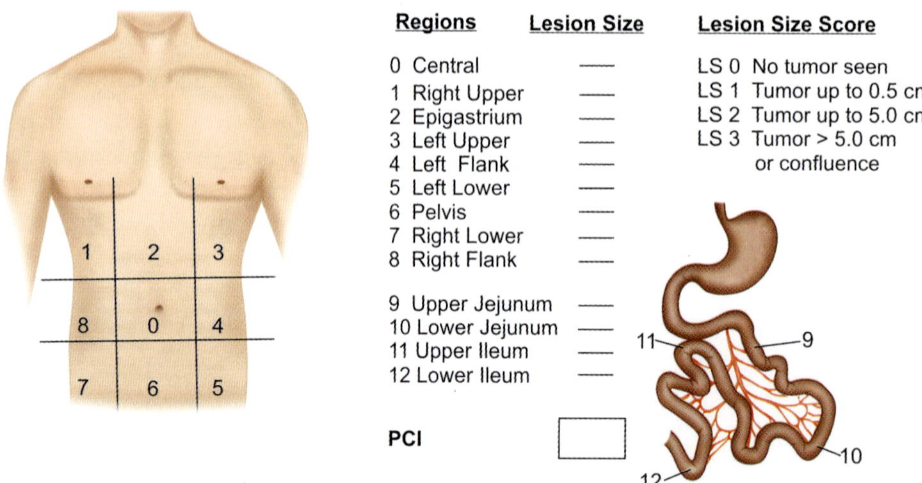

Figure 11 Peritoneal cancer index (PCI). Two transverse planes and two sagittal planes divide the abdomen into nine regions. The upper transverse plane is located at the lowest aspect of the costal margin and the lower transverse plane is placed at the anterior superior iliac spine. The sagittal planes divide the abdomen into three equal sectors. The lines define the nine regions, which are numbered in a clockwise direction with 0 at the umbilicus and 1 defining the space beneath the right hemidiaphragm. Regions 9–12 divide the small bowel into upper jejunum and lower jejunum, and upper ileum and lower ileum. Lesion size score is determined after complete lysis of all adhesions and the complete inspection of all parietal and visceral peritoneal surfaces. It refers to the greatest diameter of tumor implants that are distributed on the peritoneal surfaces. Primary tumors or localized recurrences at the primary site that can be removed definitively are excluded from the lesion size assessment. If there is confluence of disease matting abdominal or pelvic structures together, this is scored as lesion size 3 even if it is a thin confluence of cancerous implants

Peritoneal Cancer Index

The peritoneal cancer index (PCI) is a quantitative prognostic indicator that is determined at the time of surgical exploration of the abdomen and pelvis.[24] The PCI is determined according to the diagram and instructions presented in Figure 11.

For mucinous appendiceal neoplasms that show the adenomucinosis histology, the PCI is of value in determining prognosis. As shown in the top portion of Figures 12A and B this noninvasive malignancy has an excellent prognosis, 94% at 20 years follow-up, if the PCI is less than 20. However, if the PCI score is greater than 20 and all of the tumor can be removed, the survival is 65% at 20 years. When the appendiceal mucinous neoplasm has an invasive component, as in the mucinous carcinomatosis histology, the PCI continues to show a statistically significant effect on the survival (bottom portion of Figs 12A and B).

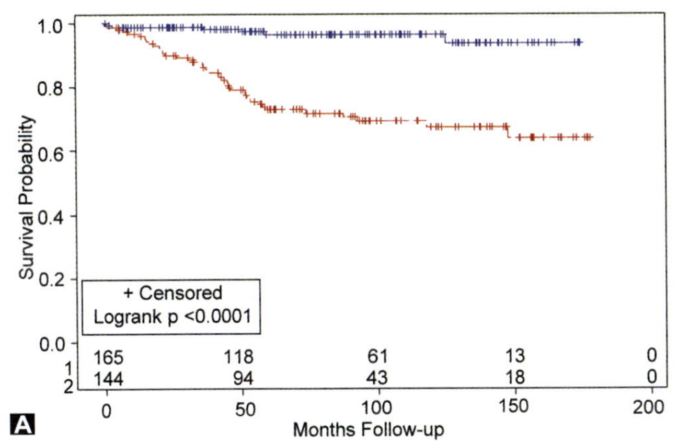

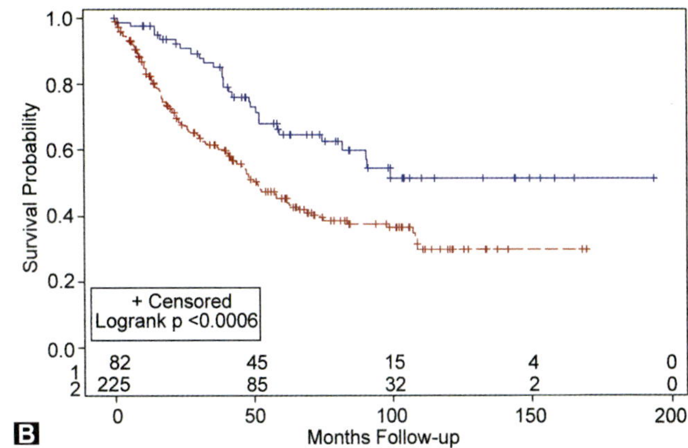

Figures 12A and B Survival by peritoneal cancer index (PCI) for mucinous appendiceal neoplasms. (A) The graph on the left shows adenomucinous patients with PCI 1–20 (blue line, N = 165) versus 21–39 (red line, N = 144); (B) The graph on the right shows mucinous adenocarcinoma patients with PCI 1–20 (blue line, N = 82) versus 21–39 (red line, N = 225)
(*Source*: Sugarbaker PH. Epithelial appendiceal neoplasms. Cancer J. 2009;15(3):225-35.)

In my opinion, these data establish a new standard of care for appendiceal mucinous neoplasms with peritoneal dissemination. The traditional "watch and wait policy" combined with "serial debulking procedures" should only be of historical interest. The definitive cytoreduction with perioperative intraperitoneal chemotherapy used in a proactive manner early in the course of this disease provides the highest likelihood of long-term survival. Figures 12A and B show that this is true for the low-grade mucinous neoplasms and the bottom portion of Figures 12A and B establishes it for mucinous adenocarcinoma.

Peritoneum as the First Line of Defense

A majority of oncologists accept the fact that the optimal treatment with a highest rate of cure, the greatest preservation of function, and the lowest morbidity and mortality is an optimal initial treatment. In treating carcinomatosis, this fact has been documented. The peritoneum is the first line of defense in carcinomatosis.[25] If extensive prior surgery with cancer cells present within the peritoneal space is performed, then these cancer cells will implant at surgical resection sites and deep to the peritoneum. Surgery in which there is disregard for the peritoneum as the first line of defense in carcinomatosis will jeopardize subsequent attempts to achieve an optimal cytoreduction. Cancer progression deep to the peritoneal surfaces and embedded within scar tissue is difficult or impossible to remove by peritonectomy or to eradicate by intraperitoneal chemotherapy.

Prior Surgical Score

Prior surgical score (PSS) quantitates the extent of surgery that was performed prior to definitive cytoreductive surgery and hyperthermic intraperitoneal chemotherapy.[18] The assessment uses a diagram similar to that for the PCI but excludes abdominopelvic regions 9–12. The PSS is a summation of the abdominopelvic regions 0–8 that have been traumatized by a prior surgery or by the additive effects of several prior surgeries. For a PSS of 0 only a biopsy was performed prior to definitive comprehensive management; PSS 1 indicates one region with prior surgery; PSS 2 indicates two to five regions previously dissected; PSS 3 indicates that five or more regions were previously dissected. This is equivalent to a prior attempt at complete cytoreduction but in the absence of perioperative intraperitoneal chemotherapy. The top of Figures 13A and B shows the statistically significant (p = 0.0005) impact of PSS on the survival of patients with DPAM. The bottom of Figures 13A and B shows the lack of significance of PSS on survival of patients with mucinous carcinoma.

The data on PSS in non-aggressive mucinous appendiceal malignancies supports the concept of respect for the peritoneum as a first line of defense. The adverse effects of prior right colectomy, prior hysterectomy and respect for the peritoneum as a first line of defense are a reality in dealing with this disease.[25] The only definitive interventions that can be supported are cytoreductive surgery with perioperative chemotherapy as the initial major treatment plan in this group of patients.

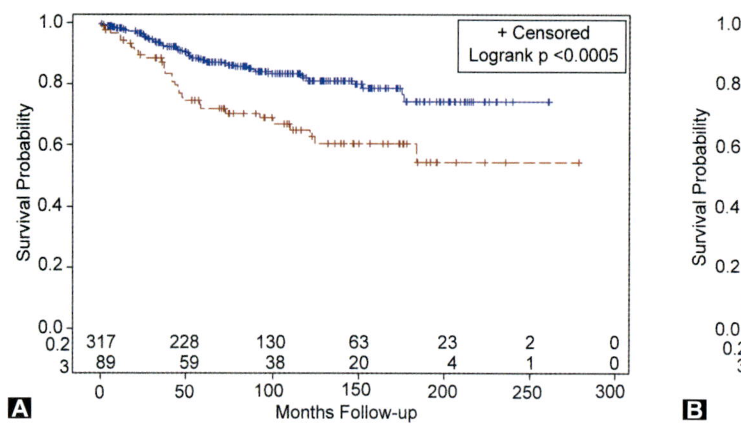

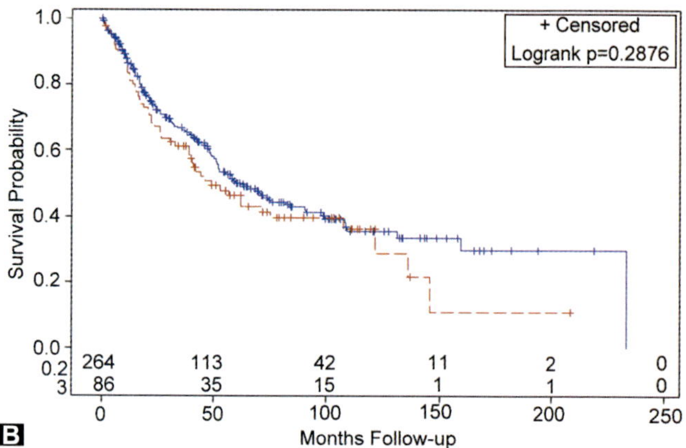

Figures 13A and B Survival of patients with mucinous appendiceal neoplasms by prior surgical score (PSS). (A) The graph on the left shows survival in patients with adenomucinosis of PSS 0–2 (blue line, N = 317) versus PSS of 3 (red line, N = 89). (B); The graph on the right shows that PSS does not have a significant impact on survival of mucinous peritoneal carcinomatosis patients. PSS 0–2 (blue line, N = 264) versus PSS of 3 (red line, N = 86)
(*Source*: Sugarbaker PH. Epithelial appendiceal neoplasms. Cancer J. 2009;15(3):225-35.)

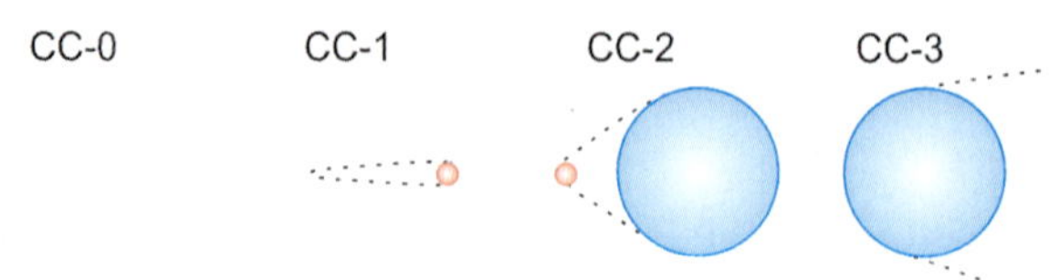

Figure 14 Completeness of cytoreduction (CC) score. A CC-0 is apparent when there is no peritoneal seeding visualized within the operative field. CC-1 indicates nodules persisting after cytoreduction less than 2.5 mm. CC-2 has nodules between 2.5 cm and 5 cm, whereas a CC-3 indicates nodules greater than 5 cm or a confluence of unresectable tumor nodule at any site within the abdomen or pelvis

Completeness of Cytoreduction

The completeness of cytoreduction score (CC score) functions as a major quantitative prognostic indicator for patients with mucinous appendiceal neoplasms. It is an assessment performed after the cytoreductive surgery is complete. Figure 14 demonstrates the CC score for mucinous appendiceal neoplasms.[24] A complete cytoreduction is defined as CC 0 or CC 1. Residual tumor nodules less than 2.5 mm with a mucinous appendiceal neoplasm are well penetrated by the intraperitoneal chemotherapy, which is always used as part of the comprehensive management plan. Therefore, tumor eradication can be predicted by removal of all tumors down to nodules less than 2.5 mm in diameter. In contrast, hard, fibrotic, non-mucinous intestinal type cancer nodules are poorly penetrated by chemotherapy solution. Only cytoreduction down to no visible evidence of disease would be expected to result in long-term survival with a tumor nodule not well penetrated by the intracavitary chemotherapy.

Also, some cancers may be remarkably more responsive to chemotherapy. This is the situation with a majority of primary ovarian cancers. Their complete response to perioperative chemotherapy is frequently seen even though tumor nodules within the CC 1 or CC 2 category remain following cytoreduction. A bidirectional chemotherapy (intraperitoneal combined with intravenous) used in the operating room may achieve a complete response in these patients despite the presence of visible disease following cytoreduction.

The survival of patients with mucinous appendiceal neoplasms by completeness of cytoreduction score is shown in Figures 15A and B. This quantitative prognostic indicator has profound predictive value in appendiceal neoplasms with peritoneal dissemination.

Survival by Presence versus Absence of Lymph Node Involvement

Lymph node metastases are unusual in patients with appendiceal mucinous neoplasms. They are seen only in patients with peritoneal mucinous carcinoma and in the intestinal type of appendiceal adenocarcinoma. Figure 16 shows the survival of these patients by the presence of regional lymph nodes versus their absence. There was a marginally significant reduced survival with positive lymph nodes.

Survival by an Interpretive Assessment of Small Bowel Regions on Computed Tomography

In these patients, a mucinous tumor is widely disseminated within the abdomen and pelvis. Using parietal

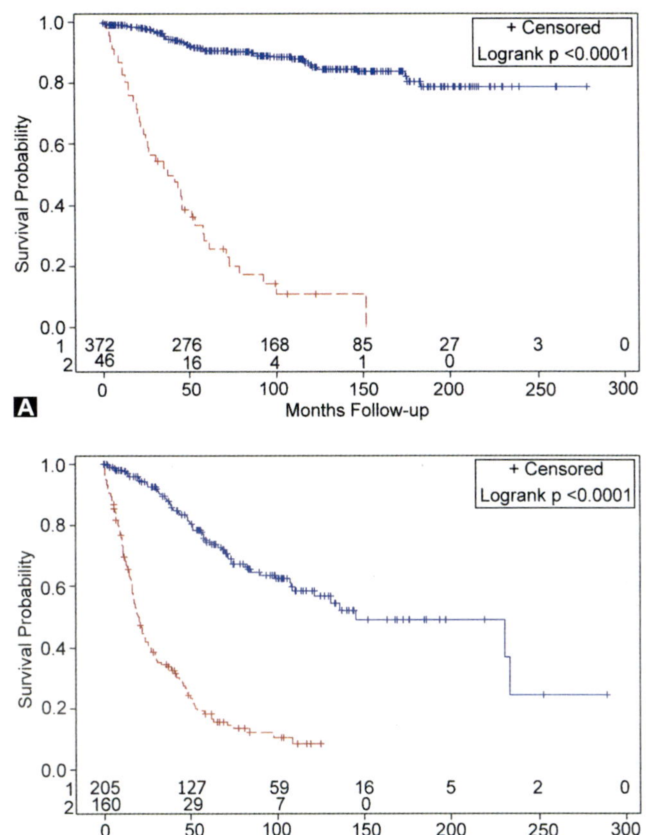

Figures 15A and B Survival of patients with mucinous appendiceal neoplasms by completeness of cytoreduction score. (A) The top graph shows adenomucinosis patients; the blue line (N = 372) indicates patients with complete cytoreduction and the red line (N = 46) indicates incomplete cytoreduction; (B) The bottom graph shows the impact of complete versus incomplete cytoreduction for mucinous carcinoma patients. The blue line indicates complete cytoreduction (N = 205) and the red line indicates incomplete cytoreduction (N = 160)

(*Source*: Sugarbaker PH. Epithelial appendiceal neoplasms. Cancer J. 2009; 15(3):225-35.)

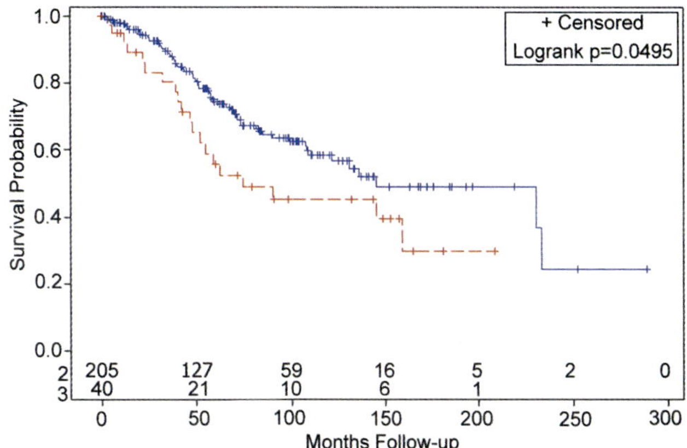

Figure 16 Survival of patients with mucinous appendiceal neoplasms by the absence of disease in regional lymph nodes (blue line, N = 205) versus its presence (red line, N = 40)

(*Source*: Sugarbaker PH. Epithelial appendiceal neoplasms. Cancer J. 2009; 15(3):225-35.)

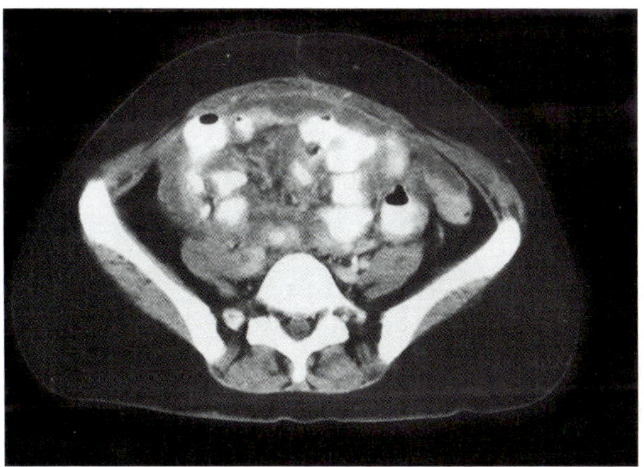

Figure 17 Computed tomography of the abdomen of a patient with appendiceal mucinous neoplasm that shows infiltration of the small bowel regions with tumor. This patient has a small or even absent likelihood of complete cytoreduction

(*Source*: Sugarbaker PH. Epithelial appendiceal neoplasms. Cancer J. 2009; 15(3):225-35.)

peritonectomy procedures, disease involving the anterior parietal peritoneum, beneath the right and left hemidiaphragm, in the paracolic sulcus and in the pelvis can be definitively resected. However, disease on small bowel and small bowel mesentery cannot be adequately removed by peritonectomy. Consequently, disease at this anatomic site can result in an incomplete cytoreduction. Data from the completeness of cytoreduction score establishes that incomplete cytoreduction in these patients is accompanied by a greatly reduced prognosis.

The CT scan performed with optimal intravenous and oral contrast can identify patients who have small bowel compartmentalization versus diffuse involvement of the small bowel.[26] In Figure 8, a CT scan shows a large volume of adenomucinosis surrounding a compartmentalized small bowel with normal contours and no apparent digestive dysfunction. This patient would have a high likelihood of complete cytoreduction. In contrast, the CT in Figure 17 shows diffuse infiltration of the spaces between small bowel regions by mucinous tumor. This patient has a small or even absent likelihood of complete cytoreduction. Although this radiologic prognostic indicator has been well described and can be completely used to predict complete versus incomplete cytoreduction, survival data to support it has not been published. Frequently, the diffuse involvement of small bowel regions by mucinous tumor is seen in patients who have had one or more attempts at cytoreduction

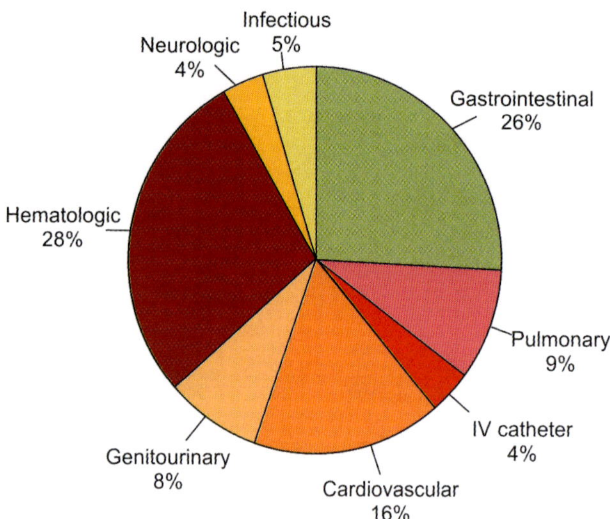

Figure 18 Grade IV adverse events occurred in 67 (19%) of 356 procedures. Because some procedures had more than a single adverse event, there were a total of 80 grade IV adverse events. The incidence of these 80 adverse events is shown

(*Source*: Sugarbaker P, Alderman R, Edwards G, et al. Prospective morbidity and mortality assessment of cytoreductive surgery plus perioperative intraperitoneal chemotherapy to treat peritoneal dissemination of appendiceal mucinous malignancy. Ann Surg Oncol. 2006;13(5):635-44.)

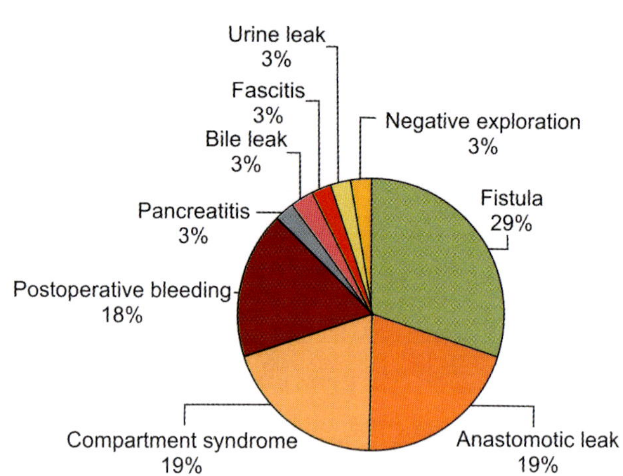

Figure 19 Cause for return to the operating room in 40 procedures (11.2%). The predominant cause for each reoperative procedure is listed

(*Source*: Sugarbaker P, Alderman R, Edwards G, et al. Prospective morbidity and mortality assessment of cytoreductive surgery plus perioperative intraperitoneal chemotherapy to treat peritoneal dissemination of appendiceal mucinous malignancy. Ann Surg Oncol. 2006;13(5):635-44.)

without complete removal of tumor and without the use of intraperitoneal chemotherapy.

Morbidity and Mortality

Sugarbaker and colleagues performed a prospective assessment of the morbidity and mortality on 356 procedures in patients who had an appendiceal mucinous neoplasm.[27] All of these patients had cytoreductive surgery with peritonectomy procedures plus heated intraoperative intraperitoneal chemotherapy. The total 30-day inhospital mortality was 2%. Nineteen percent of the procedures were accompanied by at least one grade IV adverse event (Fig. 18). Eleven percent of patients required a return to the operating room (Fig. 19). The mortality of 2% and the overall grade IV morbidity of 19% in these patients were thought to be acceptable in the light of modern standards for the management of complex gastrointestinal cancer patients.

Yan, in his systematic review of the efficacy of cytoreductive surgery and perioperative intraperitoneal chemotherapy to treat mucinous appendiceal neoplasms, surveyed the most recent updates from ten institutions.[28] This morbidity/mortality assessment involved 718 patients from eight different institutions. Two institutions did not have morbidity/mortality data available. The overall morbidity rate varied from 33–56%. The overall mortality ranged from 0–18%.

Follow-Up and Reoperative Procedures after Comprehensive Management

Following definitive treatment, these mucinous appendiceal neoplasm patients are followed regularly with CEA and CA 19–9 tumor markers and CT scan of chest, abdomen and pelvis. The CEA and CA 19–9 tumor markers, when used together, are an excellent tool for surveillance of these patients.[29] Also, the follow-up is complemented by the CT scan performed on a six monthly basis for five years after treatment. The goal of this follow-up plan is to detect recurrence in a timely fashion so that additional treatments can be initiated.

Yan and colleagues studied reoperative surgery in patients with both adenomucinosis and PMCA.[30] One hundred and eleven patients of the four hundred and two (28%) developed progressive disease. Ninety-eight patients had a repeat cytoreductive surgery with intraperitoneal chemotherapy and thirteen did not. The survival of patients who were considered poor candidates for a repeat cytoreductive effort versus those patients who had a second cytoreduction is shown in

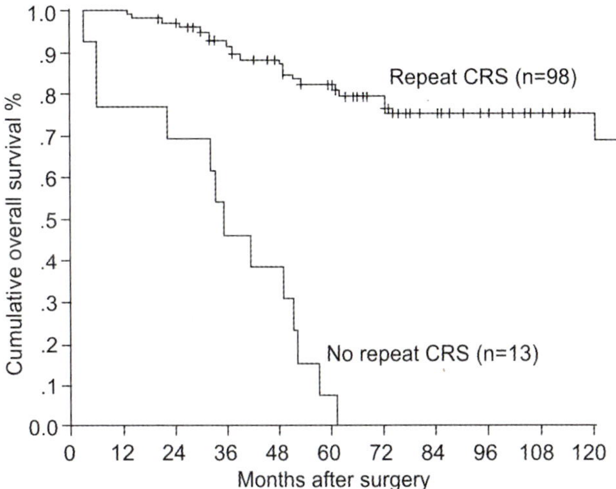

Figure 20 Survival of 111 patients who developed disease progression after initial cytoreductive surgery and perioperative intraperitoneal chemotherapy for peritoneal dissemination from appendiceal mucinous neoplasms, stratified by repeat cytoreductive surgery ($p < 0.001$)
(*Source*: Yan TD, Bijelic L, Sugarbaker PH. Critical analysis of treatment failure after complete cytoreductive surgery and perioperative intraperitoneal chemotherapy for peritoneal dissemination from appendiceal mucinous neoplasms. Ann Surg Oncol. 2007;14(8):2289-9.)

Figure 20. By these data, one is led to think that careful follow-up and reoperation, if patients can again be made disease-free, is the appropriate treatment strategy for this group of patients.

REFERENCES

1. Dhage-Ivatury S, Sugarbaker PH. Update on the surgical approach to mucocele of the appendix. J Am Coll Surg. 2006;202(4):680-4.
2. Misdraji J, Yantiss RK, Graeme-Cook FM, et al. Appendiceal mucinous neoplasms: a clinicopathologic analysis of 107 cases. Am J Surg Pathol. 2003;27(8):1089-103.
3. Sugarbaker PH, Averbach AM. Krukenberg syndrome as a natural manifestation of tumor cell entrapment. In: Sugarbaker PH (Ed.). Peritoneal carcinomatosis: principles of management. Boston: Kluwer Academic Publishers; 1996. pp. 63-191.
4. Sugarbaker PH, Ronnett BM, Archer A, et al. Pseudomyxoma peritonei syndrome. Adv Surg. 1996;30:233-80.
5. Gonzalez-Moreno S, Brun E, Sugarbaker PH. Lymph node metastasis in epithelial malignancies of the appendix with peritoneal dissemination does not reduce survival in patients treated by cytoreductive surgery and perioperative intraperitoneal chemotherapy. Ann Surg Oncol. 2005;12(1):72-80.
6. Ronnett BM, Shmookler BM, Sugarbaker PH, et al. Pseudomyxoma peritonei: new concepts in diagnosis, origin, nomenclature, relationship to mucinous borderline (low malignant potential) tumors of the ovary. In: Fechner RE, Rosen PP (Eds). Anatomic Pathology, vol. 2. Chicago: ASCP Press; 1997. pp. 197-226.
7. Ronnett BM, Kurman RJ, Shmookler BM, et al. The morphologic spectrum of ovarian metastases of appendiceal adenocarcinomas: a clinicopathologic and immunohistochemical analysis of tumors often misinterpreted as primary ovarian tumors or metastatic tumors from other gastrointestinal sites. Am J Surg Pathol. 1997;21(10):1144-55.
8. Yan H, Pestieau SR, Shmookler BM, et al. Histopathologic analysis in 46 patients with pseudomyxoma peritonei syndrome: failure versus success with a second-look operation Mod Pathol. 2001;14(3):164-171.
9. Mahteme H, Sugarbaker PH. Treatment of peritoneal carcinomatosis from adenocarcinoid of appendiceal origin. Br J Surg. 2004;91(9):1168-73.
10. González-Moreno S, Sugarbaker PH. Right hemicolectomy does not confer a survival advantage in patients with mucinous carcinoma of the appendix and peritoneal seeding. Br J Surg. 2004;91(3):304-11.
11. Varisco B, McAlvin B, Dias J, et al. Adenocarcinoid of the appendix: is right hemicolectomy necessary? A meta-analysis of retrospective chart reviews. Am Surg. 2004;70(7):593-9.
12. Morton DL, Thompson JF, Essner R, et al. Validation of the accuracy of intraoperative lymphatic mapping and sentinel lymphadenectomy for early-stage melanoma: a multicenter trial. Multicenter Selective Lymphadenectomy Trial Group. Ann Surg. 1999;230(4):453-63.
13. Sugarbaker PH. New standard of care for appendiceal epithelial neoplasms and pseudomyxoma peritonei syndrome? Lancet Oncol. 2006;7(1):69-76.
14. Sugarbaker PH. Epithelial appendiceal neoplasms. Cancer J. 2009;15(3):225-35.
15. Sugarbaker PH. Pseudomyxoma peritonei: a cancer whose biology is characterized by a redistribution phenomenon. Ann Surg. 1994;219(2):109-11.
16. Carmignani CP, Sugarbaker TA, Bromley CM, et al. Intraperitoneal cancer dissemination: mechanisms of the patterns of spread. Cancer Metastasis Rev. 2003;22(4):465-72.
17. Sugarbaker PH, Kern K, Lack E. Malignant pseudomyxoma peritonei of colonic origin. Natural history and presentation of a curative approach to treatment. Dis Colon Rectum. 1987;30(10):772-9.
18. Esquivel J, Sugarbaker PH. Clinical presentation of the pseudomyxoma peritonei syndrome. Br J Surg. 2000;87(10):1414-8.
19. Sanoff HK, Sargent DJ, Campbell ME, et al. Five-year data and prognostic factor analysis of oxaliplatin and irinotecan combinations for advanced colorectal cancer: N9741. J Clin Oncol. 2008;26(35):5721-7.
20. Sugarbaker P. Peritonectomy procedures. Ann Surg. 1995; 221(1):29-42.
21. Sugarbaker PH. Peritonectomy procedures. Surg Oncol Clin N Am. 2003;12(3):703-27.
22. Sugarbaker PH. An instrument to provide containment of intraoperative intraperitoneal chemotherapy with optimized distribution. J Surg Oncol. 2005;92(2):142-6.
23. Van der Speeten K, Stuart OA, Sugarbaker PH. Using pharmacologic data to plan clinical treatments for patients with peritoneal surface malignancy. Curr Drug Discov Technol. 2009;6(1):72-81.

24. Jacquet P, Sugarbaker PH. Current methodologies for clinical assessment of patients with peritoneal carcinomatosis. J Exp Clin Cancer Res. 1996;15(1):49-58.
25. Sugarbaker PH. Peritoneum as the first line of defense in carcinomatosis. J Surg Oncol. 2007;95(2):93-6.
26. Jacquet P, Jelinek JS, Chang D, et al. Abdominal computed tomographic scan in the selection of patients with mucinous peritoneal carcinomatosis for cytoreductive surgery. J Am Coll Surg. 1995;181(6):530-8.
27. Sugarbaker P, Alderman R, Edwards G, et al. Prospective morbidity and mortality assessment of cytoreductive surgery plus perioperative intraperitoneal chemotherapy to treat peritoneal dissemination of appendiceal mucinous malignancy. Ann Surg Oncol. 2006;13(5):635-44.
28. Yan TD, Black D, Savady R, et al. A systematic review on the efficacy of cytoreductive surgery and perioperative intraperitoneal chemotherapy for pseudomyxoma peritonei. Ann Surg Oncol. 2007;14(2):484-92.
29. Carmignani CP, Hampton R, Sugarbaker CE, et al. Utility of CEA and CA 19-9 tumor markers in diagnosis and prognostic assessment of mucinous epithelial cancers of the appendix. J Surg Oncol. 2004;87(4):162-6.
30. Yan TD, Bijelic L, Sugarbaker PH. Critical analysis of treatment failure after complete cytoreductive surgery and perioperative intraperitoneal chemotherapy for peritoneal dissemination from appendiceal mucinous neoplasms. Ann Surg Oncol. 2007;14(8):2289-9.

3

Carcinomatosis from Colon Cancer

Terence C. Chua, Jesus Esquivel

INTRODUCTION

It is estimated that about 40% of patients with colorectal cancer will develop peritoneal metastases at some point in time after initial diagnosis.[1] This clinical manifestation is universally referred to with varying terminologies that include peritoneal metastases, peritoneal carcinomatosis or diffuse intra-abdominal metastases. Carcinomatosis from colorectal cancer may occur as an isolated or combined site of treatment failure following initial curative surgery. It may also occur in individuals presented with advanced colorectal cancer with metastatic disease. Peritoneal carcinomatosis is the dominant factor of patients' symptomatology where malignant bowel obstruction and ascites leads to profound anorexia and pain. Necropsy studies have shown that the majority of patients dying of colorectal cancer have evidence of peritoneal metastases.[2-4]

The occurrence of peritoneal carcinomatosis is a result of the growth of tumor that invades through the serosal lining of the bowel lumen allowing the exfoliation and shedding of malignant cells intraperitoneally. Iatrogenic manipulation during the surgical procedure, such as transection of lymphatics or blood vessels, may also lead to seeding of tumor cells within the peritoneal cavity, hence, contributing toward the etiological origins of this clinical entity.[1,5] As described in the seed and soil hypothesis of cancer invasion and metastasis,[6,7] the implantation and establishment of a metastatic niche in the peritoneum is likely to be a result of various genes and proteins that characterize the intrinsic properties of these specific cancer cell,[8] and the cancer cell microenvironment interaction that have the propensity toward developing peritoneal metastasis.[9-11] Favored sites of the peritoneal cavity include the subphrenic region, lesser sac, bowel surfaces and mesentery, and in the pelvis due to the direction of peritoneal fluid circulation and the effects of gravitational forces.

In the last decade, tremendous progress has been made in the medical management of metastatic colorectal cancer. The addition of oxaliplatin and irinotecan to previously existing 5-fluorouracil (5-FU) and leucovorin-based therapies has improved the overall median survival that previously rarely exceeded 12 months.[12] Coupled with the addition of biological targeted therapies including bevacizumab and cetuximab, the overall median survival is now up to 24 months.[13-18] In addition, there is increasing evidence suggesting that radical surgery of metastases from colorectal cancer to sites such as the liver, lung, and peritoneum is associated with improved survival and possibly cure.[19-22] The purpose of this chapter is to provide an overview on carcinomatosis from colorectal cancer, describing the progress made in its management and the future directions that involve multimodality therapies.

NATURAL HISTORY OF CARCINOMATOSIS

Carcinomatosis from colorectal cancer was traditionally regarded a terminal condition with survival from historical patients being in the order of about 6 months. These patients often received only supportive care or palliative chemotherapy with single agent 5-FU. The terminal nature of this disease has been demonstrated in a large cohort registry study and a clinical trial.[23,24] The French multicentric EVOCAPE 1 trial, which prospectively followed 370 patients with peritoneal carcinomatosis from various primary cancers from diagnosis till death showed a mean and overall median survival of 6.0 and 3.1 months respectively.[24] Survival was often accompanied by abdominal distention, bowel obstruction and profound anorexia that occur due to the presence of malignant ascites and the peritoneal tumor burden. The ability to palliate this group of patients is often challenging. Owing to the symptomatic nature of this disease entity, patients are often not fit for chemotherapy. Medical therapy is often ineffective to manage symptoms from progressive cancer. Alternatively, nonresectional palliative abdominal surgery that includes defunctioning stoma or bypass procedures is associated with relatively high morbidity and mortality, especially when performed in an emergency setting. The Leicester Colorectal Specialist Interest Group, in their experience of 193 patients, who underwent palliative surgery, of which 169 patients had defunctioning stomas and 24 patients underwent bypass procedures, reported a 30-day mortality rate of 14% and postoperative morbidity rate of 47% in their cohort where median survival was 247 days and 1-year survival was 38%.[25] These results were similar to that reported by Krouse et al. from the Southern Arizona Veterans Affairs Health Sciences Cancer Center where postoperative 30-day mortality rate was 12%, and major and minor morbidity rates were 22% and 10% respectively.[26]

Hence, the dire survival outcome historically associated with this condition is a reflection of the failure of conventional systemic chemotherapy and palliative surgery on disease control.

SYSTEMIC CHEMOTHERAPY FOR COLORECTAL CARCINOMATOSIS

Although various novel agents have been introduced and may prove to be effective in the management of hematogenously borne metastatic colorectal cancer, the evaluation of the efficacy of these modern chemotherapy regimen, including FOLFOX and FOLFIRI, in combination with biological agents, such as cetuximab and bevacizumab, in patients with metastatic colorectal cancer specific to the peritoneum is lacking.[13,27] None of these large clinical trials evaluating modern agent systemic chemotherapy have reported the results of response and survival specific to patients with peritoneal carcinomatosis. It is likely that selecting patients with peritoneal carcinomatosis for entry into such trials is not possible due to the inability to obtain any baseline tumor size measurements on conventional computed tomography imaging scans, magnetic resonance imaging and X-ray. This highlights the difficulties of applying the RECIST criteria[28] to examine the tumor response and efficacy of systemic treatments. For example, in the trial that led toward bevacizumab becoming standard of care when used in combination with irinotecan, 5-fluorouracil and leucovorin regimen for patients with metastatic colorectal cancer,[13] patients were required to have bi-dimensionally measurable disease and if malignant ascites was present, patients were excluded from the study. Such exclusion criteria would clearly fail to capture the pool of patients with peritoneal carcinomatosis. Therefore, it is foreseeable that the majority of clinical trials would not have included patients with peritoneal carcinomatosis. For all these reasons, evidence-based data about the response and outcome of systemic treatments in this distinct subgroup of patients is very limited.

From long-term experience of managing patients with colorectal carcinomatosis, this group of patients has been observed to often be the ones with the poorest response to systemic chemotherapy when compared to patients with other sites of metastatic disease. In a collective review of published results in the literature, 14 studies included 1,955 patients with carcinomatosis from colorectal cancer treated by chemotherapy and 71% of patients underwent palliative surgery (Table 1). The median survival in this cohort was 13 months (range, 5–24 months). The median 1-, 2-, 3- and 5-year survival rates were 59% (range, 36–73%), 25% (range, 18–65%), 18% (range, 3–33%) and 6% (range, 0–22%) respectively. The majority of patients identified in this review received 5-FU and leucovorin chemotherapy only. Results of patients treated by modern chemotherapy (oxaliplatin or irinotecan) with or without biological agents were reported in four studies.[29-32] The median survival reported in these four studies ranged from 11 months to 24 months and the 5-year survival rate ranged from 0% to 13%. The best results were reported by Elias et al.,[31] where the median survival time was 24 months after palliative surgery and systemic chemotherapy. These authors reported a defined population of patients with limited isolated peritoneal metastases, the majority of which have well differentiated tumors, and excluded patients that progressed rapidly on systemic treatment. Clearly, this self-selected population represents a group of patients with reasonably minimal carcinomatosis for which treatment using modern agents, such as oxaliplatin and irinotecan, into the chemotherapy regimen might have explained the long survival outcome. A more representative population that did not undergo such stringent selection for inclusion was the study reported by Catalano et al.[29] In their study of predictors for poor response and overall survival in patients with colorectal cancer treated with first-line oxaliplatin and/or irinotecan-based chemotherapy, patients with peritoneal metastases

Table 1 Characteristics of the studies reporting outcomes of palliative surgery and/or systemic chemotherapy for carcinomatosis from colorectal cancer

Palliative Surgery and/or Systemic Chemotherapy												
First author	*Institution*	*City*	*Year*	*Level of evidence*	*Patients (n)*	*Palliative surgery*	*Type of chemotherapy*	*Median survival (months)*	*1-year survival (%)*	*2-year survival (%)*	*3-year survival (%)*	*5-year survival (%)*
Chua[30]	Multi-institutional		2011	III	114	NR	5-FU, Leucovorin, Oxaliplatin/ Irinotecan, Oxaliplatin/ Irinotecan with biological agents	11 15 23	47 62 73	NR NR NR	3 18 33	0 6 0
Lemmens[34]	Eindhoven Comprehensive Cancer Center		2010	III	395	NR	NR	8	36	18	10	0
Franko[32]	University of Pittsburgh		2010	III	38	NR	5-FU, Leucovorin, Oxaliplatin/ Irinotecan with biological agents	17	65	40	20	5
Catalano[29]	Multi-institutional		2009	III	43	Yes	5-FU, Leucovorin, Oxaliplatin, Irinotecan	11	NR	NR	NR	NR
Elias[31]	Institut Gustave Roussy	Villejuif	2009	II	48	Yes	5-FU, Leucovorin, Oxaliplatin, Irinotecan	24	NR	65	NR	13
Machida[35]	Shizuoka Cancer Center	Shizuoka	2008	III	20	Yes	5-FU, Leucovorin	12	NR	NR	NR	NR
Hasegawa[36]	Tokai University	Tokyo	2006	III	125	Yes	5-FU, Leucovorin	15	67	25	13	13
Bloemendaal[37]	Netherlands Cancer Institute	Amsterdam	2005	III	50	Yes	5-FU, Leucovorin, Irinotecan	13	55	25	19	NR
Elias[38]	Institut Gustave Roussy	Villejuif	2004	I	19	Yes	5-FU, Leucovorin	NR	NR	60	NR	22
Higashi[39]	Tokyo Kosei Nenkin Hospital	Tokyo	2003	III	21	Yes	Yes but type was NR	19	NR	NR	NR	NR
Verwaal[40]	Netherlands Cancer Institute	Amsterdam	2003	I	51	Yes	5-FU, Leucovorin	13	50	25	NR	NR
Kohne[33]	Multi-institutional		2002	III	660	NR	5-FU, Leucovorin	12	NR	NR	NR	NR
Jayne[23]	Singapore General Hospital	Singapore	2002	III	253	Yes	NR	7	NR	NR	NR	NR
Sadeghi[24]	Multi-institutional		2000	II	118	Yes	NR	5	NR	NR	NR	NR
Total	–	–	–	–	1,955	71%						
Median								13	59	25	18	6
Range			2000 to 2011					5 to 24	36 to 73	18 to 65	3 to 33	0 to 22

Abbreviations: 5-FU, 5-fluorouracil; NR, not recorded

were found to be associated with a poor overall survival on multivariate analysis, with a median overall survival of 11 months. In the largest reviewed study, Kohne et al.[33] performed a multivariate analysis of 3,825 patients with metastatic colorectal cancer treated with 5-FU to determine predictive factors for survival. The patient cohort in this study was obtained from 19 prospective randomized and three phase II trials. Similar to the previous study by Catalano et al.,[29] this study likewise identified patients with peritoneal metastases to predict for a worse outcome, with a median survival of 12 months.

These studies indicate that the survival from chemotherapy treatment remains poor; however, modern chemotherapy and biological therapy appear to be effective and may improve survival. Nonetheless, 5-year survivors in patients treated by chemotherapy were infrequently observed.

CYTOREDUCTIVE SURGERY AND HYPERTHERMIC INTRAPERITONEAL CHEMOTHERAPY TREATMENT FOR COLORECTAL CARCINOMATOSIS

A surgical approach combining cytoreductive surgery (CRS) and hyperthermic intraperitoneal chemotherapy (HIPEC) is gaining increasing acceptance in the oncological community as a treatment option for patients with carcinomatosis from colorectal cancer. This treatment was first described by Spratt et al in 1980[41] before being further developed by Dr. Paul Sugarbaker of the Washington Cancer Institute in the 1990s.[42] This procedure involves stripping of the diseased peritoneum with multiple visceral resections performed with an aim of achieving a maximal cytoreduction of all visible peritoneal lesions within the abdomen and pelvis. Following surgery, a heated chemotherapy perfusate is administered intraoperatively into the abdomen to chemically sterilize all raw peritoneal surfaces. Heated intraperitoneal chemotherapy allows a high local concentration of a cytotoxic drug to be achieved for microscopic cytoreduction to target any microscopic residual tumor volume with minimal systemic adverse effects. In addition, hyperthermia between 40°C and 44°C is cytotoxic to cancer cells and it has also been demonstrated to have a synergistic effect with the chemotherapy and can thus enhances the cytotoxicity of the drug.[43]

The survival benefits of this treatment was first reported by Verwaal et al.[40] in a randomized trial comparing systemic chemotherapy versus CRS with HIPEC which showed an almost two-fold (13 months vs. 22 months; p = 0.032) survival benefit in the arm receiving HIPEC. Subsequently, a multi-institutional registry study corroborated by the Peritoneal Surface Oncology Group of 506 patients with colorectal cancer peritoneal metastases from 28 institutions treated with CRS and HIPEC showed a median survival of 32 months in patients who had a complete cytoreduction.[44] During that time, numerous institutions reported their initial experience with this treatment modality. A systematic review elegantly summarized the results of all available studies; comprising of two randomized trials, one comparative study, the multi-institutional registry study and 10-case series demonstrated a median survival ranging from 13 months to 29 months.[45]

Recent major studies reporting the outcomes of CRS and HIPEC were reviewed (Table 2). The median survival of patients undergoing complete CRS and HIPEC was 33 months (range, 20–63 months). The median 1-, 2-, 3- and 5-year survival rates were 86% (range, 70–94%), 70% (range, 45–81%), 48% (range, 44–56%) and 42% (range, 20–51%) respectively. In highly selected patients with limited carcinomatosis, the median survival achieved may be as high as 63 months and 5-year survival of 51% as reported by Elias et al. from the Institut Gustave Roussy.[31] It must be emphasized that when we compare the opportunity for cancer control and cure, for which is commonly defined as 5-year survival, this is unlikely to be achieved when treated by palliative surgery and/or systemic chemotherapy alone. On the contrary, complete CRS and HIPEC achieves 5-year survival of 42% as shown. These data should be sufficiently strong to convince oncologists to discuss patients with colorectal carcinomatosis with a specialized unit involved in the care of patients with peritoneal surface malignancies. Clearly, a complete CRS may not be possible in every case and that the peritoneal tumor burden accepted for treatment is when the peritoneal cancer index is less than twenty. However, every effort must be made to enroll carcinomatosis patients for treatment at the earliest point in time possible, usually at the time of diagnosis.

Today, there are numerous tertiary treatment centers in every continent around the world offering this specialized treatment. In a recent meta-analysis to analyze the survival outcomes of patients with colorectal peritoneal metastases treated with CRS and perioperative intraperitoneal chemotherapy, significant improvement in survival was associated with treatment by CRS and HIPEC compared with palliative approach ($p < 0.0001$) through combining two studies that were included in this review[31,40,53] (Fig. 1).

Table 2 Characteristics of the major studies reporting outcomes of complete cytoreductive surgery and hyperthermic intraperitoneal chemotherapy for carcinomatosis from colorectal cancer

Complete Cytoreductive Surgery and Hyperthermic Intraperitoneal Chemotherapy										
First author	*Institution*	*City*	*Year*	*Level of evidence*	*Total patients (n)*	*Overall survival (months)*	*1-year survival (%)*	*2-year survival (%)*	*3-year survival (%)*	*5-year survival (%)*
Elias[46]	Multicenter		2010	III	439	32	85	60	45	30
Chua[47]	St George Hospital	Sydney	2009	III	54	33	87	70	44	NR
Elias[31]	Institut Gustave Roussy	Villejuif	2009	II	48	63	NR	81	NR	51
Shen[48]	Wake Forest University	Winston-Salem	2008	III	30	41	NR	NR	NR	NR
Franko[49]	University of Pittsburgh Medical Center	Pittsburgh	2008	III	36	20	85	NR	45	NR
Bijelic[50]	Washington Cancer Institute	Washington DC	2008	III	49	33	NR	NR	50	20
Kianmanesh[51]	Louis-Mourier University Hospital	Paris	2007	III	30	38	NR	72	NR	44
Verwaal[52]	Netherlands Cancer Institute	Amsterdam	2005	III	59	43	94	NR	56	43
Glehen[44]	Multi-institutional		2004	III	377	32	90	NR	55	40
Verwaal[40]	Netherlands Cancer Institute	Amsterdam	2003	I	39	22	70	45	NR	NR
Total	–	–	–	–	1,084					
Median						33	86	70	48	42
Range						20 to 63	70 to 94	45 to 81	44 to 56	20 to 51

Abbreviation: NR, not recorded

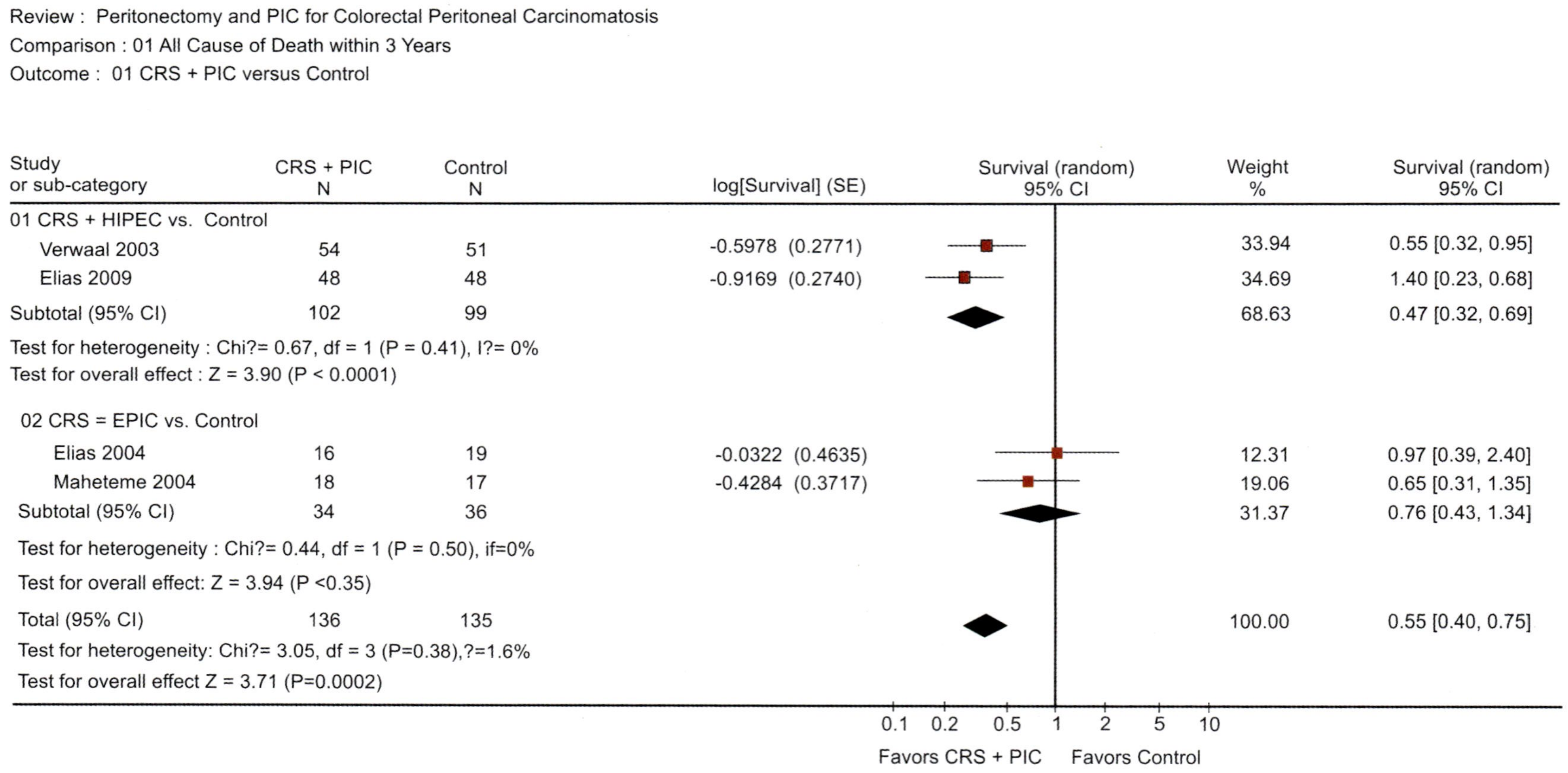

Review : Peritonectomy and PIC for Colorectal Peritoneal Carcinomatosis
Comparison : 01 All Cause of Death within 3 Years
Outcome : 01 CRS + PIC versus Control

Study or sub-category	CRS + PIC N	Control N	log[Survival] (SE)	Weight %	Survival (random) 95% CI
01 CRS + HIPEC vs. Control					
Verwaal 2003	54	51	-0.5978 (0.2771)	33.94	0.55 [0.32, 0.95]
Elias 2009	48	48	-0.9169 (0.2740)	34.69	1.40 [0.23, 0.68]
Subtotal (95% CI)	102	99		68.63	0.47 [0.32, 0.69]
Test for heterogeneity : Chi?= 0.67, df = 1 (P = 0.41), I?= 0%					
Test for overall effect : Z = 3.90 (P < 0.0001)					
02 CRS = EPIC vs. Control					
Elias 2004	16	19	-0.0322 (0.4635)	12.31	0.97 [0.39, 2.40]
Maheteme 2004	18	17	-0.4284 (0.3717)	19.06	0.65 [0.31, 1.35]
Subtotal (95% CI)	34	36		31.37	0.76 [0.43, 1.34]
Test for heterogeneity : Chi?= 0.44, df = 1 (P = 0.50), if=0%					
Test for overall effect: Z = 3.94 (P <0.35)					
Total (95% CI)	136	135		100.00	0.55 [0.40, 0.75]
Test for heterogeneity: Chi?= 3.05, df = 3 (P=0.38),?=1.6%					
Test for overall effect Z = 3.71 (P=0.0002)					

Survival (random) 95% CI: 0.1 0.2 0.5 1 2 5 10

Favors CRS + PIC Favors Control

Figure 1 Forest plot of the hazard ratio (HR) of the overall survival at three years with perioperative intraperitoneal chemotherapy versus control for colorectal peritoneal carcinomatosis where studies were analyzed according to the regimens of intraperitoneal chemotherapy used, i.e. hyperthermic intraperitoneal chemotherapy or early postoperative intraperitoneal chemotherapy. The estimate of the HR of each individual trial corresponds to the middle of the squares and horizontal line gives the 95% confidence interval. For each subgroup, the sum of the statistics, along with the summary HR is represented by the middle of the solid diamonds. A test of heterogeneity between the trials within a subgroup is given below the summary statistics[53]

Abbreviations: CI, confidence interval; CRS, combining cytoreductive surgery; EPIC, early postoperative intraperitoneal chemotherapy; HIPEC, hyperthermic intraperitoneal chemotherapy; HR, hazard ratio; PIC, perioperative intraperitoneal chemotherapy; SE, standard error

Hepatic resection for colorectal liver metastases has evolved since the early 1980s. It is now regarded as the standard of care for patients with resectable colorectal liver metastases.[54] Combining the use of systemic chemotherapy and local tumor ablation have expanded the criteria for resection.[55] This transition has taken place over a period of 20 years despite no level one evidence to support the superiority of surgical resection of colorectal liver metastases over other treatments.[56] Several studies have since also demonstrated that the survival outcome following a microscopically complete resection of colorectal liver metastases, showing that the results are similar to that of CRS and HIPEC for carcinomatosis from colorectal cancer.[57-59]

The Dutch trial by Verwaal et al.,[40] although being the only randomized trial for CRS and HIPEC to date, has been heavily criticized due to heterogeneous patient enrolment. Presently. The American College of Surgeons Oncology Group (ACOSOG) and the United States Military Cancer Institute (USMCI) had opened a multi-institutional Phase III clinical trial in which patients with limited peritoneal dissemination from colorectal cancer without distant metastases would be randomized to either best systemic chemotherapy or CRS and HIPEC followed by best systemic chemotherapy. Unfortunately the trial was closed due to poor accrual.

Although this combined treatment may achieve the prospective of long-term disease control and cure, critics have questioned the safety of this treatment.[60] The complication rate of this treatment was recently compiled through a systematic review by Chua et al.,[61] who reviewed the morbidity and mortality results from 24 treatment centers, of which 10 centers were regarded as high volume specialized centers based on the number of procedures performed. The findings of the review were that the major morbidity rate ranged from 12 to 52% and the mortality rate ranged from 0.9 to 5.8%. However, morbidity and mortality rates appeared to be lower in high volume centers. The safety of this treatment in specialized treatment center and the sound clinical judgment based on various peritoneal disease related indicators[62] used to select appropriate patients for treatment will ensure that suitable candidates are offered and treated to derive the benefits of this treatment. The maturation of this treatment strategy involves gaining of experience and mastery of the surgical procedure and decision-making skills to select appropriate patients. This necessitates a learning curve for which the successful acquisition of the technicalities will translate to improve delivery of this treatment.[63]

The treatment of patients with carcinomatosis from colorectal cancer should continue to be discussed within a multidisciplinary setting and patients who are fit surgical candidates should be referred to specialized units with expertise in peritoneal surface malignancies for further evaluation. There is a need to strive toward proper selection of patients and the need to achieve complete cytoreduction to maximize the outcomes from the surgical effort.

LIMITATIONS OF GENERAL ACCEPTANCE OF HYPERTHERMIC INTRAPERITONEAL CHEMOTHERAPY FOR CARCINOMATOSIS FROM COLORECTAL CANCER

Although demonstrating the best survival results for patients with peritoneal carcinomatosis, CRS and HIPEC have not been universally embraced by the medical community. To many, peritoneal dissemination in colorectal cancer patients represents unresectable stage IV disease and, therefore, should be treated with a combination of cytotoxic chemotherapy and biological agents.

Even though there is growing evidence that shows that just as there is a subset of patients with stage IV disease with liver metastases that have a long-term benefit from the surgical eradication of their metastatic disease, there is a subset of patients with peritoneal dissemination from colon cancer that may benefit from a complete cytoreduction and HIPEC, many important questions remain to be addressed. A review of the literature shows a wide range of HIPEC delivery, with many methodological variations including the technique, drug selection and the time of perfusion. In addition, the true added value of HIPEC to an R0 resection remains unknown.

A paucity of randomized data comparing it to modern systemic therapies, being considered "experimental" by some insurance companies, concerns about the potential morbidity of the procedure and the multiple variations on how HIPEC is delivered, are amongst the most common reasons why this multimodality approach of CRS and heated intraoperative intraperitoneal chemotherapy has not been universally accepted. Ongoing trials on both sides of the Atlantic are directed at answering some of these questions but only with a true collaboration between medical and surgical oncologists will we be able to define the most appropriate sequence of currently available therapies.

FUTURE DIRECTIONS

In conclusion, this chapter provides a broad overview of the current results of treatment for carcinomatosis from colorectal cancer, in particular, reporting the results of treatment from radical CRS with HIPEC and that of palliative surgery and/or systemic chemotherapy. The results suggest that judicious selection of patients for CRS and HIPEC to achieve a complete cytoreduction is necessary and is superior over the current best systemic chemotherapy. There is a body of evidence to support the treatment of CRS and HIPEC for carcinomatosis from colorectal cancer. A randomized trial that replicates and confirm these early results will establish and cement the position of this treatment as first line therapy for patients with resectable disease. In addition, trials directed at maximizing the efficacy of HIPEC will be needed as we know that the current method fails to maintain the complete surgical response achieved by CRS in the vast majority of patients.

To the best of our knowledge, ongoing future trials such as a neoadjuvant trial by the Dutch group to investigate the role of preoperative chemotherapy prior to CRS and HIPEC compared to upfront CRS and HIPEC may elucidate further findings that potentially allow us to determine whether preoperative chemotherapy may facilitate surgery through down staging of the peritoneal tumor burden and improve progression-free and overall survival. In addition, there are two groups, Institut Gustave Roussy and the United States National Cancer Institute, who are investigating the role of prophylactic HIPEC for patients who are at high risk for developing carcinomatosis from colorectal cancer. Both these trials will serve to allow an early intervention as a primary preventive measure through early treatment of patients at a time point close to the initial diagnosis of colorectal cancer to improve survival.

REFERENCES

1. Koppe MJ, Boerman OC, Oyen WJG, et al. Peritoneal carcinomatosis of colorectal origin: incidence and current treatment strategies. Ann Surg. 2006;243(2):212-22.
2. Welch JP, Doanldson GA. The clinical correlation of an autopsy study of recurrent colorectal cancer. Ann Surg. 1979; 189(4):496-502.
3. Gilbert JM. Distribution of metastases at necropsy in colorectal cancer. Clin Exp Metastasis. 1983;1(2):97-101.
4. Weiss L, Grundmann E, Torhorst J, et al. Haematogenous metastastic patterns in colonic carcinoma: an analysis of 1541 necropsies. J Pathol. 1986;150(3):195-203.
5. Sugarbaker PH, Yu W, Yonemura Y. Gastrectomy, peritonectomy, and perioperative intraperitoneal chemotherapy: the evolution of treatment strategies for advanced gastric cancer. Semin Surg Oncol. 2003;21(4):233-48.
6. Paget S. The distribution of secondary growths in cancer of the breast. Lancet. 1889;133(3421):571-3.
7. Hart IR, Fidler IJ. Role of organ selectivity in the determination of metastatic patterns of B16 melanoma. Cancer Res. 1980; 40(7):2281-7.
8. Kawajiri H, Yashiro M, Shinto O, et al. A novel transforming growth factor beta receptor kinase inhibitor, A-77, prevents the peritoneal dissemination of scirrhous gastric carcinoma. Clin Cancer Res. 2008;14(9):2850-60.
9. Furuya M, Kato H, Nishimura N, et al. Down-regulation of CD9 in human ovarian carcinoma cell might contribute to peritoneal dissemination: morphologic alteration and reduced expression of beta1 integrin subsets. Cancer Res. 2005;65(7): 2617-25.
10. Takatsuki H, Komatsu S, Sano R, et al. Adhesion of gastric carcinoma cells to peritoneum mediated by alpha 3 beta 1 integrin (VLA-3). Cancer Res. 2004;64(17):6065-70.
11. Yonemura Y, Fujimura T, Ninomiya I, et al. Prediction of peritoneal micrometastasis by peritoneal lavaged cytology and reverse transcriptase-polymerase chain reaction for matrix metalloproteinase-7 mRNA. Clin Cancer Res. 2001;7(6): 1647-53.
12. Saltz LB, Cox JV, Blanke C, et al. Irinotecan plus fluorouracil and leucovorin for metastatic colorectal cancer. Irinotecan Study Group. N Engl J Med. 2000;343(13):905-14.
13. Hurwitz H, Fehrenbacher L, Novotny W, et al. Bevacizumab plus irinotecan, fluorouracil, and leucovorin for metastatic colorectal cancer. N Engl J Med. 2004;350(23):2335-42.
14. Colucci G, Gebbia V, Paoletti G, et al. Phase III randomized trial of FOLFIRI versus FOLFOX4 in the treatment of advanced colorectal cancer: a multicenter study of the Gruppo Oncologico Dell'Italia Meridionale. J Clin Oncol. 2005;23(22): 4866-75.
15. Cassidy J, Clarke S, Diaz-Rubio E, et al. Randomized phase III study of capecitabine plus oxaliplatin compared with fluorouracil/folinic acid plus oxaliplatin as first-line therapy for metastatic colorectal cancer. J Clin Oncol. 2008;26(12): 2006-12.
16. Porschen R, Arkenau H-T, Kubicka S, et al. Phase III study of capecitabine plus oxaliplatin compared with fluorouracil and leucovorin plus oxaliplatin in metastatic colorectal cancer: a final report of the AIO Colorectal Study Group. J Clin Oncol. 2007;25(27):4217-23.
17. Saltz LB, Clarke S, Diaz-Rubio E, et al. Bevacizumab in combination with oxaliplatin-based chemotherapy as first-line therapy in metastatic colorectal cancer: a randomized phase III study. J Clin Oncol. 2008;26(12):2013-9.
18. Falcone A, Ricci S, Brunetti I, et al. Phase III trial of infusional fluorouracil, leucovorin, oxaliplatin, and irinotecan (FOLFOXIRI) compared with infusional fluorouracil, leucovorin, and irinotecan (FOLFIRI) as first-line treatment for metastatic colorectal cancer: the Gruppo Oncologico Nord Ovest. J Clin Oncol. 2007;25(13):1670-6.
19. Pfannschmidt J, Dienemann H, Hoffmann H. Surgical resection of pulmonary metastases from colorectal cancer: a systematic review of published series. Ann Thorac Surg. 2007; 84(1):324-38.

20. Carpizo DR, D'Angelica M. Liver resection for metastatic colorectal cancer in the presence of extrahepatic disease. Lancet Oncol. 2009;10(8):801-9.
21. Tomlinson JS, Jarnagin WR, DeMatteo RP, et al. Actual 10-Year Survival After Resection of Colorectal Liver Metastases Defines Cure. J Clin Oncol. 2007;25(29):4575-80.
22. Verwaal VJ, Bruin S, Boot H, et al. An eight year follow-up of randomized trial: cytoreduction and hyperthermic intraperitoneal chemotherapy versus systemic chemotherapy in patients with peritoneal carcinomatosis of colorectal cancer. Ann Surg Onco. 2008;15(9):2426-32.
23. Jayne DG, Fook S, Loi C, et al. Peritoneal carcinomatosis from colorectal cancer. Br J Surg. 2002;89(12):1545-50.
24. Sadeghi B, Arvieux C, Glehen O, et al. Peritoneal carcinomatosis from non-gynecologic malignancies: results of the EVOCAPE 1 multicentric prospective study. Cancer. 2000; 88(2):358-63.
25. Mann CD, Norwood MG, Miller AS, et al. Nonresectional palliative abdominal surgery for patients with advanced colorectal cancer. Colorectal Dis. 2010;12(10):1039-43.
26. Krouse RS, Nelson RA, Farrell BR, et al. Surgical Palliation at a Cancer Center: Incidence and Outcomes. Arch Surg. 2001;136(7):773-8.
27. Cunningham D, Humblet Y, Siena S, et al. Cetuximab monotherapy and cetuximab plus irinotecan in irinotecan-refractory metastatic colorectal cancer. N Engl J Med. 2004; 351(4):337-45.
28. Therasse P, Arbuck SG, Eisenhauer EA, et al. New guidelines to evaluate the response to treatment in solid tumors. European Organization for Research and Treatment of Cancer, National Cancer Institute of the United States, National Cancer Institute of Canada. J Natl Cancer Inst. 2000;92(3):205-16.
29. Catalano V, Loupakis F, Graziano F, et al. Mucinous histology predicts for poor response rate and overall survival of patients with colorectal cancer and treated with first-line oxaliplatin-and/or irinotecan-based chemotherapy. Br J Cancer. 2009; 100:881-7.
30. Chua TC, Morris DL, Saxena A, et al. Influence of modern systemic therapies as adjunct to cytoreduction and perioperative intraperitoneal chemotherapy for patients with colorectal peritoneal carcinomatosis: a multicenter study. Ann Surg Oncol. 2011;18(6):1560-7.
31. Elias D, Lefevre JH, Chevalier J, et al. Complete cytoreductive surgery plus intraperitoneal chemohyperthermia with oxaliplatin for peritoneal carcinomatosis of colorectal origin. J Clin Oncol. 2009;27(5):681-5.
32. Franko J, Ibrahim Z, Gusani NJ, et al. Cytoreductive surgery and hyperthermic intraperitoneal chemoperfusion versus systemic chemotherapy alone for colorectal peritoneal carcinomatosis. Cancer. 2010;116(16):3756-62.
33. Kohne CH, Cunningham D, Di Costanzo F, et al. Clinical determinants of survival in patients with 5-fluorouracil-based treatment for metastatic colorectal cancer: results of a multivariate analysis of 3825 patients. Ann Oncol. 2002;13(2): 308-17.
34. Lemmens VE, Klaver YL, Verwaal VJ, et al. Predictors and survival of synchronous peritoneal carcinomatosis of colorectal origin: a population-based study. Intl J Cancer. 2010; 128(11):2717-25.
35. Machida N, Yoshino T, Boku N, et al. Impact of baseline sum of longest diameter in target lesions by RECIST on survival of patients with metastatic colorectal cancer. Jpn J Clin Oncol. 2008;38(10):689-94.
36. Hasegawa S, Mukai M, Sato S, et al. Long-term survival and tumor 5-FU sensitivity in patients with stage IV colorectal cancer and peritoneal dissemination. Oncol Rep. 2006;15(5):1185-90.
37. Bloemendaal ALA, Verwaal VJ, van Ruth S, et al. Conventional surgery and systemic chemotherapy for peritoneal carcinomatosis of colorectal origin: a prospective study. Eur J Surg Oncol. 2005;31(10):1145-51.
38. Elias D, Delperro JR, Sideris L, et al. Treatment of peritoneal carcinomatosis from colorectal cancer: impact of complete cytoreductive surgery and difficulties in conducting randomized trials. Ann Surg Oncol. 2004;11(5):518-21.
39. Higashi H, Shida H, Ban K, et al. Factors affecting successful palliative surgery for malignant bowel obstruction due to peritoneal dissemination from colorectal cancer. Jpn J Clin Oncol. 2003;33(7):357-9.
40. Verwaal VJ, van Ruth S, de Bree E, et al. Randomized trial of cytoreduction and hyperthermic intraperitoneal chemotherapy versus systemic chemotherapy and palliative surgery in patients with peritoneal carcinomatosis of colorectal cancer. J Clin Oncol. 2003;21(20):3737-43.
41. Spratt JS, Adcock RA, Muskovin M, et al. Clinical delivery system for intraperitoneal hyperthermic chemotherapy. Cancer Res. 1980;40:256-60.
42. Sugarbaker PH. Peritonectomy procedures. Ann Surg. 1995; 221(1):29-42.
43. Sugarbaker P. Peritoneal Carcinomatosis: Drugs and Diseases. Boston: Kluwer Academic Publishers; 1996.
44. Glehen O, Kwiatkowski F, Sugarbaker PH, et al. Cytoreductive surgery combined with perioperative intraperitoneal chemotherapy for the management of peritoneal carcinomatosis from colorectal cancer: a multi-institutional study. J Clin Oncol. 2004;22(16):3284-92.
45. Yan TD, Black D, Savady R, et al. Systematic review on the efficacy of cytoreductive surgery combined with perioperative intraperitoneal chemotherapy for peritoneal carcinomatosis from colorectal carcinoma. J Clin Oncol. 2006;24(24):4011-9.
46. Elias D, Gilly Fo, Boutitie F, et al. Peritoneal colorectal carcinomatosis treated with surgery and perioperative intraperitoneal chemotherapy: retrospective analysis of 523 patients from a multicentric French study. J Clin Oncol. 2010;28(1): 63-8.
47. Chua TC, Yan TD, Ng KM, et al. Significance of lymph node metastasis in patients with colorectal cancer peritoneal carcinomatosis. World J Surg. 2009;33(7):1488-94.
48. Shen P, Thai K, Stewart JH, et al. Peritoneal surface disease from colorectal cancer: comparison with the hepatic metastases surgical paradigm in optimally resected patients. Ann Surg Oncol. 2008;15(12):3422-32.
49. Franko J, Gusani NJ, Holtzman MP, et al. Multivisceral resection does not affect morbidity and survival after cytoreductive surgery and chemoperfusion for carcinomatosis from colorectal cancer. Ann Surg Oncol. 2008;15(11):3065-72.

50. Bijelic L, Yan TD, Sugarbaker PH. Treatment failure following complete cytoreductive surgery and perioperative intraperitoneal chemotherapy for peritoneal dissemination from colorectal or appendiceal mucinous neoplasms. J Surg Oncol. 2008;98(4):295-9.
51. Kianmanesh R, Scaringi S, Sabate JM, et al. Iterative cytoreductive surgery associated with hyperthermic intraperitoneal chemotherapy for treatment of peritoneal carcinomatosis of colorectal origin with or without liver metastases. Ann Surg. 2007;245(4):597-603.
52. Verwaal VJ, van Ruth S, Witkamp A, et al. Long-term survival of peritoneal carcinomatosis of colorectal origin. Ann Surg Oncol. 2005;12(1):65-71.
53. Cao C, Yan TD, Black D, et al. A systematic review and meta-analysis of cytoreductive surgery with perioperative intraperitoneal chemotherapy for peritoneal carcinomatosis of colorectal origin. Ann Surg Oncol. 2009;16(8):2152-65.
54. Petrelli NJ, Abbruzzese J, Mansfield P, et al. Hepatic resection: the last surgical frontier for colorectal cancer. J Clin Oncol. 2005;23(20):4475-7.
55. Khatri VP, Petrelli NJ, Belghiti J. Extending the frontiers of surgical therapy for hepatic colorectal metastases: is there a limit? J Clin Oncol. 2005;23(33):8490-9.
56. Kaido T. Verification of evidence in surgical treatment for colorectal liver metastasis. Hepatogastroenterology. 2008; 55(82-83):378-80.
57. Cao CQ, Yan TD, Liauw W, et al. Comparison of optimally resected hepatectomy and peritonectomy patients with colorectal cancer metastasis. J Surg Oncol. 2009;100(7): 529-33.
58. Gertsch P. A historical perspective on colorectal liver metastases and peritoneal carcinomatosis: similar results, different treatments. Surg Oncol Clin N Am. 2003;12(3): 531-41.
59. Varban O, Levine EA, Stewart JH, et al. Outcomes associated with cytoreductive surgery and intraperitoneal hyperthermic chemotherapy in colorectal cancer patients with peritoneal surface disease and hepatic metastases. Cancer. 2009;115(15):3427-36.
60. Lo CH, Bohmer RD, Blomfield PI. An evidence-based approach: Sugarbaker protocol and pseudomyxoma peritonei of appendiceal origin. ANZ J Surg. 2008;78(5):327-8.
61. Chua TC, Yan TD, Saxena A, et al. Should the treatment of peritoneal carcinomatosis by cytoreductive surgery and hyperthermic intraperitoneal chemotherapy still be regarded as a highly morbid procedure? a multi-institutional review of morbidity and mortality. Ann Surg. 2009;249(6):900-7.
62. Pelz JO, Stojadinovic A, Nissan A, et al. Evaluation of a peritoneal surface disease severity score in patients with colon cancer with peritoneal carcinomatosis. J Surg Oncol. 2009;99(1):9-15.
63. Moradi III BN, Esquivel J. Learning curve in cytoreductive surgery and hyperthermic intraperitoneal chemotherapy. J Surg Oncol. 2009;100(4):293-6.

4

Malignant Peritoneal Mesothelioma (MPM)

Haroon A. Choudry, David L. Bartlett

BACKGROUND AND EPIDEMIOLOGY

Malignant mesothelioma (MM) is a rare but aggressive primary malignancy that develops from the serosal lining of the pleural cavity, peritoneal cavity and, rarely, from the pericardium or tunica vaginalis testis.[1] According to the most recent update of the United States, surveillance, epidemiology and end results (SEER) program data for mesothelioma, the annual estimated incidence of MM in males and females is 2,000 and 560 cases respectively.[2] By far malignant pleural mesothelioma (MPlM) is more prevalent (80–90%), while the peritoneum (MPM) accounts for 10–20% of the cases (250–500 cases per year).

Malignant mesothelioma was first described by Miller and Wynn in 1908, and was rarely diagnosed prior to the 1950s. Subsequently, the incidence of MM over the last half-century has closely mirrored exposure patterns to asbestos. There was a dramatic increase in exposure to asbestos from 1930 to 1960 as asbestos use exponentially increased, through asbestos mining, manufacture and use in industries where factory workers, carpenters, electricians, shipfitters, boilermakers, insulation manufacturers and rail-road workers were involved, including that of the automobile brake systems industry. Barring a latency period of 20–40 years, the incidence of mesothelioma increased in the 1970s through 1990s, and continues to do so presently in underdeveloped countries where strict regulations against asbestos use have not yet been implemented. Conversely, following strict asbestos regulation by the US Occupational Safety and Health Administration (OSHA) starting in the early 1970s, incidence of MM appears to have peaked in the United States and is expected to peak in other developed nations within the next 5–10 years (Fig. 1). The age-adjusted incidence of mesothelioma has been consistently higher in males than in females with a progressive rise over time in males, and a virtually constant baseline rate in females. In general, this disparity reflects the higher occupational workplace exposure to asbestos in males compared to the lower environmental exposure in females.[2] Epidemiologically, administration of polio vaccines contaminated with Simian Virus 40 (SV40) in the 1950s and 1960s was also implicated in the subsequent steep rise in MM cases in the United States; however, the recent SEER database analysis does not corroborate this hypothesis.

ETIOLOGY AND PATHOGENESIS

Asbestos exposure is the predominant etiological factor for MM, responsible for an estimated 80% of the cases. MM was rarely diagnosed prior to the 1950s, followed by an exponential rise in incidence starting in the 1970s due to a rapid growth in asbestos-related industries during World War II and the industrial revolution. Oncogenicity of asbestos is determined by the size, shape and solubility of the fibers. Only 5% of the asbestos-exposed individuals develop MM, and multiple secondary events that include genetic and environmental factors are presumed to be required for augmenting malignant transformation. Malignant transformation from asbestos related MM may involve four major pathways; direct pleural irritation leading to a repetitive cycle of damage, inflammation and scarring; asbestos fibers may disrupt mitotic spindles, leading to aneuploidy and chromosomal damage;

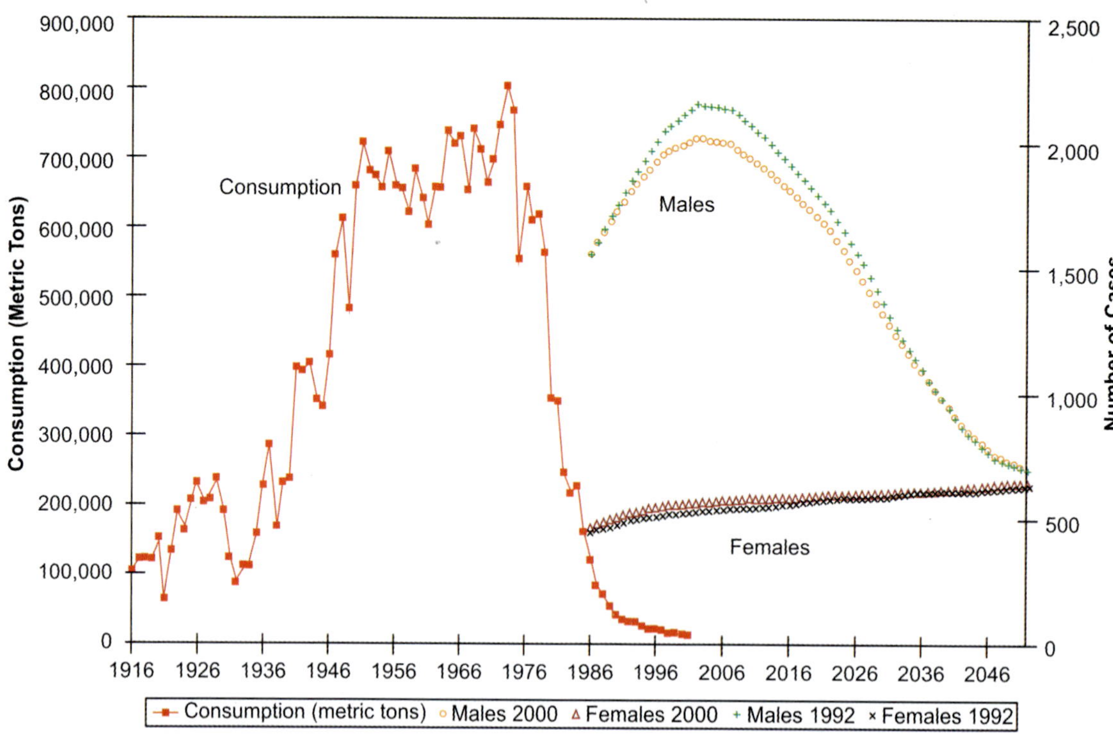

Figure 1 Asbestos use (consumption) in the US, and projected numbers of male and female mesothelioma cases based on a birth-cohort and age model estimated from surveillance, epidemiology, and end results (SEER) program data for two periods; 1973–1992 and 1973–2000[2]

DNA damage through asbestos-induced free radical synthesis and asbestos induces phosphorylation of the mitogen-activated protein kinase (MEK); extracellular signal-regulated kinase 1/2 (ERK1/2) pathways leading to mesothelial proliferation.[3]

Losses of tumor suppressor genes through segmental chromosomal deletions at chromosome 1, 3p (Ras associated domain family 1; RASSF1A gene), 6q, 9p (CDKN2A or p16 gene, MTAP gene), 13q, 15q and 22 (Neurofibromatosis 2; NF2 gene) have been described. Loss of p16^{INK4a} gene product is universal in MM, and leads to inactivation of the retinoblastoma (Rb) gene and the *p53* which are important cell cycle regulatory proteins.[4-7] Krasinskas and colleagues demonstrated a strong correlation between CDKN2A-MTAP deletions and poor prognosis.[8]

DNA sequences of Simian Virus 40 (SV40), a potent oncogenic virus that blocks tumor suppressor genes, have been isolated from MM, although its role in malignant progression is controversial. Polio vaccine stocks (prepared in monkey kidney cells) in the 1950s and 1960s were inadvertently contaminated with SV40 and were temporally related to the rise in MM cases through the 1970s to the 1990s. Although the role of SV40 in MM transformation has been debated, recent evidence demonstrates that SV40 induces activation of Met and Notch1 oncogenes, methylation and silencing of RASSF1A gene, inhibition of Rb and *p53* proteins, thus implying a role in malignant transformation.[4,9-11]

Other putative risk factors for MM include exposure to ionizing radiation (thorotrast),[12] chronic/recurrent peritonitis[13] and exposure to erionite in Turkey.[14]

CLINICAL PRESENTATION

Malignant peritoneal mesothelioma (MPH) is an aggressive locoregionally invasive disease that rarely involves lymph nodes (LNs) (5–10%) or metastasizes extra-abdominally (3–5%). Compressive symptoms occur due to progressive accumulation of tumor and ascites in the abdomen, which leads to organ-dysfunction, morbidity and eventual mortality. The median age of diagnosis is 50–55 years; males account for approximately 55–60% of the cases, and women tend to present at an earlier stage with nonspecific gynecological complaints. MM grossly presents as numerous whitish tumor nodules of variable sizes as well as consistency that may coalesce to form plaques, masses or layer out to uniformly cover the serosal surface. The initial symptoms and signs of MPM are non-specific, leading to a delay in diagnosis in most patients. The most common presenting symptoms of MPM include abdominal pain (40%) and abdominal distention (40%) whereas constitutional symptoms, like weight loss and fever, are less common initial symptoms (20%), and usually signify advanced disease. Frequently encountered features on physical examination include abdominal ascites (70%), abdominal or pelvic mass (30%), and less commonly abdominal wall hernia (10%), tenderness (10%) and pleural effusion (5%).[1]

DIAGNOSIS

Diagnostic Imaging

Computed tomography (CT) scan is considered the imaging modality of choice for MPM. Yan and colleagues provided a detailed interpretive CT scan-based analysis of the unique distribution pattern of MPM in 33 patients. This was based on preoperative distribution of MPM in 13 specific abdominopelvic regions, 16 abdomino-pelvic anatomic sites, CT-based classification of small bowel and mesentery distribution and quantification of ascites (Table 1). They described classic findings that should raise the level of suspicion for MPM including diffuse disease distribution throughout the peritoneal cavity with large tumor volume in the central abdominal and pelvic regions, lack of a primary site and no LN or extra-abdominal metastasis.[15] This unique pattern of distribution provides diagnostic differentiation from other peritoneal surface malignancies. Subsequently, Yan and colleagues showed that the preoperative CT scan assessment of the extent of tumor at specific anatomic sites could accurately predict the likelihood of adequate cytoreductive surgery (CRS). According to their analysis, large tumor volume in the epigastrium, and along the small bowel and its mesentery is particularly difficult to cytoreduce adequately. Preoperative CT scan findings of tumor size greater than 5 cm in the epigastrium, and Class III appearance of the small bowel and its mesentery have a 100% probability of inadequate cytoreduction, whereas a lack of both these features is associated with a 94% probability of adequate cytoreduction.[16]

Table 1 MPM: Preoperative CT interpretation[16]

Class	*Ascites*	*SB/Mesentery involvement*	*Loss of mesenteric vessel clarity*	*CT interpretation*
0	No	No	No	Normal
I	Yes	No	No	Ascites only
II	Yes	Thickening, Enhancing	No	Solid tumor
III	Yes	Nodular thickening, Obstruction	Yes	Loss of normal architecture

The role of MRI and PET scan in MPM is still unclear. Compared to CT scanning, MRI may be beneficial in visualizing invasion of the diaphragm in patients with contraindication to intravenous iodinated contrast material or in patients with questionable areas of local tumor invasion on CT scan. PET scan may provide useful information regarding occult extra-abdominal metastatic disease, recurrent disease, directing appropriate biopsy site based on high metabolic activity not apparent on CT scanning, and may have prognostic value.[17] A recent study in MPlM demonstrated poorer survival in patients with higher FDG-uptake.[18]

Serology

The role of serum markers in mesothelioma management is still unclear. Traditionally CA-125 level has shown promising results as a tumor marker in MPM. New serum markers, including mesothelin, soluble mesothelin-related proteins (SMRP) and osteopontin, have been studied in pleural mesothelioma so far, and have been shown to correlate with disease burden before and after CRS.

Serum CA-125 is frequently elevated in patients with MPM, and levels tend to correlate with response to chemotherapy. CEA and CA 19-9 tend to remain normal in MPM. Baratti et al. evaluated tumor markers in 60 consecutive patients with MPM undergoing cytoreductive surgery (CRS) and hyperthermic intraperitoneal (HIPEC). Baseline CA-125 levels were elevated in 53% of the patients overall, and 65% of the patients not previously treated with systemic chemotherapy. Higher CA-125 levels significantly correlated with high grade tumors; PCI greater than 25, and no preoperative systemic chemotherapy. Adequate CRS with HIPEC was associated with normalization of elevated preoperative CA-125 levels at 3 month follow-up in all, but one patient who had a coexisting autoimmune disorder. Sensitivity of CA-125 in assessing subsequent disease progression after adequate CRS + HIPEC was 100%, with no cases of false-positive marker elevation during postoperative follow-up. However, in this study, elevated CA-125 level did not correlate with survival in a multivariate Cox-regression analysis.[19]

Mesothelin is expressed by normal mesothelial cells and is highly overexpressed in various cancers including MPM, pancreas and ovarian carcinomas. It is a 40 KD cell surface glycoprotein anchored to the cell membrane by phosphatidylinositol, and is involved in cell-to-cell adhesion, recognition and signaling. SMRP is related to the mesothelin family of molecules, and is thought to be released from membrane-bound mesothelin into serum or pleural effusion after abnormal splicing events or proteolytic cleavage. Serum and pleural effusion levels of SMRP have been found to be significantly elevated in patients with MPlM (sensitivity 84%; specificity 100%) as compared to patients with other pulmonary malignancies, benign mesothelial lesions or prior asbestos exposure. SMR levels have been shown to correlate with the size and stage of MPlM but not with survival.[20-22]

Osteopontin is a glycoprotein that is overexpressed in a number of cancers; is involved in cell-matrix interactions, and cell signaling proteins related to asbestos-induced carcinogenesis. Serum osteopontin levels are significantly elevated in MPlM compared to patients with asbestos exposure alone, and absolute osteopontin levels are higher with prolonged exposure to asbestos. Osteopontin has also shown to be useful in early detection of MPlM.[23]

Cytology, Biopsy and Histopathology

Tissue diagnosis of MPM may involve cytologic specimens from paracentesis or tissue biopsy specimens from image-guided biopsy techniques, laparoscopic or open biopsy. MPM cells have a strong propensity for implantation in biopsy needle-tracts, laparoscopic port sites and surgical incisions, therefore every effort should be made to perform these procedures through the midline so that complete *en bloc* excision of these areas may be performed at the time of definitive surgery. Preoperative diagnosis is vital for the subsequent planning and implementation of a multimodality therapeutic approach in MPM patients. Patients suspected of having MPM should undergo laparoscopic exploration to assess the extent of disease, disease resectability, and to obtain tissue biopsy prior to definitive surgery while those incidentally discovered at surgical exploration should be biopsied only, and referred to specialized centers for multidisciplinary planning.

Cytologic analysis of ascites fluid is often inconclusive. Pathologists are frequently unable to differentiate between benign mesothelial proliferations, MPM and adenocarcinomas based on routine staining, and often require a series of immunohistochemical markers. MPM is characterized by positive calretinin, epithelial membrane antigen (EMA, aka CA15-3, aka MUC1), cytokeratin 5/6, Wilms' tumor 1 antigen (WT-1), human mesothelial cell 1 (HBME-1), thrombomodulin and mesothelin staining, accompanied by negative glycoprotein B72.3, carcinoembryonic antigen (CEA), MOC-31, thyroid transcription factor (TTF-1), CD15, Leu-M1 and BER-EP4 staining. However, in general, positive calretinin coupled with EMA staining with negative CEA staining is highly suggestive of MPM. Calretinin and WT-1 markers identify the tissue as mesothelial in origin. Markers, like EMA, identify the tissue as malignant in nature. Cytokeratin staining helps to confirm invasion, and differentiates MPM from sarcoma and melanoma.[1,3,24]

Table 2 MPM: Pathologic classification[25]

Tumor type	*Histology*	*Incidence (%)*	*Biological behavior*
Malignant DMPM	Epithelial (Tubulo-papillary, Solid non-glandular)	75%	Intermediate prognosis
	Sarcomatous	13%	Poor prognosis
	Biphasic (Mixed)	6%	Poor prognosis
	Undifferentiated	6%	Poor prognosis
Borderline/ Low Malignant DMPM	Well-differentiated Papillary	Rare	Good prognosis
	Multicystic	Rare	Good prognosis

Diffuse MPM is the most common primary peritoneal tumor; however, localized forms occasionally occur and tend to be less clinically aggressive. MPM have a diverse spectrum of histopathologic patterns as described by Battifora and McCaughey, and categorized in the WHO classification (Table 2). The most common histologic form of MPM is the epithelial variant (75–90%), which is of intermediate biological aggressiveness, and can be further sub-categorized into a single or mixed subtypes including tubulopapillary, solid, deciduoid, storiform-like, fascicular-type, multicystic, papillary, microcystic and granular. The sarcomatoid form of MPM is less common (10–15%), has an aggressive biological behavior and may contain a diverse mixture of osteoid, sarcomatoid or cartilaginous differentiation patterns. Less common types include biphasic (mixed) variant of MPM (5–10%), which contains a mixture of malignant epithelial and sarcomatoid elements, and undifferentiated variant (5–10%), both of which are clinically aggressive forms of the disease.[25]

Histomorphologic features of MPM may be prognostic as demonstrated by Cerruto and colleagues in 62 patients treated with CRS and perioperative intraperitoneal chemotherapy (PIC). They assessed the histologic types and subtypes of all the tumors in addition to nuclear and nucleolar size categories, chromatin pattern, nuclear to cytoplasmic ratio, pleomorphism, stroma, lymphovascular invasion, depth

Table 3 MPM: Prognostic variables affecting overall survival using multivariate analysis

PI	Feldman[28]	Deraco[29]	Yan[30]	Cerruto[26]	Yan[31]	Yan[27]	Baratti[32]	Yan[33]
Year	2003	2006	2006	2006	2007	2009	2010	2010
# of patients	49	49	100	62	62	401	83	294
Age > 60 y	Yes							
Female			Yes					
Prior CRS	Yes							
Histology			Yes	Yes		Yes	Yes	Yes
LN metastasis					Yes	Yes	Yes	
Deep tissue invasion	Yes							
Nuclear size				Yes	Yes			
Mitoses/HPF		Yes					Yes	
Proposed TNM Stage								Yes
CCR	Yes (≤ 1 cm)	Yes (≤ 2.5 mm)	Yes (≤ 2.5 mm)			Yes (≤ 2.5 mm)	Yes (≤ 2.5 mm)	Yes (≤ 2.5 mm)
HIPEC						Yes		

of bowel invasion, mitotic index, necrosis, differentiation and LN involvement. The nuclear size was categorized into Nuclear size I (10–20 μm), Nuclear size II (21–30 μm), Nuclear size III (31–40 μm) and Nuclear size IV (> 40 μm). In their multivariate Cox-regression analysis, biphasic histology and nuclear-nucleolar size category IV were associated with a dismal prognosis and they recommended neoadjuvant and adjuvant therapy protocols for these patients.[26]

Prognostic Variables and Proposed Preoperative Staging System

Prognostic factors for overall and disease-free survival (DFS) in MPM have been extensively studied and published in the literature (Table 3). The most consistent prognostic factors for improved survival include epithelial histology, negative LN disease, small nuclear size (I/II), adequate CRS (CC-0/CC-1) and less than or equal to 5 mitoses/50 HPF. Other prognostic factors associated with improved survival include age less than or equal to 60 years, female gender, prior surgical debulking, lack of deep tissue invasion, hyperthermic intraperitoneal chemoperfusion (HIPEC) and early stage of disease (Stage I/II).[26-33]

In 2010, the peritoneal surface oncology group proposed a TNM-based clinicopathologic staging system through the identification of prognostic factors in a large multicenter cohort of patients, with MPM treated uniformly with CRS and HIPEC (Fig. 2). The overall median survival in this cohort was 67 months, with a 5-year survival of 52%. Intraoperative PCI score was categorized into four groups: (1) T1 (PCI 1–10); (2) T2 (PCI 11–20); (3) T3 (PCI 21–30) and (4) T4 (PCI 31–39) with 5-year survival rates of 85%, 52%, 48% and 30% respectively. Intraoperatively or postoperatively diagnosed LN status was categorized into N0 (negative LN status) and N1 (positive LN status) diseases, with 5-year survival rates of 54% and 30% respectively. Preoperatively diagnosed extra abdominal metastatic disease was categorized into M0 (no metastasis) and M1 (metastasis) diseases, with 5-year survival rates of 54% and 0% respectively. Based on homogeneity of survival curves, T1N0M0 was considered stage I (87% 5-year survival), T2T3N0M0 was considered stage II (53% 5-year survival) and T4N1M1 was considered stage III (29% 5-year survival). This staging system has not been validated, and is only applicable to epithelial type MPM since outcomes for non-epithelial MPM are uniformly poor.[33]

TREATMENT

In the past, MPM was treated with a combination of systemic chemotherapy, palliative surgery and, occasionally, total abdominal radiation. Although no randomized controlled trials compared these treatment endeavors to the natural history of the disease, patients rarely responded to treatment, with median survival of 12 months, and rare long-term survivors.[34-36] The locoregional nature of the disease lends itself to aggressive locoregional therapies. Recent success with CRS and PIC (HIPEC ± EPIC) in other peritoneal surface malignancies has led to a number of centers publishing their experience with this treatment strategy in MPM, showing median survival

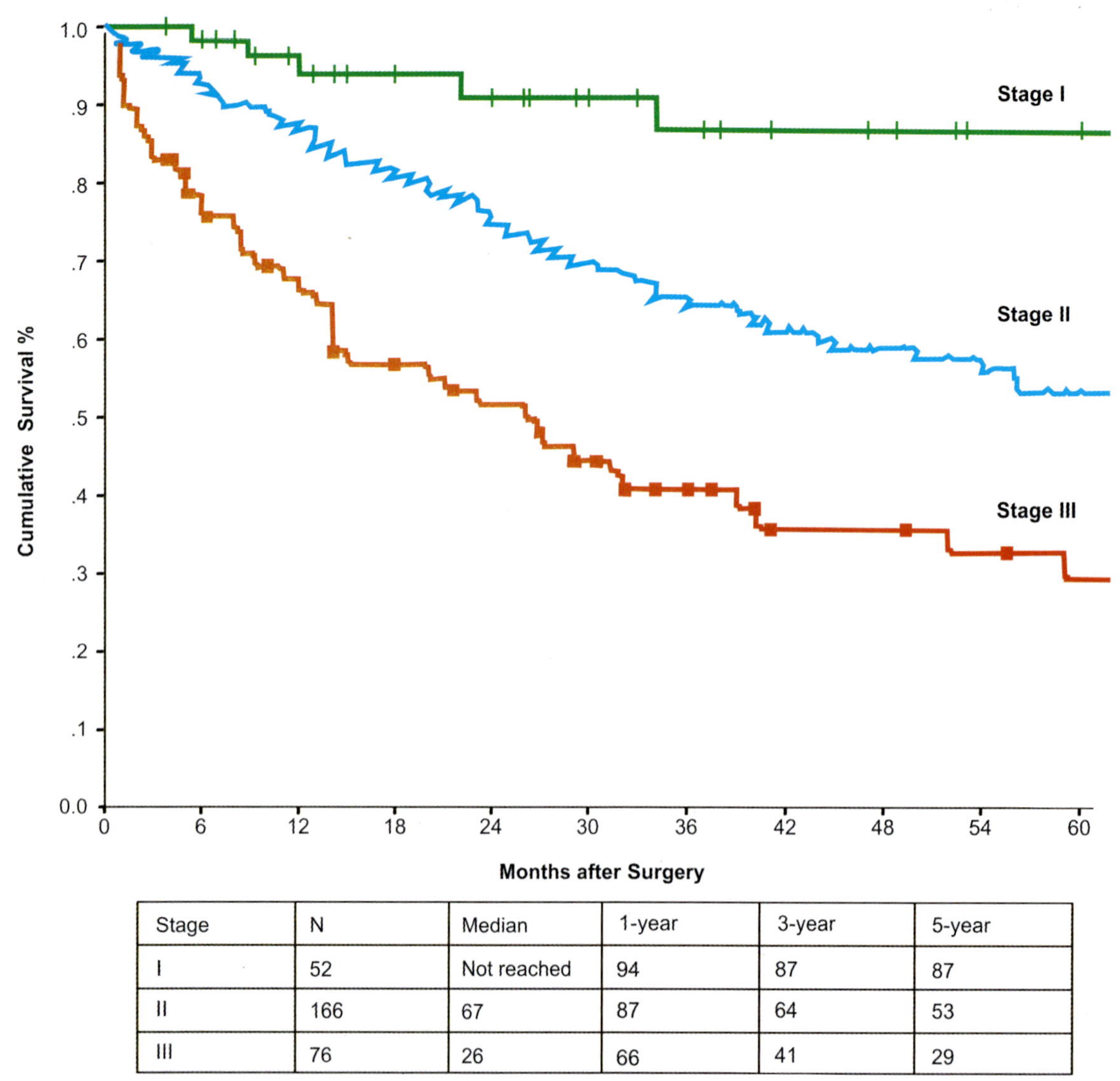

Stage	N	Median	1-year	3-year	5-year
I	52	Not reached	94	87	87
II	166	67	87	64	53
III	76	26	66	41	29

Figure 2 MPM: Kaplan-Meier survival curves demonstrating overall survival stratified, according to proposed TNM staging system[33]

of 60 months and 50% 5-year survival rates, which is far superior to the 12 months median survival with palliative therapies (Table 4).[27-29,31-33,37-39]

Biologic Rationale for Intraperitoneal Chemoperfusion

The rationale for intraperitoneal chemotherapy in peritoneal surface malignancies has been extensively published in the literature. Systemic chemotherapy has little effect on peritoneal surface metastases since the doses required to see an effect are toxic. Surgery is focused at eradicating macroscopic disease while intraperitoneal chemotherapy targets microscopic disease. Intra-abdominal chemotherapy was initially introduced by Weissberger in 1955, with the purpose of allowing local exposure to higher doses of drugs. Subsequently, in 1978, Dedrick and colleagues demonstrated penetration of intraperitoneal chemotherapy up to a maximum depth of 1–3 mm. Therefore, surgical lysis of adhesions and CRS to less than or equal to 2.5 mm deposits is considered ideal (CC-0/CC1) in order to maximize the effective surface area exposed to intraperitoneal chemotherapy, and minimize the required depth of penetration of the chemotherapy.[40]

Sugarbaker introduced the concept of specific peritonectomy procedures to perform systematic maximal cytoreduction. These specific peritonectomy procedures include omentectomy with or without splenectomy, left hemidiaphragm peritoneal stripping, right hemidiaphragm peritoneal stripping, pelvic peritonectomy with or without rectosigmoid resection or colectomy, lesser omentectomy with or without cholecystectomy and total anterior parietal peritonectomy.[41]

Hyperthermic intraperitoneal chemotherapy (HIPEC) was first developed and studied in a canine

Table 4 MPM: Literature review of cytoreductive surgery and perioperative intraperitoneal chemotherapy

Treatment center	# of patients	Residual disease status	HIPEC technique	PIC agents	HIPEC duration (min)	HIPEC Temp (°C)	Mortality (%)	5 yr OS (%)	Median Survival (months)	Grade III/IV Morbidity (%)
Multicenter[33]	294	47% < 2.5 mm	Variable	Variable	Variable	Variable	–	52	67	–
Milan, Italy[32]	83	80% < 2.5 mm	Closed	Cisplatin, MMC	90	42.5	2.4	50	44	28
Multicenter[27]	401	46% < 2.5 mm	Variable	Variable	Variable	Variable	2	47	53	31
New York, NY[37]	27	1st surgery: 44% < 5 mm 2nd surgery: 48% < 5 mm	Open	Cisplatin, Doxorubicin, γINF, MMC	60	41	0	67 (3y)	70	30
Washington, DC[31]	62	37% < 2.5 mm	Open	Cisplatin, Doxorubicin, EPIC: Paclitaxel	90	41.5	3	50	79	41
Lyon, France[38]	15	73% < 2.5 mm	Closed	Cisplatin, MMC	90	42	0	29	36	40
Milan, Italy[29]	49	82% < 2.5 mm	Closed	Cisplatin, Doxorubicin, MMC	90	42.5	0	57	Not reached	27
NCI, Bethesda, MD[28]	49	88% < 1cm; 33% < 5 mm	Open	Cisplatin, EPIC: Paclitaxel	90	41	0	59	92	25
Wake Forest, NC[39]	12	60% < 2.5 cm	Closed	MMC	120	42.5	8	33	34	–

Table 5 Characteristics of common drugs used during HIPEC and EPIC[40,42]

Drug	AUC ratio	Heat synergy	Depth of penetration	Cell-cycle specific	MTD
MMC	23.5	Yes	2000 μ	No	35 mg/m^2
Cisplatin	7.8	Yes	1-3 mm	No	300 mg/m^2
Doxorubicin	230	Yes	4-6 cell layers	No	–
Oxaliplatin	16	Yes	1-2 mm	No	460 mg/m^2
Paclitaxel	1000	No	> 80 cell layers	No	–
5FU	250	No	0.2 mm	Yes	–

model by Spratt and colleagues, and subsequently carried out in a human patient with pseudomyxoma peritonei in 1979. It is defined as the administration of chemotherapy at temperatures greater than 41°C into the peritoneal cavity. Synergy between hyperthermia and drug cytotoxicity starts at 39°C, and decreases after 43°C; therefore, most centers perfuse at 42°C. Hyperthermia causes direct toxic effects through impaired DNA repair, denatures proteins, induces heat-shock proteins that may serve as receptors for NK-cells, induces apoptosis and inhibits angiogenesis. The cytotoxic effect of hyperthermia is temperature-dependent as well as related to exposure time and has a synergistic effect with specific cytotoxic drugs. Hyperthermia increases cell membrane permeability of tumor tissue to drugs, alters the pharmacokinetics of drugs to enhance transport and reduces systemic toxicity by increasing their metabolism and excretion since the transport of large molecule drugs across the peritoneal-plasma barrier is slower than the rate of systemic clearance of the drug. Optimum drugs include those with larger molecular weight, hydrophilic properties, rapid systemic clearance, cytotoxic synergism with hyperthermia and non-cell cycle specificity since they act rapidly. Mitomycin C (MMC), cisplatin, melphalan, mitroxantrone, bleomycin and doxorubicin are ideal drugs that show synergism with hyperthermia, and are non-cell cycle specific, whereas taxanes show no synergism with hyperthermia but are non-cell cycle specific while 5FU has none of the attributes, and is least effective. Currently, combination of cisplatin and doxorubicin is considered the regimen of choice (Table 5).[40,42] In a recently published retrospective study of 34 patients with MPM, clinical outcomes were compared after treatment with CRS and HIPEC with MMC or cisplatin. In this study, median survival for patients treated with cisplatin was 40.8 months against 10.8 months after MMC treatment, and survival at 1, 2 and 3 years was significantly better in patients treated with cisplatin.[43]

The pharmacokinetics and efficacy of HIPEC may be effected by a number of parameters that include type of drugs, concentration of drugs, combination of drugs, carrier solution, volume of perfusate, temperature, duration of exposure and perfusion technique.

Technical Aspects of Intraperitoneal Chemoperfusion

Perioperative intraperitoneal chemotherapy refers to the application of chemotherapy directly into the peritoneal cavity during the surgical procedure or in the immediate postoperative period. It may refer to HIPEC, early postoperative intraperitoneal chemotherapy (EPIC) or a combination of both.[44]

Hyperthermic intraperitoneal chemoperfusion refers to the delivery of heated chemotherapy into the peritoneal cavity using a closed continuous circuit with a pump, heater, heat exchanger and real-time temperature monitoring. Optimal intra-abdominal temperature and the duration are controversial; however, 41.5–43°C for 30–120 minutes is considered standard. This requires an inflow perfusate temperature of 46–48°C. Higher drug concentration may be perfused for a shorter exposure time with equivalent efficacy to a lower drug concentration for a prolonged duration. There is no definitive evidence for any additional surgical complications related to hyperthermia, although there are also no randomized trials to show additional benefit of hyperthermic chemoperfusion over CRS alone. Documented systemic toxicity to HIPEC includes renal failure related to cisplatin perfusion, and hematologic toxicity related to MMC perfusion.

Early postoperative intraperitoneal chemotherapy (EPIC) refers to the intra-abdominal delivery of normothermic chemotherapy via a Tenckhoff catheter or subcutaneous port usually for the first five postoperative days. The chemotherapy is allowed to bathe the abdominal cavity for 24 hours, and then evacuated via closed suction drains placed during the initial operative procedure. Increased systemic absorption as a result of prolonged exposure time is minimized by selecting drugs, like 5-FU, with high first-pass effect through the portal system. Some of the drawbacks of EPIC include catheter related complications, increased systemic drug toxicity, limited efficacy due to adhesions that develop early in the postoperative period and lack of synergistic benefit of hyperthermia.

The open abdominal technique or "Coliseum" technique involves securing a silastic sheet to a Thompson retractor, and the edges of the abdominal incision. Subsequently an opening is made in the center of the silastic sheet over the incision for access to the peritoneal cavity, and a smoke evacuator is used to minimize exposure to aerosolized chemotherapy. Perfusion and drainage catheters are placed into the abdominal cavity while manual agitation allows thermal homogeneity. Drawbacks to this technique include loss of heat and increased exposure to chemotherapeutic drugs.

The closed abdominal technique involves placement of inflow and outflow catheters followed by temporary or definitive closure of the abdominal incision and subsequent hyperthermic perfusion. Manual agitation of the abdomen is performed to uniformly dissipate heat and perfusate. Advantages of this technique include easy maintenance of hyperthermia, and minimal exposure to chemotherapeutic agents while potential drawbacks include inhomogeneous heat dissipation, pooling of perfusate leading to non-uniform peritoneal surface exposure, increased systemic absorption and thermal injury.

Peritoneal cavity expander refers to an acrylic cylinder filled with heated perfusate and placed into the abdominal cavity to allow the bowel to float freely in it. Inflow and outflow catheters enter as well as exit the cylinder, and manual manipulation of the bowel allows dissipation of perfusate. Complexity of the system and lack of exposure of the peritoneal surface are the major drawbacks.

Semi-open abdominal technique is a hybrid of the open Coliseum and the closed abdominal techniques; however, the complexity of the system is unpopular (Figs 3A to D).

Cytoreductive Surgery and HIPEC

Combined CRS and PIC is a potentially morbid procedure therefore, appropriate patient selection is vital. Generally, candidates must have an adequate performance status, be free of extra-abdominal metastatic disease and have surgically resectable disease to less than or equal to 2.5 mm (CC-0/CC-1) based on preoperative imaging or laparoscopic exploration. Retrospective studies have demonstrated overall median survival, ranging from 36 months to 92 months, and overall 5-year survival rates ranging from 29 to 59%. Mortality rates range from 0 to 8%, and Grade III/IV morbidity rates range from 25 to 41%.

Recently Yan and colleagues published results of a large multi-institutional experience in treating 401 patients with MPM. Adequate cytoreduction (CC-0/CC-1) was achieved in 46% of the patients; HIPEC was performed in 92% of the patients while 23% received EPIC. Overall median survival was 53 months with 5-year survival rate at 47%. Mortality rate was 2%, and 31% of the patients had Grade III/IV morbidity. In their multivariate Cox-regression analysis, epithelial histology, absence of LN involvement, CC-0/CC-1 resection and HIPEC were associated with improved survival.[27]

Baratti and colleagues assessed the prognostic significance of LN metastasis in 83 patients, with MPM treated uniformly with CRS and HIPEC. LN assessment was made in 38 patients overall, with 20 patients deemed to have clinically suspicious LN at the time of surgical resection; positive LN disease was documented in 13% of the patients overall (11/83), and 29% of the patients in whom LN were actually assessed (11/38). Internal, external and common iliac LN were most commonly involved. Overall 5-year survival was 82.5% for patients with negative LN disease, and 16.7% for LN positive disease. In their multivariate Cox-regression analysis, epithelial histology, mitotic count less than or equal to 5/50 HPF, absence of LN involvement, and CC-0/CC-1 resection were associated with improved survival.[32]

The Columbia experience involves a combination of CRS (≤ 5 mm residual disease); prolonged postoperative intraperitoneal multi-agent chemoimmunotherapy via two portacath peritoneal access catheters placed intraoperatively (schedule: weekly IP-cisplatin

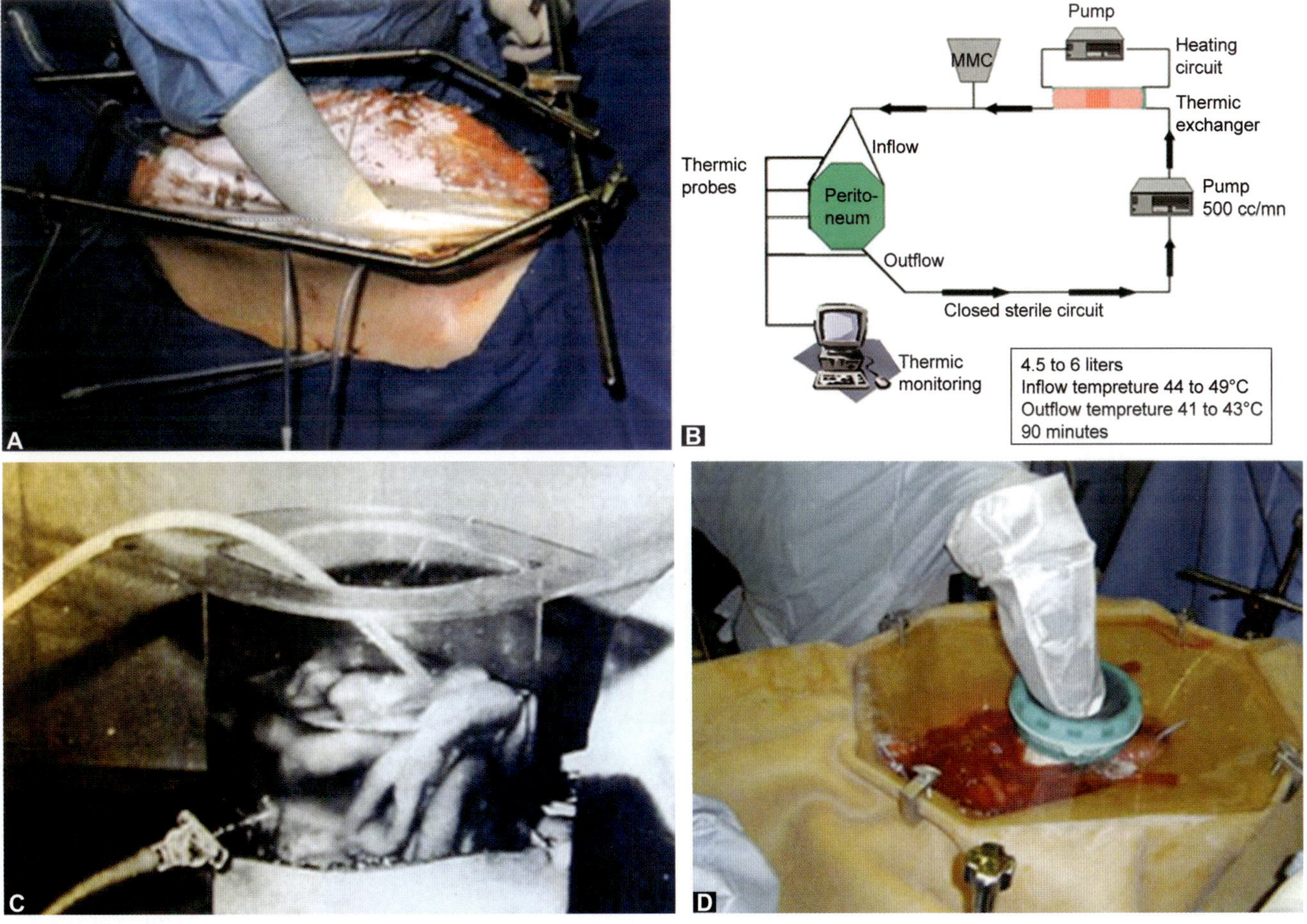

Figures 3A to D (A) Open abdominal technique (Coliseum apparatus); (B) Closed abdominal technique; (C) Peritoneal cavity expander; (d) Abdominal cavity expander[44]

alternating with IP-doxorubicin; 4 cycles each for a total of 8 courses; followed by IP-γ-INF1b weekly for 4 weeks); a second look surgery, and further debulking for persistent disease with HIPEC (MMC + Cisplatin, 60 minutes, 41C) in the presence of minimal or no disease; followed by whole abdominal radiation (RTX alone if no gross disease or initial systemic cyclophosphamide and doxorubicin, followed by RTX for gross disease). In 2008, Hesdorffer et al. published their phase I/II feasibility trial documenting their experience with this technique to treat 27 patients with MPM. In the first surgery, 3 patients were unresectable, and 12 had bulky disease left behind. In the second surgery, 5 additional patients were unresectable, and 6 patients had small volume disease left behind. The median overall survival was 70 months, with a 3-year survival rate at 67%. Median DFS was 30 months with 3-year DFS at 50%. Patients with sarcomatous histology did poorly (median survival 11 months), with no long-term survivors. Bulky disease and the findings of pleural disease were poor prognostic factors. Patients tolerated this prolonged therapeutic course well. Second-look surgery repeatedly showed that long-term multimodality therapy can eradicate or mitigate widespread peritoneal disease.[37]

Section 1

A systematic review of published peer-reviewed articles on using CRS and PIC in combination (HIPEC or combined HIPEC and EPIC) for MPM has been published. Seven manuscripts comprising of a total of 240 patients met their inclusion criteria, and were reviewed. All articles were prospective observational studies without control groups. No randomized control trials (RCT), comparative studies, prior systematic reviews or meta-analyses were identified. Only one of the seven studies included patients with extra-abdominal disease or positive LN disease. The median survival range for the studies was 34 months to 92 months, with 5-year and 7-year survival rates at 29–59% and 33–39% respectively. The overall morbidity rate ranged from 25–40%; hematologic toxicity varied from 8–26%; mean blood loss was 590 ml; mean operative time ranged from 6.5 hours to 9.6 hours; median hospital stay ranged from 16 days to 23 days; reoperative rates varied from 4–11% and overall mortality rates ranged from 0–8%.[45]

Sugarbaker et al. published their experience of 123 CRS for MPM in 100 patients; 65 patients received both HIPEC (cisplatin 50 mg/m^2 and doxorubicin 15 mg/m^2 for 90 minutes at 42°C) and EPIC (paclitaxel, daily for the first 5 postoperative days). The overall median survival was 50 months, and 5-year survival rate was 44%; whereas the median survival for the 65 patients receiving both HIPEC and EPIC was 79 months. In evaluating 18 potential prognostic clinical and surgical factors, multivariate Cox-regression analysis demonstrated female gender, epithelial histologic type and adequacy of cytoreduction as being independent predictors of improved survival. Postoperative mortality rate was 5%. Grade III morbidity occurred in 24% of the patients, most commonly involving pleural effusion and Grade IV morbidity developed in 11% of the patients was predominantly postoperative bleeding.[46]

In 2007, Yan et al. published their prospective experience with 62 patients undergoing CRS and PIC. They assessed clinical, radiologic and histopathologic prognostic indicators for survival in order to propose a staging system, and improve preoperative patient selection. All the patients were treated uniformly with CRS followed by HIPEC (cisplatin 50 mg/m^2 and doxorubicin 15 mg/m^2 for 90 minutes at 42°C) as well as EPIC (paclitaxel daily for the first 5 postoperative days). CC-0/CC-1 was achieved in 37% of the patients, and CC-2 in 34% of the patients. Median survival was 79 months with a 5-year survival rate at 50%. In a univariate analysis, female gender, PCI score less than or equal to 24, CC-score 0/1/2, interpretive CT scan classification of small bowel and mesentery involvement 0/I/II, epithelial histology, nuclear size I/II, normal nuclear/cytoplasmic ratio, less than or equal to 4 mitoses/10 HPF, no atypical mitoses, uniform or granular chromatin pattern, no cellular necrosis, no perineural invasion, fibrous or myxoid stroma pattern and depth of invasion limited to the subserosa were associated with improved survival. In a multivariate Cox-regression analysis, only nuclear size was independently predictive of improved survival. The authors proposed a histopathologic staging system for MPM based on nuclear size that when applied to preoperative biopsy specimens may be used to select patients for CRS based on tumor biology.[31]

In 2006, Yan et al. published their prospective experience with 70 patients undergoing initial major CRS and PIC, and assessed preoperative and operative factors associated with postoperative morbidity and mortality in order to improve patient selection. All the patients were treated uniformly with CRS followed by HIPEC (cisplatin 50 mg/m^2 and doxorubicin 15 mg/m^2 for 90 minutes at 42°C) only, and a combination of HIPEC and EPIC (paclitaxel daily for the first 5 postoperative days) in 66% of the patients. Forty-seven adverse events were categorized into eight organ systems, and Graded I–IV. Mean preoperative PCI was 23; mean EBL was 590 ml, and mean OR duration was eight hours. Overall median survival was 59 months with 5-year survival rate at 49%. Overall 59% and 3% of the patients suffered postoperative morbidity and mortality respectively. Grades III and IV morbidity rates were 27% (most commonly, anemia and line sepsis) and 14% (most commonly, bleeding requiring reoperation and respiratory distress) respectively. Factors associated with Grade III/IV morbidity on univariate analysis included colonic anastomosis, greater than 4 peritonectomy procedures, and OR duration greater than 7 hours.[47]

Yan and colleagues assessed the significance of positive LN disease on survival using their prospective experience of 100 patients undergoing initial major CRS and PIC for MPM. The initial nine patients were treated with induction intraperitoneal chemotherapy (cisplatin 15 mg/m^2/day and doxorubicin 6 mg/m^2/day) for 5 days before CRS and then they received EPIC using the same regimen. The next 24 patients underwent CRS and HIPEC (cisplatin 50 mg/m^2 and doxorubicin 15 mg/m^2 at 42°C for 90 minutes). The remaining 67 patients were to receive CRS, HIPEC and EPIC (paclitaxel postoperative day 1–5); however, 11 patients did not receive EPIC for a variety of reasons. Enlarged or firm LNs were excised and sent for histopathologic analysis separately. For a tumor nodule to be interpreted as a metastatic LN, it had to be removed from an anatomic site containing LNs, be an encapsulated mass and have some residual lymphoid tissue remaining. LNs were sampled and documented in pathology reports in 21 patients; 15 of whom had suspicious looking LNs intraoperatively. Seven patients were found to have positive LN disease, and all of these patients had clinically suspicious appearing LNs intraoperatively. Overall median survival was 52 months, and 5-year survival rate was 46%. In a univariate and multivariate analysis positive LN disease adversely affected survival. All seven patients with positive LNs died of their disease, and had a median survival of 6 months, with no 2-year survivors. Median survival of the 93 patients without LN disease was 59 months with 5-year survival rate at 50%. Most common sites of positive LN disease were external, internal and common iliac LNs; ileocolic and gastrohepatic LNs that may be related to active phagocytic activity at the ileocolic area, and the documented tendency of peritoneal fluid to flow along the root of the mesentery to these locations. The authors recommended routine iliac and ileocolic LN sampling and advocated adjuvant systemic therapy in this high risk group of patients.[30]

A prospective phase II French study assessed outcomes in 15 patients with MPM treated with CRS and HIPEC. All patients underwent CRS in combination with HIPEC (MMC 0.5 mg/kg and cisplatin 0.7 mg/kg for 90 minutes at 42°C). Eleven patients were considered to have CC-0/CC-1 resection. There were no perioperative deaths, and 6 patients had a postoperative complication but no reoperations were required. Median survival was 35.6 months, and 5-year survival rate was 28.9%. In a univariate analysis, CC-0/CC-1 resection and Gilly peritoneal carcinomatosis score 1/2 were associated with improved survival.[38]

The Italian group involving Deraco and colleagues analyzed prognostic factors affecting survival in 49 patients with MPM treated with CRS and HIPEC. Fifty percent of the patients had received systemic chemotherapy prior to the index procedure. All the patients received CRS in combination with HIPEC (cisplatin 25 mg/m^2/L + MMC 3.3 mg/m^2/L; or cisplatin 25 mg/m^2/L + doxorubicin 7 mg/m^2/L at 42.5°C for 60–90 minutes). Grade III complications occurred in 15% of the patients; Grade III/IV toxicity occurred in 12% of patients, and there were no perioperative deaths. Median PFS was 39.7 months with 5-year PFS, and OS rate being 31% and 57% respectively. Multivariate Cox-regression analysis revealed inadequate cytoreduction and mitotic count greater than 5/50 HPF as predictors of OS, and performance status 0 and mitotic count greater than 5/50 HPF as predictors of PFS.[29]

Feldman and colleagues at the NIH published a phase II study of 49 patients treated with CRS and HIPEC (cisplatin 250 mg/m^2 for 90 minutes at 41°C) followed by a single dose of EPIC (fluorouracil 800 mg/m^2 and paclitaxel 125 mg/m^2 between 7–10 days postoperatively) in 35 patients. Prior systemic chemotherapy had been given to 16% of the patients. Postoperative complications occurred in 25% of the patients. Median PFS and OS were 17 months and 92 months respectively with 5-year PFS and OS rates were 14% and 59% in the same order. Multivariate Cox-regression analysis revealed that no prior debulking and deep invasion adversely affected PFS; whereas age greater than 60 years, no prior debulking, deep invasion and residual tumors greater than 1cm in size adversely impacted OS.[28]

Systemic Chemotherapy

Patients with biologically aggressive variants of MPM (biphasic and sarcomatoid) should be strongly considered for multimodality therapeutic strategies including neoadjuvant or adjuvant chemotherapy protocols in addition to CRS and PIC. Most of the trials of systemic therapy have been performed in MPlM. Response rates to conventional chemotherapeutic drugs or drug combinations rarely exceed 20%. Combination therapy has provided better response rates than single-agent therapy (26% vs 8%; $p < 0.001$), although median survival is similar (10 months vs 8 months). Three-drug combinations are no more effective than two-drug combination therapies. Platinum-containing regimens have a greater activity than non-platinum containing combinations, with cisplatin and doxorubicin showing the highest response rates.[48,49]

More recently, preclinical studies have shown that third-generation multitargeted antifolates like pemetrexed (Alimta) and raltitrexed (Tomudex) are concentrated in mesothelioma cells, and specifically inhibit one or several key enzymes involved in the synthesis of purines and pyrimidines. Combination therapy of cisplatin with these third-generation antifolates—pemetrexed and raltitrexed—has demonstrated 40% response rates; 10% mortality risk reduction in 1 year, and corresponding improvement in survival by 6–8 weeks. This combination is currently considered the standard of care in patients with good performance status and unresectable disease and should be administered for a median of 4–6 cycles unless progression or severe toxicity occurs.[50]

In 2006, Berhmans et al. published a meta-analysis of all prospective trials using various chemotherapy regimens (cisplatin, doxorubicin, cisplatin + doxorubicin, other regimens) to treat pleural or peritoneal MM. About 2,300 patients included in 80 single-arm studies, and 3 randomized phase II trials were taken into account. Overall response rates ranged from 11.3 to 28.5%; cisplatin/doxorubicin combined had the highest response rate (28.5%) and overall cisplatin was more active than doxorubicin alone (23% vs 11%).[49]

In 2003, Vogelzang and colleagues published encouraging data from a phase III RCT of unresectable pleural mesothelioma patients treated with pemetrexed 500 mg/m2 and cisplatin 75 mg/m2 versus cisplatin alone, and demonstrated significant improvement in response rates as well as median survival with respect to combination treatment versus cisplatin alone (combination: median survival at 12.1 months, response rate at 41.3%; against cisplatin alone: median survival at 9.3 months, response rate at 16.7%; $p = 0.002$).51

Subsequently, in 2008, the EORTC lung cancer group conducted a phase III RCT of cisplatin alone versus combination cisplatin/raltitrexed in advanced unresectable pleural mesothelioma patients. Combination therapy demonstrated a trend toward improved response rates (24% vs 14%; $p = 0.06$), and median survival (11.2 m vs 8.8 m; $p = 0.056$).[52]

Success with combination therapy using third-generation antifolate drugs prompted the FDA to expand access to allow the use of pemetrexed in a non-randomized fashion alone or in combination with cisplatin or carboplatin in MM of all origins. In 2005, Janne et al. published the results of the combination pemetrexed and cisplatin administered once every 21 days for 6 cycles in unresectable chemotherapy naïve patients with MPM; whereas pemetrexed alone was given to patients who had received cisplatin in the recent past. There were 98 patients with MPM with evaluable response rates by RECIST in 73 patients. Overall response rate was 26%; complete response 5.5%; partial response 20.5%; stable disease 45.2% and disease progression 28.8%. Combination therapy demonstrated improved median survival in patients who had received prior chemotherapy regimens (13.1 m vs 8.7 m) as well as chemotherapy naïve patients (Not reached vs 13.1 m).[53]

Immunotherapy and Molecular Targeted Therapy

Although MM displays a low metastatic efficiency, it is highly invasive to surrounding tissues. The invasive properties of MM cells are related to high levels of expression of matrix metalloproteinases that are able to degrade basement membranes and stromal extracellular matrix components. Molecular therapies targeting various pathways involved in tumor invasion and metastasis have been tested in MPlM. Proliferation, spread and invasion of MM cells is highly dependent on the aberrant activation of a number of growth factor receptors, including EGFR (ErbB1), PDGFR, VEGFR, HGFR, TGFβR, IGFR. With the exception of TGFβ, which is a serine/threonine kinase receptor, all the other growth factor receptors involved are tyrosine kinase receptors. Strategies to inhibit growth factor receptor signaling are based on blocking antibodies that target growth factor ligands or receptors, and on small molecule receptor tyrosine kinase inhibitors that compete for ATP binding sites in the receptor catalytic domain (Table 6).[54]

Table 6 MPM: Targeted therapies in clinical trials[54]

Molecular target	Therapeutic agent	Clinical trial
EGFR	Gefitinib	Phase II[55]
	Erlotinib	Phase II[56]
PDGFR	Dasatinib	Phase II (NCT00509041)
Flt-1, KDR, Flt-4, PDGFR	Sunitinib	Phase I/II (NCT00392444)
	Sorafenib	Phase I/II (NCT00107432)
VEGF	Bevacizumab	Phase II (NCT00027703, NCT00137826, NCT00295503, NCT00407459)
mTOR	Rapamycin	Phase I (NCT00375245)
Proteasome	Bortezumib	Phase II (NCT00513877)
HDAC	SAHA	Phase I/III (NCT00128102)
Mesothelin	SS1P	Phase I (NCT00006981)
	MORAb-009	Phase I (NCT00325494)

EGFR Inhibitors

Preclinical studies with gefitinib and erlotinib have shown that they inhibit growth of cultured MM cells and MM xenograft models; however, clinical studies as single agents have been unsuccessful. A phase II trial on combination therapy of erlotinib with anti-VEGF humanized monoclonal antibody bevacizumab is underway.

PDGFR Inhibitors

Preclinical studies of the combination—imatinib, gemcitabine and pemetrexed—have shown synergy in inhibiting MM cell growth, and tumor-bearing mice. A phase-I trial treating MM patients with this combination is underway. A phase-II study of dasatinib is also underway in MM patients.

VEGFR Inhibitors

A phase II study of single agent sunitinib and a phase I study of the combination—sunitinib and pemetrexed—are underway. Sorafenib is being studied in a phase II trial of MM. Bevacizumab, a recombinant humanized monoclonal antibody that targets VEGF-A, and sterically blocks its binding to VEGFR, demonstrated prolonged survival in MM-bearing mice when used in combination with pemetrexed. Currently a multicenter phase II trial of cisplatin and gemcitabine with or without bevacizumab is underway in systemic chemotherapy naïve MM patients.

PTEN/PI3K/AKT Pathway Inhibition

Elevated AKT activity has been observed in more than two-thirds of MM tissues. Inhibition of PI2K/AKT pathway can induce growth arrest, apoptosis, reduce migration and invasion and sensitize MM cells to various anticancer drugs. The downstream effector of this pathway—mTOR—is expressed at high levels in MM cells. PI3K/AKT inhibitors like perifosine and celebrex and mTOR inhibitors, like rapamycin, have shown promising results in xenograft models and in vitro studies of MM, and are currently being tested in combination therapy regimens.

Ubiquitin-Proteasome Degradation Pathway Inhibition

Proteasomes are responsible for regulated degradation of cytoplasmic and nuclear proteins as well as control of orderly progression of cell cycle, apoptosis, transcription, differentiation, adhesion, angiogenesis and antigen presentation. Inhibition of proteasomes is more toxic to transformed cells than normal cells lending itself to cancer therapy. Based on encouraging pre-clinical data, phase II trials using bortezumib in MM patients are underway.

HDAC Inhibitors

Several HDAC inhibitors have been shown to have cytostatic and cytotoxic effects on cultured MM cells. A phase I trial of SAHA (vorinostat) showed partial responses in patients with MM and is currently being tested in a phase III trial.

Mesothelin

Mesothelin is regarded as a differentiation antigen and is highly expressed in a number of cancers including MM, ovarian cancer, pancreatic cancer and some squamous cell carcinomas. It is only expressed in the epithelial variant of MM or the epithelial component of the biphasic variant and not in the sarcomatoid variant. Immunotherapy using antibodies developed against mesothelin have been tested in preclinical and phase I/II clinical trials with some success.

CONSENSUS STATEMENT: MANAGEMENT ALGORITHM FOR MPM

A consensus statement was published in 2008 providing the following guidelines for the management of resectable and unresectable MPM.[25] Patients with resectable low malignant potential mesothelioma (multicystic and papillary well-differentiated) should undergo complete CRS (CC-0/CC-1) and HIPEC. Patients with resectable mesothelioma of epithelial subtype should receive complete CRS, HIPEC and EPIC with the consideration for adjuvant or neo-adjuvant systemic chemotherapy; whereas patients with biphasic and sarcomatoid subtypes should undergo complete CRS and HIPEC in combination with adjuvant or neo-adjuvant systemic chemotherapy. In the case of unresectable disease, maximal debulking procedure was recommended for low malignant potential mesothelioma (multicystic and papillary well-differentiated). Unresectable epithelial, biphasic and sarcomatoid mesothelioma patients should undergo primary systemic chemotherapy with subsequent re-staging for CRS and HIPEC in select cases with significant therapeutic response.

REFERENCES

1. Munkholm-Larsen S, Cao CQ, Yan TD. Malignant peritoneal mesothelioma. World J Gastrointest Surg. 2009;1(1):38-48.
2. Price B, Ware A. Mesothelioma trends in the United States: an update based on surveillance, epidemiology, and end results program data for 1973 through 2003. Am J Epidemiol. 2004; 159(2):107-12.
3. Robinson BW, Musk AW, Lake RA. Malignant mesothelioma. Lancet. 2005;366(9483):397-408.
4. Gazdar AF, Carbone M. Molecular pathogenesis of malignant mesothelioma and its relationship to simian virus 40. Clin Lung Cancer. 2003;5(3):177-81.
5. Hirao T, Bueno R, Chen CJ, et al. Alterations of the p16(INK4) locus in human malignant mesothelial tumors. Carcinogenesis. 2002;23(7):1127-30.
6. Balsara BR, Bell DW, Sonoda G, et al. Comparative genomic hybridization and loss of heterozygosity analyses identify a common region of deletion at 15q11.1-15 in human malignant mesothelioma. Cancer Res. 1999;59(2):450-4.
7. Murthy SS, Testa JR. Asbestos, chromosomal deletions, and tumor suppressor gene alterations in human malignant mesothelioma. J Cell Physiol. 1999;180(2):150-7.
8. Krasinskas AM, Bartlett DL, Cieply K, et al. CDKN2A and MTAP deletions in peritoneal mesotheliomas are correlated with loss of p16 protein expression and poor survival. Mod Pathol. 2010;23(4):531-8.
9. Bocchetta M, Di Resta I, Powers A, et al. Human mesothelial cells are unusually susceptible to simian virus 40-mediated transformation and asbestos cocarcinogenicity. Proc Natl Acad Sci U S A. 2000;97(18):10214-9.
10. Shivapurkar N, Wietheqe T, Wistuba II, et al. Presence of simian virus 40 sequences in malignant mesotheliomas and mesothelial cell proliferations. J Cell Biochem. 1999;76(2): 181-8.
11. Engels EA, Katki HA, Nielsen NM, et al. Cancer incidence in Denmark following exposure to poliovirus vaccine contaminated with simian virus 40. J Natl Cancer Inst. 2003; 95(7):532-9.
12. Comin CE, de Klerk NH, Henderson DW. Malignant mesothelioma: current conundrums over risk estimates and whither electron microscopy for diagnosis? Ultrastruct Pathol. 1997;21(4):315-20.
13. Gentiloni N, Febbraro S, Barone C, et al. Peritoneal mesothelioma in recurrent familial peritonitis. J Clin Gastroenterol. 1997;24(4):276-9.
14. Baris I, Simonato L, Artvinli M, et al. Epidemiological and environmental evidence of the health effects of exposure to erionite fibres: a four-year study in the Cappadocian region of Turkey. Int J Cancer. 1987;39(1):10-7.
15. Yan TD, Haveric N, Carmignani CP, et al. Computed tomographic characterization of malignant peritoneal mesothelioma. Tumori. 2005;91(5):394-400.
16. Yan TD, Haveric N, Carmignani CP, et al. Abdominal computed tomography scans in the selection of patients with malignant peritoneal mesothelioma for comprehensive treatment with cytoreductive surgery and perioperative intraperitoneal chemotherapy. Cancer. 2005;103(4):839-49.
17. Wang ZJ, Reddy GP, Gotway MB, et al. Malignant pleural mesothelioma: evaluation with CT, MR imaging, and PET. Radiographics. 2004;24(1):105-19.
18. Flores RM, Akhurst T, Gonen M, et al. Positron emission tomography predicts survival in malignant pleural mesothelioma. J Thorac Cardiovasc Surg. 2006;132(4):763-8.
19. Baratti D, Kusamura S, Martinetti A, et al. Circulating CA125 in patients with peritoneal mesothelioma treated with cytoreductive surgery and intraperitoneal hyperthermic perfusion. Ann Surg Oncol. 2007;14(2):500-508.
20. Pass HI, Wali A, Tang N, et al. Soluble mesothelin-related peptide level elevation in mesothelioma serum and pleural effusions. Ann Thorac Surg. 2008;85(1):265-72.
21. Robinson BW, Creaney J, Lake R, et al. Soluble mesothelin-related protein—a blood test for mesothelioma. Lung Cancer. 2005;49(Suppl. 1):S109-11.
22. Robinson BW, Creaney J, Lake R, et al. Mesothelin-family proteins and diagnosis of mesothelioma. Lancet. 2003;362 (9396):1612-6.
23. Pass HI, Lott D, Lonardo F, et al. Asbestos exposure, pleural mesothelioma, and serum osteopontin levels. N Engl J Med. 2005;353(15):1564-73.
24. Robinson BW, Lake RA. Advances in malignant mesothelioma. N Engl J Med. 2005;353(15):1591-603.
25. Deraco M, Bartlett D, Kusamura S, et al. Consensus statement on peritoneal mesothelioma. J Surg Oncol. 2008;98(4):268-72.
26. Cerruto CA, Brun EA, Chang D, et al. Prognostic significance of histomorphologic parameters in diffuse malignant peritoneal mesothelioma. Arch Pathol Lab Med. 2006;130(11):1654-61.
27. Yan TD, Deraco M, Baratti D, et al. Cytoreductive surgery and hyperthermic intraperitoneal chemotherapy for malignant peritoneal mesothelioma: multi-institutional experience. J Clin Oncol. 2009;27(36):6237-42.
28. Feldman AL, Libutti SK, Pingpank JF, et al. Analysis of factors associated with outcome in patients with malignant peritoneal mesothelioma undergoing surgical debulking and

intraperitoneal chemotherapy. J Clin Oncol. 2003;21(24):4560-7.
29. Deraco M, Nonaka D, Baratti D, et al. Prognostic analysis of clinicopathologic factors in 49 patients with diffuse malignant peritoneal mesothelioma treated with cytoreductive surgery and intraperitoneal hyperthermic perfusion. Ann Surg Oncol. 2006;13(2):229-37.
30. Yan TD, Yoo D, Sugarbaker PH. Significance of lymph node metastasis in patients with diffuse malignant peritoneal mesothelioma. Eur J Surg Oncol. 2006;32(9):948-53.
31. Yan TD, Brun EA, Cerruto CA, et al. Prognostic indicators for patients undergoing cytoreductive surgery and perioperative intraperitoneal chemotherapy for diffuse malignant peritoneal mesothelioma. Ann Surg Oncol. 2007;14(1):41-9.
32. Baratti D, Kusamura S, Cabras AD, et al. Lymph node metastases in diffuse malignant peritoneal mesothelioma. Ann Surg Oncol. 2010;17(1):45-53.
33. Yan TD, Deraco M, Elias D, et al. A novel tumor-node-metastasis (TNM) staging system of diffuse malignant peritoneal mesothelioma using outcome analysis of a multi-institutional database. Cancer. 2010.
34. Markman M, Kelsen D. Efficacy of cisplatin-based intraperitoneal chemotherapy as treatment of malignant peritoneal mesothelioma. J Cancer Res Clin Oncol. 1992; 118(7):547-50.
35. Neumann V, Muller KM, Fischer M. Peritoneal mesothelioma—incidence and etiology. Pathologe. 1999;20(3):169-76.
36. Eltabbakh GH, Piver MS, Hempling RE, et al. Clinical picture, response to therapy, and survival of women with diffuse malignant peritoneal mesothelioma. J Surg Oncol. 1999; 70(1):6-12.
37. Hesdorffer ME, Chabot JA, Keohan ML, et al. Combined resection, intraperitoneal chemotherapy, and whole abdominal radiation for the treatment of malignant peritoneal mesothelioma. Am J Clin Oncol. 2008;31(1):49-54.
38. Brigand C, Monneuse O, Mohamed F, et al. Peritoneal mesothelioma treated by cytoreductive surgery and intraperitoneal hyperthermic chemotherapy: results of a prospective study. Ann Surg Oncol. 2006;13(3):405-12.
39. Loggie BW, Fleming RA, McQuellon RP, et al. Prospective trial for the treatment of malignant peritoneal mesothelioma. Am Surg. 2001;67(10):999-1003.
40. Witkamp AJ, de Bree E, Van Goethem R, et al. Rationale and techniques of intra-operative hyperthermic intraperitoneal chemotherapy. Cancer Treat Rev. 2001;27(6):365-74.
41. Sugarbaker PH. Peritonectomy procedures. Ann Surg. 1995; 221(1):29-42.
42. Kusamura S, Dominique E, Baratti D, et al. Drugs, carrier solutions and temperature in hyperthermic intraperitoneal chemotherapy. J Surg Oncol. 2008;98(4):247-52.
43. Blackham AU, Shen P, Stewart JH, et al. Cytoreductive surgery with intraperitoneal hyperthermic chemotherapy for malignant peritoneal mesothelioma: mitomycin versus cisplatin. Ann Surg Oncol. 2010;17(10):2720-7.
44. Glehen O, Cotte E, Kusamura S, et al. Hyperthermic intraperitoneal chemotherapy: nomenclature and modalities of perfusion. J Surg Oncol. 2008;98(4):242-6.
45. Yan TD, Welch L, Black D, et al. A systematic review on the efficacy of cytoreductive surgery combined with perioperative intraperitoneal chemotherapy for diffuse malignancy peritoneal mesothelioma. Ann Oncol. 2007;18(5):827-34.
46. Sugarbaker PH, Yan TD, Stuart OA, et al. Comprehensive management of diffuse malignant peritoneal mesothelioma. Eur J Surg Oncol. 2006;32(6):686-91.
47. Yan TD, Edwards G, Alderman R, et al. Morbidity and mortality assessment of cytoreductive surgery and perioperative intraperitoneal chemotherapy for diffuse malignant peritoneal mesothelioma—a prospective study of 70 consecutive cases. Ann Surg Oncol. 2007;14(2):515-25.
48. Garcia-Carbonero R, Paz-Ares L. Systemic chemotherapy in the management of malignant peritoneal mesothelioma. Eur J Surg Oncol. 2006;32(6):676-81.
49. Berghmans T, Paesmans M, Lalami Y, et al. Activity of chemotherapy and immunotherapy on malignant mesothelioma: a systematic review of the literature with meta-analysis. Lung Cancer. 2002;38(2):111-21.
50. Fennell DA, Gaudino G, O'Byrne KJ, et al. Advances in the systemic therapy of malignant pleural mesothelioma. Nat Clin Pract Oncol. 2008;5(3):136-47.
51. Vogelzang NJ, Rusthoven JJ, Symanowski J, et al. Phase III study of pemetrexed in combination with cisplatin versus cisplatin alone in patients with malignant pleural mesothelioma. J Clin Oncol. 2003;21(14):2636-44.
52. van Meerbeeck JP, Gaafar R, Manegold C, et al. Randomized phase III study of cisplatin with or without raltitrexed in patients with malignant pleural mesothelioma: an intergroup study of the European Organisation for Research and Treatment of Cancer Lung Cancer Group and the National Cancer Institute of Canada. J Clin Oncol. 2005;23(28):6881-9.
53. Janne PA, Wozniak AJ, Belani CP, et al. Open-label study of pemetrexed alone or in combination with cisplatin for the treatment of patients with peritoneal mesothelioma: outcomes of an expanded access program. Clin Lung Cancer. 2005; 7(1):40-6.
54. Palumbo C, Bei R, Procopio A, et al. Molecular targets and targeted therapies for malignant mesothelioma. Curr Med Chem. 2008;15(9):855-67.
55. Govindan R, Kratzke RA, Herndon JE, et al. Gefitinib in patients with malignant mesothelioma: a phase II study by the Cancer and Leukemia Group B. Clin Cancer Res. 2005; 11(6):2300-4.
56. Garland LL, Rankin C, Gandara DR, et al. Phase II study of erlotinib in patients with malignant pleural mesothelioma: a Southwest Oncology Group Study. J Clin Oncol. 2007; 25(17):2406-13.

Section 2

Gynecological Malignancies

5 Intraperitoneal Chemotherapy for Ovarian Cancer

Anne Garrison, Sarah H. Hughes

INTRODUCTION

Epithelial ovarian cancer (EOC) is the second most common gynecologic malignancy diagnosed in the United States, and it is the leading cause of death from gynecologic cancer. In 2007, there were approximately 22,000 new cases, and 1,500 deaths from ovarian cancer.[1]

The majority of women with ovarian cancer present with stage III disease with bulky intraperitoneal disease (Figs 1A to C). Despite high response rates

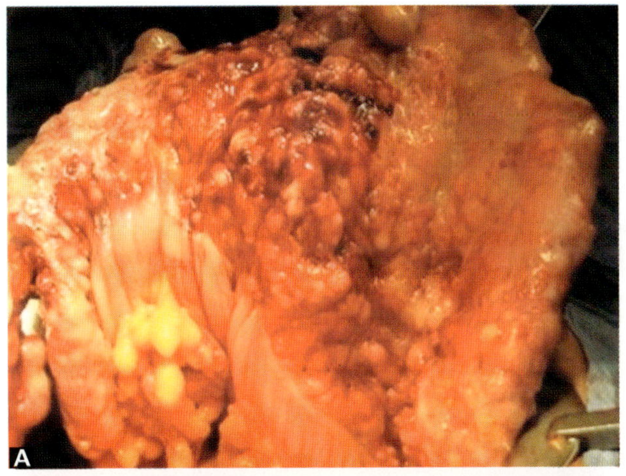

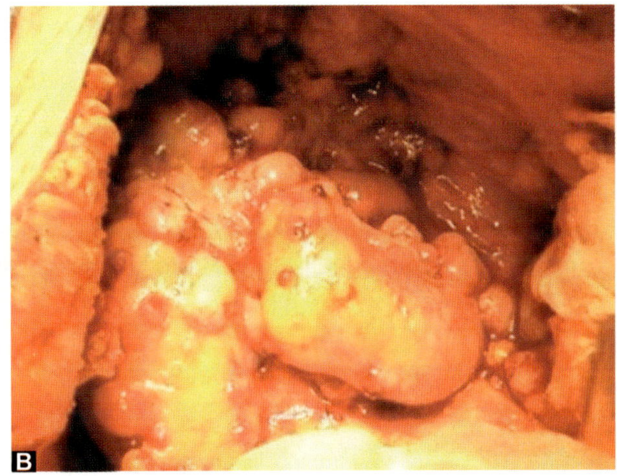

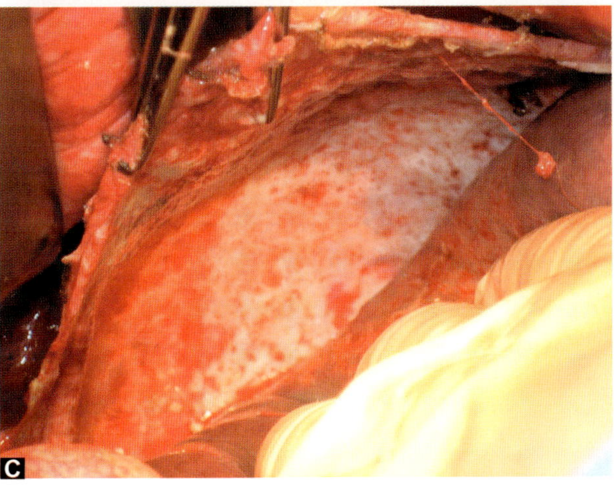

Figures 1A to C: Extensive tumor implants in the abdomen and pelvis. Optimal tumor cytoreductive surgery includes removal of all tumor so that residual disease is < 1cm. This can include omentectomy, bowel resection and stripping of peritoneal and diaphragmatic surfaces. This improves tumor penetration by intraperitoneal chemotherapy. (A) Omental cake in Stage IIIC ovarian cancer; (B) Pelvic Carcinomatosis in Stage IIIC ovarian cancer; (C) Diaphragmatic tumor plaque in Stage IIIC ovarian cancer

to conventional first-line treatment, overall survival (OS) rates remain low, with 5-year survival rates of approximately 40% for stage III and approximately 20% for stage-IV disease. The majority of patients with ovarian cancer undergo comprehensive surgical staging to both identify spread and to direct adjuvant therapy. Surgical cytoreduction plays an important role in therapy, with the goal of achieving optimal tumor reduction (defined as either no residual disease or residual disease < 1 cm at completion of surgery).

The standard of care for first-line postoperative adjuvant treatment of ovarian cancer remains combination chemotherapy with a platinum and taxane. Traditionally chemotherapy has been given intravenously (IV). The Gynecologic Oncology Group (GOG) study #158 established the standard of care to be IV carboplatin and IV paclitaxel.[2] However, there is a growing body of evidence that shows improved rates of progression free survival (PFS) and overall survival (OS) with the use of intraperitoneal (IP) chemotherapy. In 2006, the results of GOG 172 were published. This study compared IV cisplatin and IV paclitaxel (the standard of care at the time the study was begun) to IP paclitaxel and cisplatin, and IV paclitaxel. Median PFS was significantly longer in the IP arm (23.8 vs 19.3 months), and OS was also significantly longer in the IP group (65.6 vs 49.7 months) (Figs 2A and B). The GOG concluded that IV paclitaxel plus IP cisplatin and paclitaxel improves survival in patients with optimally debulked stage-III ovarian cancer.[3] The results of GOG 172 and the six other randomized trials available at the time prompted the National Cancer Institute (NCI) to issue a clinical announcement pertaining to IP chemotherapy for EOC.[4]

This chapter reviews the historical development, recent trials and current practice standards for the use of intraperitoneal chemotherapy in the treatment of EOC.

THEORY

The theory behind intraperitoneal chemotherapy as a chemotherapeutic strategy started in the 1970s, and was based on pharmacokinetic studies.[5] The concept of intraperitoneal chemotherapy makes sense for several reasons. Ovarian cancer spreads by seeding the abdominal cavity and peritoneal surface, and recurrences most commonly occur in the abdominal cavity. From a pharmacokinetic standpoint, based on the studies from the 1970s, the amount of the bioavailable drug in contact with tumor is much higher when administered into the peritoneal cavity. The concentration of chemotherapy that can be achieved in the peritoneal cavity with IP chemotherapy is greater, and a high systemic plasma concentration can be achieved with a relatively low peak plasma concentration. This leads to less toxicity associated with cisplatin such as tinnitus, hearing loss and bone marrow suppression.[6] In addition, the half-life of the agent in the peritoneal cavity also appears to be longer, leading to increased exposure of cancer cells to chemotherapeutic agents. Despite this regional advantage of IP chemotherapy, studies have shown that penetration into tumor tissue is limited to a few millimeters of tumor

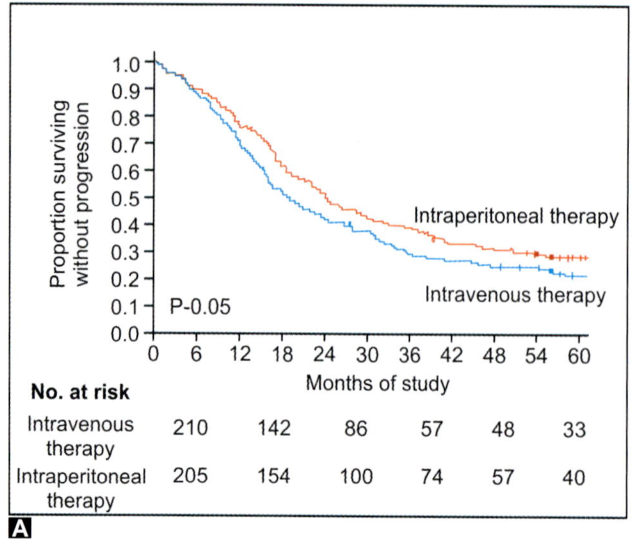

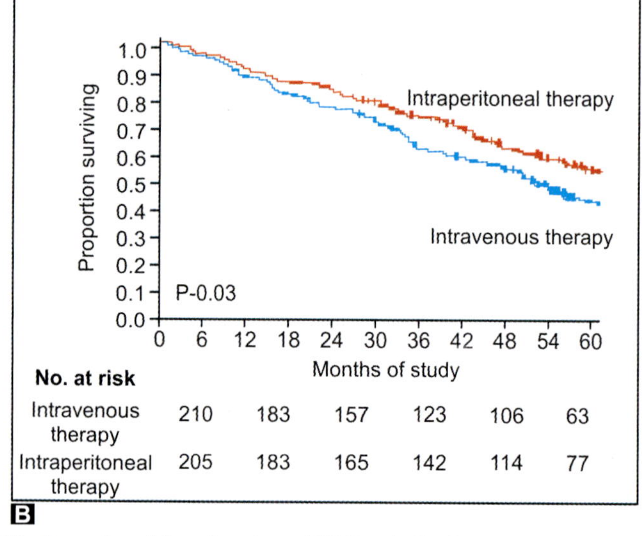

Figures 2A and B: Progression free and overall survival in GOG 172. Reproduced from Armstrong DK, Bundy B, Wenzel L, et al. Intraperitoneal cisplatin and paclitaxel in ovarian cancer. N Engl J Med. 2006; 354 (1): 34-43.

on the peritoneal surface layers.[7] This has led to the concept that IP chemotherapy is best suited to patients with minimal residual disease after surgical cytoreduction.

FIRST-LINE TREATMENT

Randomized clinical trials of IP versus IV chemotherapy began over 30 years ago. Since 1978, seven prospective randomized studies have been published comparing IP chemotherapy with IV chemotherapy in first-line treatment for advanced stage EOC. In all studies, IP chemotherapy was administered only if the patient underwent optimal cytoreductive or debulking surgery. Over time, the definition of optimal debulking has changed from less than 2 cm to less than 1 cm to the recently proposed microscopic residual disease; therefore, the various trials have different definitions of optimal debulking.

Trials

Over time the development of clinical trials for IP chemotherapy have been based on the concurrent IV regimen considered as the standard of care for ovarian cancer. Studies began in the 1970s and reported on the use of 5-fluorouracil and cisplatin. IV cisplatin and cyclophosphamide were the standard chemotherapies used prior to the publication in 1996 of GOG 111 which showed an improved PFS and OS in patients who received paclitaxel and cisplatin. Two studies compared IV and IP cisplatin and cyclophosphamide. Kirmaini et al. compared IP cisplatin and IP etoposide to IV cisplatin and IV cyclophosphamide, and found no difference in response rates, survival (PFS or OS) or toxicities.[8] However, the results of a Southwestern Oncology Group (SWOG) 8501 and GOG 104 study randomized women to IV cyclophosphamide and either IV or IP cisplatin. The median survival was significantly longer in the IP cisplatin group (49 months vs 41 months), and the risk of death was lower in the IP group. Patients who received IV cisplatin had more frequent tinnitus, loss of hearing and neuromuscular toxicity.[9] In addition, the Gruppo Oncologico Nord Ovest trial was published in 2000. They evaluated 113 women with optimally debulked (< 2 cm) stage-III or stage-IV ovarian cancer. They randomized them to receive IP cisplatin and IV epidoxorubicin and cyclophosphamide, or IV cisplatin, epidoxorubicin and cyclophosphamide. No significant differences in pathologic response rate in hematologic and nonhematologic toxicities were seen between the two arms. Also, there was no difference in PRS or OS.[10] Yen et al. found a similar median OS between patients treated with IP cisplatin-based chemotherapy, and those treated with IV cisplatin-based chemotherapy (43 vs 48 months). In the IP arm, catheter blockade and catheter related infections were reported in 13% and 25.5% of the cases, and only 25% of the IP arm patients were able to complete the assigned therapy.[11]

In the 1980s, it was shown that paclitaxel had activity as a single agent in platinum resistant ovarian cancer.[12] Two randomized trials—GOG 111 and OV-10—were begun in the 1990s, and established that IV paclitaxel and cisplatin combination therapy prolonged progression-free and OS.[2,13]

Cisplatin has many toxicities that make administration challenging. Neurotoxicity, gastrointestinal toxicity and hematologic toxicity can limit therapy. In the 1990s, studies were begun to investigate if carboplatin, which has a more favorable side effect profile, was equivalent to cisplatin in treating ovarian cancer. After phase-I and phase-II studies supported this, GOG 158 was designed as a noninferiority trial comparing cisplatin and paclitaxel versus carboplatin and paclitaxel. The results supported substituting carboplatin for cisplatin. Several studies have also explored the use of carboplatin as an IP agent.[14]

In 2001, the GOG in conjunction with SWOG and Eastern Cooperative Oncology Group (ECOG) (SWOG9227/GOG114) compared PFS and OS in women with small volume residual ovarian cancer. Patients were randomized to receive either IV paclitaxel and IV cisplatin or IV carboplatin and IV paclitaxel followed by IP cisplatin. Progression free survival was superior in the IP group (28 months vs 22 months), and OS (63 months vs 52 months). They concluded that because of borderline improvement (P: 0.05), and increased toxicity in IP arm; further research was necessary before concluding that IP regimen should be routinely used.[15]

Polyzos et al. conducted another study that compared the effectiveness and toxicity of carboplatin administration either IV or IP plus cyclophosphamide IV. Women were randomized to receive either IV carboplatin/cyclophosphamide or IP carboplatin and IV cyclophosphamide. There was no difference in response rate or time to progression between the two groups.[16]

In 2006, the results of GOG 172 were published. This was a randomized phase-III trial comparing IV paclitaxel and IV cisplatin with IV paclitaxel plus IP cisplatin and IP paclitaxel in patients with optimally debulked stage-

III ovarian cancer. Only 42% of the patients in the IP arm completed the assigned therapy. Median PFS was significantly longer in the IP arm (23.8 months vs 19.3 months), and OS was also significantly longer in the IP group (65.6 months vs 49.7 months) (Figs 2A and B). The GOG concluded that IV paclitaxel plus IP cisplatin and paclitaxel improves survival in patients with optimally debulked stage-III ovarian cancer.[3]

The results of GOG 172 and the six other randomized trials available at the time prompted the National Cancer Institute (NCI) to issue a clinical announcement pertaining to IP chemotherapy for EOC.[4]

Meta-Analyses

A meta-analysis of eight randomized trials (including GOG 172) compared standard intravenous therapy with chemotherapy that included a component of IP administration following primary cytoreductive surgery. Overall, the analysis revealed a significantly improved progression free and overall survival for patients treated with IP chemotherapy, with a 21.6% reduction in risk of death. Progression-free interval was also significantly prolonged.[17] Another meta-analysis demonstrated a similar HR for PFS and OS advantage favoring IP delivery.[18]

Acceptance of the IV/IP regimen is further complicated because the IV-only regimen used in GOG Protocol 172 was not the current preferred treatment of IV administration of paclitaxel; 175 mg/m^2 over 3 hours, and IV administration of carboplatin (area under the curve, 7.5). Intravenous administration of paclitaxel, 175 mg/m^2 over 3 hours, and IV administration of carboplatin (area under the curve, 7.5) was one of the treatments compared with 24-hour IV administration of paclitaxel and cisplatin in GOG Protocol 158. The paclitaxel (given over 3 hours) and carboplatin treatment arm of GOG Protocol 158 demonstrated improved survival as compared with 24-hour IV administration of paclitaxel and cisplatin, which was the IV-only regimen used in GOG Protocol 172.[6] Women in GOG Protocol 172 and GOG Protocol 158 had optimally debulked stage-III ovarian cancer. Robust exploratory cross-trial comparisons of IV administration of carboplatin and IV administration of paclitaxel compared with IV/IP regimens suggest similar efficacy.[17,19]

Ongoing Studies

Two large multicentric randomized trials are presently ongoing to further evaluate IP chemotherapy. One is led by the National Cancer Institute of Canada, and one by the GOG. Both use strict criteria with similar dosages and schedules of chemo administration, and include the evaluation of carboplatin compared with cisplatin, the addition of weekly paclitaxel, and the use of bevacizumab (OV.21 and GOG 252).

Complications

The major reluctance to comply with the data presented above is related to the increased complexity of providing IP chemotherapy, and the increased morbidity related to the administration route.

For example, in GOG 172, the complication rate of the IP regimen was significantly greater than the complication rate of IV therapy alone. The IP group had more severe toxicities, which included pain, fatigue, hematologic, gastrointestinal, metabolic and neurologic toxicities. In addition, only 42% of the patients randomized to IV/IP chemotherapy completed the recommended six cycles. The most common reason for discontinuation of IP therapy was catheter-related problems (34%). This leads to cross over to IV therapy, which complicates the results of the data supporting improved outcome with IP treatment. Nine percent of the patients refused additional IP treatment. There has not been widespread acceptance of IV/IP therapy because of toxicities, catheter problems and a complicated treatment regimen. Not all oncologists are familiar with IP catheters, and, if administration is done according to GOG 172, patients must be hospitalized overnight for treatment. This is an added inconvenience as well as cost incurring.

The GOG 172 data was analyzed in a separate health-related quality of life analysis, and patients in the IP arm experienced significantly worse physical and functional well-being, abdominal discomfort and neurotoxicity during treatment while on therapy. Overall quality of life one year after treatment was equivalent, and only neurotoxicity remained significantly greater after therapy[20] (Fig. 3).

Because of the risk of catheter-related complications, especially infection—patients with bowel resection during cytoreductive surgery have been studied. If bowel resection has been complicated by gross contamination of the peritoneal cavity, delayed insertion of IP catheter devices is recommended because of the increased risk of catheter-related complications including infection. However, the requirement for bowel resection during debulking surgery is not an absolute contraindication to IP chemotherapy.

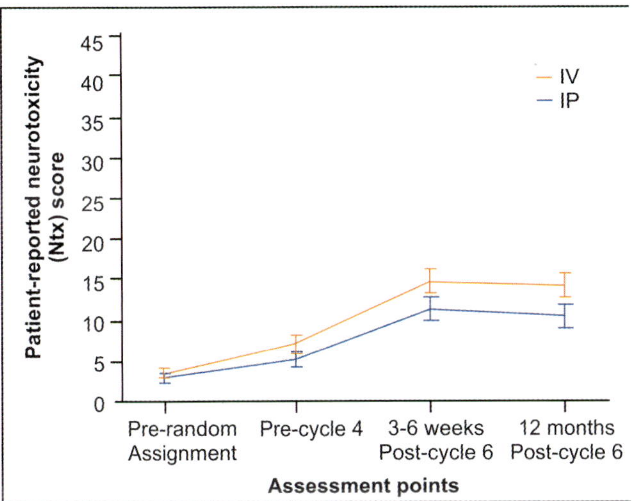

Figure 3: Increased persistent neurotoxicity in patients enrolled in GOG 172. Reproduced from Wenzel LB, Huang HQ, Armstrong DK, et al. Health related quality of life during and after intraperitoneal versus intravenous chemotherapy for optimally debulked ovarian cancer : a Gynecologic Oncology Group Study. J Clin Oncol 2007;24(4):437-43.

Alternative Regimens

The clinical trials on IP platinum-based chemotherapy are dominated by cisplatin. However, carboplatin has become the mainstay of IV chemotherapy because of the ease of administration, and the reduction in neuro and nephrotoxicities. In animal studies, carboplatin penetrates into tumor cells at far lower rates than cisplatin. In a retrospective analysis by Markman et al., IP cisplatin was compared to IP carboplatin for salvage therapy of patients with small volume residual disease.[21] IP cisplatin was shown to have better response and survival rates. Other studies have shown IP carboplatin to have similar survival rates as cisplatin with lower toxicity. On the basis of the available data, cisplatin should be considered the standard of care of IP chemotherapy in EOC, but IP carboplatin deserves to be compared with IP cisplatin with three-weekly and weekly regimens.

The Gynecology Oncology Group is currently evaluating other IV/IP chemotherapy regimens to identify a less toxic, more tolerable and less complicated treatment regimen.

Neoadjuvant/Second-Line/Salvage

Although several large, phase-III, randomized control studies have been published showing PFS and OS benefits in women with optimally debulked stage-III ovarian cancer, the same is not true for the role of IP therapy after neoadjuvant chemotherapy followed by surgery or for salvage chemotherapy. One phase-II study looked at women with stage-III/IV EOC who had three cycles of IV carboplatin and paclitaxel, who then underwent cytoreductive surgery. The women who were optimally debulked, were then treated with IV paclitaxel followed by IP carboplatin and paclitaxel. Only 18 of the 31 patients completed therapy, and 11/26 who were treated developed grade 3/4 neutropenia. Survival was no different for women who completed therapy as compared to the entire cohort, and did not compare well with results from GOG 172 (66 months vs 34 months).[22] Clearly, further studies are needed to evaluate the utility of IP chemotherapy in this subset of women.

In the past two decades, several phase-II trials have shown that IP cisplatin-based chemotherapy could achieve objective responses including surgically documented complete responses in patients with persistent disease after first-line systemic chemotherapy, with potential (although not proven) improvement of their clinical outcome.[23-25] Response rates and survival were mainly dependent on the size of residual disease at the start of IP chemotherapy and the sensitivity to prior systemic cisplatin-based chemotherapy. Other studies have shown less favorable results, and results similar to less toxic IV-based chemotherapy regimens. Despite multiple trials, the role of IP chemotherapy as salvage treatment for recurrent or persistent disease remains controversial and unclear.

CURRENT PRACTICE STANDARDS

Combination IP/IV chemotherapy is an option for carefully selected patients with optimally debulked stage-III EOC. These patients should be well counseled regarding the risks and benefits of IV plus IP chemotherapy versus IV chemotherapy alone. Ideally such patients will be enrolled in current studies exploring the role of IV versus IP carboplatin and paclitaxel. To date, it is unclear if IP cisplatin with IP and IV paclitaxel is superior to the standard IV therapy comprising of carboplatin and paclitaxel. Given the more favorable side effect profile of carboplatin, patients would benefit from this data.

Following the results of GOG 172, the NCI issued a clinical announcement supporting IP chemotherapy for advanced ovarian cancer. This stated that despite the positive findings of the trials, the ideal combination of drugs for IV/IP therapy had not been identified. Because of the uncertainty as to the best treatment approach, standard IV regimens of paclitaxel and carboplatin remain acceptable alternatives to IP therapy, especially given its increased toxicity. Some patients may be too medically frail to tolerate the intensity of side effects produced by IP therapy. The Society of Gynecologic Oncologists (SGO) has neither endorsed nor discouraged the use of IP chemotherapy. Their statement, released on January 3, 2006 in response to the NCI alert, emphasizes that no consensus exists as to what constitutes the "standard" IP regimen. Ongoing studies may identify more tolerable IP regimens for further consideration. The GOG is currently enrolling patients in a study comparing IP/IV cisplatin/paclitaxel versus IP carboplatin/weekly IV/IP paclitaxel versus all IV carboplatin/weekly paclitaxel.

REFERENCES

1. American Cancer Society. Cancer facts and figures 2007. Atlanta (GA): ACS; 2007. Available at: http://www.cancer.org/downloads/STT/CAFF 2007 PWSecured.pdf. Retrieved August 22, 2007.
2. McGuire WP, Hoskins WJ, Brady MF, et al. Cyclophosphamide and cisplatin compared with paclitaxel and cisplatin in patients with stage III and stage IV ovarian cancer. N Engl J Med. 1996;334:1-6.
3. Armstrong DK, Bundy B, Wenzel L, et al. Gynecologic Oncology Group. Intraperitoneal cisplatin and paclitaxel in ovarian cancer. N Engl J Med. 2006;354:34-43.
4. NCI Clinical Alert available online at www. Nlm.nih.gov/databases/alerts/ovarian_ip_chemo.html (accessed January 16, 2006).
5. Dedrick RL, Myers CE, Bungay PM, et al. Pharmacokinetic rationale for peritoneal drug administration in the treatment of ovarian cancer. Cancer Treat Rep. 1978;62(1):1-11.
6. Alberts DS, et al. Intraperitoneal therapy for stage III ovarian cancer: a therapy whose time has come! J Clin Oncol. 2002; 20(19):3944-6.
7. Los G, Mutsaers PH, van der Vijgh WJ, et al. Direct diffusion of cis-diamminedichloroplatinum(II) in intraperitoneal rat tumors after intraperitoneal chemotherapy: a comparison with systemic chemotherapy. Cancer Res. 1989;49:3380-4.
8. Kirmani S, Braly PS, McClay EF, et al. A comparison of intravenous versus intraperitoneal chemotherapy for the initial treatment of ovarian cancer. Gynecol Oncol. 1994;54: 338-44.
9. Alberts DS, Liu PY, Hannigan EV, et al. Intraperitoneal cisplatin plus intravenous cyclophosphamide versus intravenous cisplatin plus intravenous cyclophosphamide for stage III ovarian cancer. N Engl J Med. 1996;335:1950-5.
10. Gadducci A, Carnino F, Chiara S, et al. Intraperitoneal versus intravenous cisplatin in combination with intravenous cyclophosphamide and epidoxorubicin in optimally cytoreduced advanced epithelial ovarian cancer: a randomized trial of the Gruppo Oncologico Nord-Ovest. Gynecol Oncol. 2000;76(2):157-62.
11. Yen MS, Juang CM, Lai CR, et al. Intraperitoneal cisplatin-based chemotherapy vs. intravenous cisplatin-based chemotherapy for stage III optimally cytoreduced epithelial ovarian cancer. Int J Gynaecol Obstet. 2001;72:55-60.
12. Thigpen JT, Blessing JA, Ball H, et al. Phase II trial of paclitaxel in patients with progressive ovarian carcinoma after platinum-based chemotherapy: a Gynecologic Oncology Group study. J Clin Oncol. 1994;12:1748-53.
13. Piccart MJ, Bertelsen K, James K, et al. Randomized intergroup trial of cisplatin-paclitaxel versus cisplatin-cyclophosphamide in women with advanced epithelial ovarian cancer: three-year results. J Natl Cancer Inst. 2000;92(9):699-708.
14. Ozols R, Bundy BN, Greer BE, et al. Phase III trial of carboplatin and paclitaxel compared with cisplatin and paclitaxel in patients with optimally resected stage III ovarian cancer: a Gynecologic Oncology Group study. J Clin Oncol. 2003;21(17):3194-200.
15. Markman M, Bundy BN, Alberts DS, et al. Phase III trial of standard-dose intravenous cisplatin plus paclitaxel versus moderately high-dose carboplatin followed by intravenous paclitaxel and intraperitoneal cisplatin in small-volume stage III ovarian carcinoma: an intergroup study of the Gynecologic Oncology Group, Southwestern Oncology Group, and Eastern Cooperative Oncology Group. J Clin Oncol. 2001;19(4):1001-7.
16. Polyzos A, Tsavaris N, Kosmas C, et al. A comparative study of intraperitoneal carboplatin versus intravenous carboplatin with intravenous cyclophosphamide in both arms as initial chemotherapy for stage III ovarian cancer. Oncology. 1999; 56(4):291-6.
17. Jaaback K, Johnson D. Intraperitoneal chemotherapy for the initial management of primary epithelial ovarian cancer. Cochrane Database Syst Rev. 2006.
18. Hess LM, Benham-Hutchins M, Herzog TJ, et al. A meta-analysis of the efficacy of intraperitoneal cisplatin for the front line treatment of ovarian cancer. Int J Gynecol Cancer. 2007;17:561.
19. Ozols RF, Bookman MA, du Bois A, et al. Intraperitoneal cisplatin therapy in ovarian cancer: comparison with standard intravenous carboplatin and paclitaxel. Gynecol Oncol. 2006; 103(1):1-6.
20. Wenzel LB, Huang HQ, Armstrong DK, et al. Gynecologic Oncology Group. Health-related quality of life during and after intraperitoneal versus intravenous chemotherapy for optimally debulked ovarian cancer: a Gynecologic Oncology Group Study. J Clin Oncol. 2007;25(4):437-43.
21. Markman M, Reichman B, Hakes T, et al. Evidence supporting the superiority of intraperitoneal cisplatin compared to intraperitoneal carboplatin for salvage therapy of small-volume residual ovarian cancer. Gynecol Oncol. 1993; 50(1):100-04.
22. Tiersten AD, Liu PY, Smith HO, et al. Phase II evaluation of neoadjuvant chemotherapy and debulking followed by intraperitoneal chemotherapy in women with stage III and IV epithelial ovarian, fallopian tube or primary peritoneal cancer: Southwest Oncology Group Study S0009. Gynecol Oncol. 2009;112(3):444-9.
23. Braly PS, Berek J, Blessing J, et al. Intraperitoneal administration of cisplatin and 5-fluorouracil in residual ovarian cancer: a Phase II Gynecologic Oncology Group trial. Gynecol Oncol. 1993;56:164-8.
24. Markman M. Salvage therapy in ovarian cancer: is there a role for intraperitoneal drug delivery? Gynecol Oncol. 1993;51: 86-9.
25. Kirmani S, Lucas WE, Kim S, et al. A phase II trial of intraperitoneal cisplatin and etoposide as salvage treatment for minimal residual ovarian carcinoma. J Clin Oncol. 1991; 9(4): 649-57.

6

Hyperthermic Intraperitoneal Chemotherapy (HIPEC) for Ovarian Cancer

C. William Helm

INTRODUCTION AND BACKGROUND

Epithelial ovarian carcinoma (EOC) is a classic peritoneal surface malignancy that arises from the ovarian surface epithelium, derived from the lining of the celomic cavity in the embryo which develops into the peritoneum. Although EOC is an invasive cancer, it remains within the confines of the peritoneum for much of its natural history. Its major initial route of spread is by exfoliation of cells into peritoneal fluid and implantation on peritoneal surfaces where it is slow to invade deeply.

Worldwide, EOC affects 200,000 new women annually causing 125,000 deaths;[1] in the USA, affecting over 21,000 women annually, and being responsible for 14,600 deaths.[2] As Table 1 shows, overall survival (OS) for women with EOC is much worse than for those with other types of solid cancers.

Any improvement in the outcome for women suffering from EOC has been slow, with mortality declining by only 0.3% in the USA in the years 1997–2006.[3] Primarily, this is because of ineffective treatment for advanced disease beyond the short term. Unfortunately, most women with the disease that has spread widely in the abdominal cavity, 60% of them having the FIGO stage IIIB and C [T3b, T3c and/or any T:N1, IV (any T:any N:M1)][4,5] stages are most likely to include peritoneal carcinomatosis (PC) (Table 2).

Epithelial ovarian carcinoma (EOC) has two "sister" cancers which are less common but behave similarly; share a common histologic subtype; both are serous as well as treated identically, resulting in equivalent outcomes. The first—primary peritoneal carcinoma—is thought to arise directly from the peritoneum outside of the ovaries and the second—Fallopian tube carcinoma—arises from the epithelium of the distal (fimbrial) end of the Fallopian tube. The percentage contribution of each of these types of EOC is 91.8% for ovary, 5.3% for

Table 1 Relative 5-year survival of solid tumors in females

Primary site	*5-year survival (%)*
Breast	90.6
Endometrium	83.6
Bladder	76.2
Colon/Rectum	67.9
Ovary	44.4
Lung/Bronchus	18.8

(*Source:* For women diagnosed in the year 2002; based on data from Reference 3)

Table 2 FIGO and TNM stages at presentation

TNM Stage	*FIGO Stage*		*Proportion (%)*
T1, N0, M0	I		28.3
T2, N0, M0	II		8.4
T3a, N0, M0		A	2.6
T3b, N0, M0	III	B	5.6
T3c and/or any T:N1		C	42.0
Any T, any N, M1	IV		13.0

Abbreviations: FIGO = International Federation of Gynecology and Obstetrics[4]; TNM = Tumor Node Metastasis[5]

(*Source:* Based on data from Reference 4)

peritoneum and 2.8% for Fallopian tube.[6] In this chapter, EOC is referred to all three types as a single entity.

There is a type of epithelial carcinoma of the ovary called "low malignant potential" (LMP) or, sometimes, either "borderline" or "atypical proliferative tumor".[7] LMP tumors are a very distinct form of EOC, occurring at a young age; at an early stage, characterized by a much less aggressive behavior and much better prognosis. A ten year relative OS for LMP carcinomas is 95%, and for stages I, II, III and IV, it is 97%, 90%, 88% and 69% respectively.[8] Data from FIGO (the International Federation of Gynecology and Obstetrics) show an overall 5-year survival of 87.3% compared with 49.7% for invasive EOC.[4] LMP tumors do not respond to chemotherapy, although it may be used in those tumors which are associated with invasive peritoneal implants or advanced disease.[8] LMP carcinoma, although requiring surgical resection, is not a candidate for HIPEC and will not be considered further.

CURRENT STANDARD TREATMENT FOR ADVANCED OVARIAN CARCINOMA

Primary cytoreductive surgery (CRS) became the accepted initial modality of treatment after reports pertaining to the prognosis for patients with EOC was related to the amount of residual disease (RD) remaining at the end of surgery—the less the amount, the longer the survival.[9,10] Clarification of the precise aim of CRS has been a gradual process. In the gynecologic oncology literature, the extent of CRS is assessed by the greatest dimension of the largest lesion remaining at the end of CRS. Initially, surgery leaving behind disease up to 2 cm as the greatest dimension used to be considered "optimal" surgery (as opposed to "suboptimal") but the consensus evolved to be that, this be no greater than 1 cm.[11-13] Currently, many gynecologic surgeons believe that the goal should be to remove all visible disease since this is associated with the best prognosis.[14,15] The term "optimal" when applied to the extent of CRS remains ill-defined.

Unfortunately, even maximal surgery that removes all visible disease is ineffective on its own, surgery has to be used in conjunction with chemotherapy and/or supplementary treatment of some kind. In a classic paper, Rubin et al. reported that after a complete pathologic response confirmed at second look laparotomy following front-line treatment of stages III and IV EOC, 60% recurred in 5 years and 66% in 10 years.[16] This suggests that residual and initially, undetectable disease is left behind after surgery.

The aim of this chapter is to present and discuss the possible role of HIPEC in improving outcomes at the natural history time-points for EOC.

RATIONALE OF HIPEC AND IP THERAPY

The essence of regional therapy is a focus on treatment on the originating site of a cancer as well as the sites of regional spread by simultaneously achieving higher exposure to cytotoxic drugs without increasing systemic toxicity. Since EOC is confined to the peritoneal cavity, the biological barrier of the peritoneum (and adjacent tissues) can be used to advantage. The rationale for intraperitoneal (IP) therapy has already been discussed by Dr. Garrison and Hughes.

The characteristics of the "ideal" drug for IP delivery were defined by Dedrick,[17] and the peritoneal/plasma ratios for peak concentration and area under the concentration (AUC) versus time curve for some chemotherapy agents are given in Table 3.

The IP requirements for maximum drug effect are firstly, the absence of any adhesions between IP organs and structures that would prevent the distribution of drug to all surfaces (and tumors) and secondly, the minimum volume of any tumors present. In comparison with large tumors, smaller tumors theoretically are better oxygenated; have a greater percentage of proliferating cells susceptible to chemotherapy and, because of the limited depth of penetration into tumors, they will have a greater percentage of their cells exposed to chemotherapy.

Cisplatin and its analog carboplatin are the most active agents in EOC and have been the principal agents in treatment since their introduction. The cytotoxicity of cisplatin and many other chemotherapeutic agents has been shown to be enhanced by hyperthermia in both human cell culture and animal models[18-35] and may

Table 3 Peritoneal/plasma ratios for peak concentration and area under the concentration (AUC) versus time curve of chemotherapy agents whose activity is enhanced by hyperthermia

Drug	Peak	AUC	Drug	Peak	AUC
Cisplatin	20	12	Gemcitabine		500
Carboplatin	18	18	Melphalan	93	65
Oxaliplatin	25	16	Doxorubicin	474	230
Docetaxel	120	552	Mitoxantrone	57	115
Paclitaxel	> 1,000	> 1,000	Mitomycin	71	23

(*Source:* Adapted from Reference 18)

partially reverse cisplatin resistance.[36] Cellular effects include increased DNA cross-linking and increased DNA adduct formation.[20,37] Cisplatin penetrates deeper into peritoneal tumor implants when delivered intraperitoneally with hyperthermia.[37]

The two major rationales for HIPEC are that heat will enhance the activity of IP-delivered chemotherapy agents and secondly, that this effect itself will be enhanced by giving the combined treatment at the time of surgery when there are no adhesions and tumor volume is at its lowest.

TIME-POINTS FOR TREATMENT OF EOC

The natural history of EOC lends itself to discussion of treatment at distinct time-points. For this discussion, treatment at the time of initial presentation is "front-line". Traditionally, surgery is performed first—"initial surgery"—followed by chemotherapy delivered intravenously (IV) or IV and IP combined. Some patients are managed with initial "neoadjuvant" chemotherapy (NAC) followed by surgery (interval debulking: ID) after 3–4 courses. Following a complete response to front-line treatment, "consolidation" chemotherapy may be given to try to reduce the chance of recurrence. Recurrence occurs following complete response to front-line or some other therapy. Recurrent disease is sometimes, loosely used to include "persistent" disease following front-line therapy as well as disease recurring following complete response. These may both be referred to as "front-line failure".

DEFINITIONS OF PLATINUM RESPONSE

Prognosis for patients with EOC is defined by response to platinum[38-40] and disease can be divided into two relatively distinct groups depending on prior response to platinum-containing chemotherapy. Those that are platinum-sensitive, recur after more than 6 months following a complete response to platinum-containing chemotherapy while those that are platinum-resistant, recur after less than 6 months following response to treatment. Platinum-resistant tumors also include those that had only partial or no response to front-line platinum. This is called "persistent" disease. Disease that progresses on front-line cisplatin is called "platinum refractory" (Table 4).

Table 4 The time-points of treatment of EOC

Front-line	(A) Initial surgery then IV or IV/IP chemotherapy
	(B) Neoadjuvant IV chemotherapy (NAC) (3–4 cycles) then interval debulking surgery (ID) then IV/IP chemotherapy
Consolidation	(C) Treatment given following complete response to front-line therapy
Front-line failure	Persistent disease at the end of front-line therapy
Recurrence	Following complete response to front-line therapy

(**Abbreviations:** IV = intravenous; IP = intraperitoneal)

FRONT-LINE TREATMENT OF EOC

Initial Surgery Then Chemotherapy

The standard management for patients who present with EOC in the USA is CRS, with the aim of achieving a minimum of RD—either none or at most, a largest lesion size of 1 cm or less. This is followed by IV chemotherapy for a minimum of 6 cycles.

A Gynecologic Oncology Group study (GOG 172), in 2006,[41] reported significantly improved progression-free survival (PFS) and OS for patients treated with a combination of IV and IP chemotherapy. The median OS for patients treated with IV/IP chemotherapy was 65.6 months versus 49.7 months for patients treated with CRS and IV chemotherapy only. This was the first large study of EOC that reported a median survival of greater than 5 years. A Cochrane Collaboration meta-analysis of all randomized studies utilizing IP therapy for EOC, including this one, confirmed a significant survival advantage.[42]

Unfortunately, no less than 65% of the patients in the experimental arm of GOG 172 experienced recurrence within the follow-up period of the study, and recurrence in EOC is usually ultimately fatal. These days, although many gynecologic oncologists will offer women with small volume RD following initial CRS a "modified" GOG 172 regimen, IP therapy has not been widely adopted in the oncology community for reasons that include the toxicity of the IP chemotherapy itself and the morbidity associated with IP delivery. So the question is what can be done to enhance initial response and to prevent or further delay recurrence?

There are good theoretical reasons why HIPEC could be added at the time of initial surgery to help achieve these aims. The reason, EOC recurs after front-line treatment is most likely the isolated single or multiple cell deposits left behind at initial surgery

Table 5 Reports of HIPEC at the time of initial surgery for EOC

Authors	*Year*	*Type of Study*	*Time-point*	*n*	*n at initial surgery*	*Agent*
Stellar[45]	1999	Phase I	FL/ID	6	5	Carboplatin
Look [46]	2004	Retrospective	FL/R/P	28	*	Carboplatin, MMC
Piso[47]	2004	Retrospective	FL/R	19	8	Cisplatin mitoxantrone
Yoshida[48]	2005	Retrospective	FL/ID/C	10	2	Cisplatin, MMC, etoposide
Rufian[49]	2006	Retrospective	FL/R	33	19	Paclitaxel
Lentz[50]	2007	Phase I	FL/C	17	11	Carboplatin
Digiorgio[51]	2008	Prospective	FL/ID/R	47	18	Cisplatin
Lim[52]	2009	Phase II	FL	30	16	Cisplatin
HYPERO*[53]	2010	Retrospective	FL	141	26	Various including cisplatin, carboplatin, doxorubicin

(**Abbreviations:** FL = front-line 'initial' surgery (not interval debulking); R = recurrence; P = progression; C = consolidation; MMC = mitomycin)
*including 141 patients with HIPEC some of whom were included in published reports

Table 6 Progression-free survival and overall survival for patients treated with initial CRS and HIPEC

Authors	*Year*	*n*	*PFS*		*OS*	
			Median (months)	*% (5-year)*	*Median (months)*	*% (5-year)*
Rufian[49]	2006	19			38*	37
Digiorgio[51]	2008	18	25.5		27	
HYPERO*[53]	2010	26	24.8	19.7	41.7	33.3

(**Abbreviations:** PFS = progression-free survival; OS = overall survival)
*mean only given

Section 2

which do not succumb to front-line chemotherapy. They remain undetectable by current clinical, biochemical and radiological methods of detection until they re-grow at an interval from treatment, and become large enough to be detected.

At the time of initial surgery, when the abdomen is open, the tumor is found to be at its lowest volume, and adhesions will have been divided allowing for exposure of all peritoneal lined surfaces to the chemotherapy solution. Cytoreductive surgery inevitably releases cancer cells into the operative field, and these "floaters" may increase the chance for persistence and then recurrence. There is interesting animal data suggesting that normothermic chemotherapy alone instilled at the time of surgery will reduce the tumor burden.[43]

With regard to the aim of CRS prior to HIPEC, 90% of the members of the Ovarian Consensus Panel convened for the 5th International Workshop on Peritoneal Surface Malignancy held in Milan, Italy in 2007,[44] considered that it should be a residual lesion size of less than or equal to 2.5 mm.

Clinical Experience with HIPEC Front-Line

The first report of HIPEC used at the time of initial surgery was published in 1999.[45] Working at the National Cancer Institute of the USA, Steller and his colleagues assessed the feasibility, toxicity and pharmacokinetics of carboplatin given as HIPEC in a phase I study of six stage IIc or III patients—five with biopsy-proven EOC; five of whom were chemotherapy naïve and five, who had no macroscopic RD prior to HIPEC. Two of the patients underwent HIPEC at the same surgery as the CRS whereas four had their CRS performed in the preceding weeks. The maximum tolerated dose of carboplatin was defined as 800 mg/m^2. Systemic chemotherapy started 3–5 weeks following HIPEC. Since that paper, there have been several other reports as well (Table 5).

As with the use of HIPEC in other situations, these studies were non-randomized and the data is heterogeneous making it difficult to interpret, and it is often difficult to tease out results for specific subgroups. Several studies do not report survival data because of their phase I design or lack of sufficient follow-up at the time of publication.[50,52] The largest single-center series from Spain[49] reported on 19 patients with stage III treated at the time of initial surgery with paclitaxel for 60 minutes at 41–43°C. The mean 5-year OS was 37% but for those patients with a resection to no macroscopic disease, the median OS was 66 months (Table 6).

Table 7 Progression-free survival and overall survival for patients treated with initial CRS only

Authors	Year	N	PFS		OS	
			Median (months)	% (5-year)	Median (months)	% (5-year)
Eisenkop[54]	2003	408	*	*	58.2	49
Panici[55]	2005	189	27.4	31.2	62.1	49.5
Armstrong[41]	2006	205	23.8	*	65.6	*
Chi[56]	2009	210	20**	31	54	47

*data not given
**data estimated from data given

By way of contrast, results for large series reporting either maximal initial CRS[54-56] or resection to less than 1 cm largest residual lesion size followed by treatment with combined IP and IV chemotherapy (GOG 172)[41] are given in Table 7. Eisenkop[54] reported a median OS of 58.2 months (5-year OS at 49%) in 408 patients; most with advanced disease, and 98.9% of whom underwent a complete CRS followed by standard chemotherapy. Benedetti-Panici[55] reported a median OS of 62.1 months (5-year OS at 49.5%) for patients with stage IIIB and C or IV treated with maximal CRS and systematic lymphadenectomy.

It is interesting to mention that the results for two sub-groups in the studies of HIPEC used front-line. Rufian[49] reported that the median OS and 5-year OS for patients with EOC who underwent a complete resection to no visible disease followed by HIPEC were 66 months and 63% respectively. Within the HYPERO initial report dataset,[53] there were 20 patients who fitted entry criteria for GOG 172 by virtue of having RD of less than 1 cm at front-line CRS prior to HIPEC delivery. Although some data from GOG 172 had to be estimated by extrapolation from data presented therein,[41] there was no significant difference in the OS (HIPEC's 57.5 months vs GOG's 65.6 months, and 2-year OS at 66.4% and 82% respectively) and 2-year PFS (47.6% vs 53% respectively)—unpublished data. Although the patients reported in the studies including those of the HYPERO registry received HIPEC, they did receive further systemic chemotherapy following the HIPEC. However, it is unlikely that this included repeated courses of normothermic IP chemotherapy. These all suggest that further research on HIPEC at the time of initial surgery is warranted including the use of normothermic IP chemotherapy post HIPEC.

There is a dearth of specific data with regard to morbidity of HIPEC given at the time of initial surgery for EOC. However, in an extremely well conducted and reported study, Lim and colleagues at the National Cancer Center of Korea reported a phase I study in which HIPEC cisplatin 75 mg/m^2 at approximately 41.5°C for 90 minutes was delivered using a closed method to 30 patients following CRS to less than 1 cm (16 at initial CRS and 14 at the time of ID), and following intestinal anastomoses.[52] Postoperative events were common but mostly grade I (self-limiting) or grade II, requiring only medical treatment for resolution; specifically, 22 of 30 (73%) experienced grade I events including transient nausea and vomiting, diarrhea, line sepsis, thrombocytopenia and pleural effusion. Twenty-seven patients (90%) experienced one or more grade II events including nausea and vomiting, cardiac arrhythmia, hypertension, diarrhea, pleural effusion, line sepsis and raised creatinine. Twelve patients (40%) experienced one or more grade III complication that required invasive intervention including anemia, pleural effusion, pneumothorax, fascial dehiscence, diarrhea, ileus and pancreatic leakage. There were no grade IV events that would have required definitive urgent intervention such as reoperation or a return to the intensive care unit, and there were no deaths. The authors argue that the events can mostly be ascribed to the CRS. The three cases of thrombocytopenia, all occurred before postoperative day three followed large blood transfusions. No case of leukopenia was reported and no intestinal/anastomotic leak as well. These data suggest that HIPEC can be delivered at the completion of initial CRS without significant additional toxicity.

INTERVAL DEBULKING

When patients with EOC are treated with initial "neoadjuvant"chemotherapy (NAC) for 3–4 courses followed by CRS, the surgery is frequently referred to as "interval debulking" (ID). The question as to whether this approach results in equivalent outcome to initial surgery followed by chemotherapy has been debated for years.

This question is not pertinent to a patient who is temporarily unfit for a major initial CRS because of co-morbidities such as acute heart or pulmonary disease associated with high risk for perioperative medical complications. NAC at this time has a good chance of reducing the disease burden while the medical condition is given time to improve. The reduction in disease burden alone (including reduction in the amount of ascites) may significantly improve a patient's general condition. The benefit of CRS following a response to NAC is that the surgery is often of shorter duration requiring less procedures, and having less morbidity and quicker recovery for the patient.[57,58] A recent meta-analysis reported that NAC and ID were associated with a higher chance of optimal cytoreduction than initial CRS.[59]

However, despite the potential for a greater percentage of patients undergoing optimal CRS, the effect on OS is disputed. Two major contributions lead the arguments on both sides. In a systematic review of 26 studies including 1336 patients undergoing NAC in lieu of initial CRS, Bristow[60] found that the survival outcome was inferior to initial CRS followed by chemotherapy. In contrast, a randomized and controlled trial organized by the European Organization for Research and Treatment of Cancer (EORTC) randomized 632 women with mostly stage IIIC and stage IV disease to either initial CRS followed by IV chemotherapy or NAC followed by ID surgery, and then further IV chemotherapy. Survival and PFS was similar in both arms.[61]

Whatever the exact timing of the front-line surgery is, there is debate about the value of a major CRS that does not manage to reduce the disease burden to less than 1 cm residual and about the value of HIPEC in the presence of larger RD. Most of the data on the efficacy of IP therapy relates to small volume disease and so, if HIPEC is contemplated, and resources are not available to affect a maximal attempt at CRS, then it might well be worth waiting until NAC has reduced the tumor burden and increased the chances for optimal surgery. Figure 1 shows the preoperative criteria to defer an attempt at CRS until after NAC considered by the Ovarian Consensus Panel convened for the 5th International Workshop on Peritoneal Surface Malignancy held in Milan, Italy, in 2007.[44] The panel considered these as relative contraindications with every case needing to be considered individually.

Whatever the real answer to the debate about the efficacy of ID is, this would be an excellent time for HIPEC. The patient's performance status is optimized prior to surgery, and the extent of necessary CRS would be reduced. HIPEC given at the time of ID has the advantage of allowing lead-time for preparation of the patient, the operating team, and the perfusion equipment and team. It has all the other theoretic advantages of HIPEC in the surgical setting.

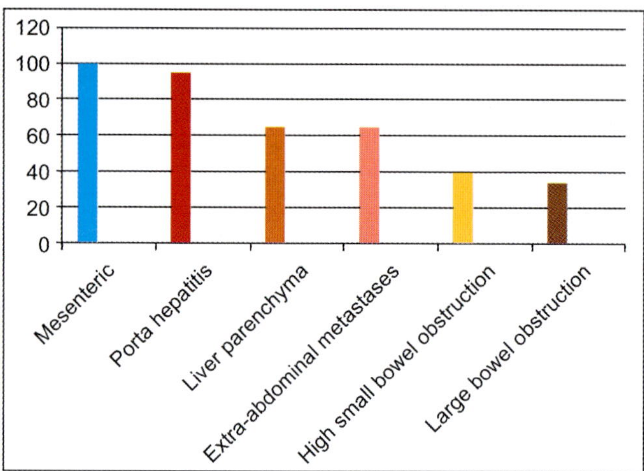

(**Abbreviations**: CRS = cytoreductive surgery; NAC = neoadjuvant IV chemotherapy)

Figure 1 Preoperative criteria to defer attempt at CRS until after NAC (*Source*: Opinion of the Ovarian Consensus Panel convened for the 5th International Workshop on Peritoneal Surface Malignancy held in Milan, Italy, in 2007. Adapted from Reference 44)

There are reports in the literature of HIPEC being given at the time of ID but they are few, and the data is not separately analyzed. Steller included a single case and three other reports included only 17 patients in total.[48,62,63] de Bree reported on four patients who had between six and eight courses of chemotherapy prior to CRS, which is too many to fall within the accepted optimum of 3–4 cycles prior to ID.[60,64] Ryu reported a non-randomized series of 117 patients with different types of ovarian cancer; 57 of whom were treated with either (A) initial CRS followed by IV chemotherapy (6–8 cycles) which was followed by a further surgery combined with HIPEC or (B) 3–4 cycles of NAC, followed by ID and HIPEC.[65] Carboplatin and interferon-α were the agents given in combination as HIPEC. The historical 'control' arm included 60 patients treated by traditional CRS followed by IV chemotherapy. There were 74 patients with stage III disease who received HIPEC in arms A or B. In the whole group, there was no significant difference in survival between the HIPEC groups and controls. However, within stage III, the median disease-free survival of 39 patients undergoing HIPEC was 26.4 months in comparison to 6.1 months for 39 historical controls. When only those patients within stage III with a RD at the second CRS of less than 1 cm were considered, both the median disease-free survival and 5-year survival were significantly better;

40.6 months versus 13.2 months, and 65.6% versus 40.7%. Although the difference in outcome appears impressive, the study contained some major confounding issues. It was non-randomized while the control arm had an unusually poor survival of only 6.1 months, and there was no separate analysis of patients undergoing HIPEC at ID or second look laparotomy. In addition, the stage III control arm included patients with dysgerminoma, choriocarcinoma and granulosa cell carcinoma, and the stage III group undergoing HIPEC included patients with choriocarcinoma, endodermal sinus tumor and squamous cell carcinoma.

The HYPERO initial report included 19 patients who were treated by NAC followed by ID. The median OS was 68.6 months with 2-year and 5-year survivals of 80.4 months and 50.2 months respectively. Although the numbers are too small to come to any meaningful conclusion, these survivals were not significantly different from the 26 patients treated with front-line surgery and HIPEC followed by chemotherapy where the median OS was 41.7 months, and 2-year and 5-year survivals were 57.0 months and 33.3 months respectively.[53]

RECURRENT DISEASE

Despite the good news that 70% of EOC are inherently sensitive to platinum and that most patients can achieve a complete clinical response at the end of front-line therapy, the bad news is that the majority will recur[12] and the outcome for most women experiencing recurrence is poor.

The traditional approach to recurrent disease has been to deliver further IV chemotherapy with the type of agent(s) used being guided by the time-interval from (i) completion and response to primary therapy and (ii) to recurrence.[38-40] Clinical trials of chemotherapy alone for recurrent EOC report survival periods of between 15 months and 18 months,[66-71] and only a few studies report survival of close to 30 months.[69,72,73]

For the subgroup with platinum-resistant and platinum-refractory disease, median survival of about 12 months is reported.[66,67] In general, such patients should be offered non-platinum chemotherapy and entry onto clinical trials of novel treatments.

Only a small minority of patients with recurrent EOC is likely to have been treated with CRS, and this would usually be followed by further IV chemotherapy. Traditionally, those selected for CRS would have single or few isolated recurrences in sites that are more easily resected, with the recurrence occurring at a significant interval (12 months or more) from prior treatment. No randomized studies have been performed for either CRS for recurrent disease with or without chemotherapy versus chemotherapy alone for recurrence. Bristow reported a meta-analysis of studies that included over 2,000 women undergoing surgical treatment for recurrent disease with or without chemotherapy, and reported a mean weighted median post-recurrence survival of 30.3 months (Table 8).[69] The most important prognostic factor was the amount of RD at the end of surgery for recurrence. Another review reported that survival of 40–60 months was possible with CRS in selected patients.[74]

Unfortunately, most women with recurrent EOC do not have the localized and easily resectable disease that would make them traditional surgical candidates. To the contrary, two-thirds of those with recurrence will have PC.[76] It is in this situation that HIPEC may have a significant role to play in conjunction with CRS.

Table 8 compares the OS for patients treated with surgery for recurrent disease. The German collaborative group, Arbeitsgemeinschaft Gynäkologische Onkologie (AGO) performed a study of 250 women in German centers to determine the effect of CRS for recurrent EOC on survival.[75] This study is remarkable for its detailed prospective data collection and analysis. Patients with non-epithelial ovarian cancer and LMP tumors were excluded, as were patients undergoing primarily symptom-related and palliative surgery. In the 125 women with PC, the treatment-free interval was less than 6 months in 17.6%. Complete resection of all visible disease was possible in 74% of those without PC, and only 26% with PC. The overall median survival was 29.5 months for the 250 patients but for those with or without PC, it was 45.3 months and 19.9 months respectively. Interestingly, 2-year survival for those with PC undergoing complete resection to no RD was not significantly different from those without PC undergoing a similar complete resection—77% versus 81%. In the

Table 8 Median overall survival for surgery for recurrent ROC

Authors		n	OS Median (months)
Bristow[69]		2,019	30.3
Harter[75]	Overall	250	29.5
	With PC	125	19.9
HYPERO[53]		83	23.5

(**Abbreviations:** OS = overall survival; PC = peritoneal carcinomatosis)

Table 9 Reports of HIPEC for EOC including patients treated for recurrence

Authors	Year	Type	Situation	N	Agent	Dose	Time (min)	Temp (°C)
Loggie[77]	1994	Pilot	Advanced	1	MMC	30 mg	120	39–40.5
van der Vange[78]	2000	Pilot	P/R	5	Cisplatin	50/75 mg/m²	90	40
Cavaliere[79]	2000	Retro	P/R	20	Cisplatin	25 mg/m²/L	90	41.5–42.5
Deraco[80]	2001	Phase II	P/R	27	Cisplatin	25 mg/m²/L	60	42.5
Panteix[81]	2002	PK	R	16	Cisplatin	60/80/100 mg	90	41–43
de Bree	2003	Pro	P/R	19	Docetaxel	75 mg/m²	120	41–43
Chatzigeorgiou[83]	2003	Pro	P/R	20	Cisplatin	50-75 mg/m²	120	39–40
Zanon[84]	2004	Phase II	P/R	30	Cisplatin	100/150 mg/m²	60	41.5–42.5
Look[46]	2004	Retro	FL/P/R	12[E]	Cisplatin/MMC	*	60	41.5–42.5
Piso[47]	2004	Retro	FL/R	19	Cisplatin or mitoxantrone	75 mg/m² 15 mg/m²	90	41.5
Reichman[63]	2005	Retro	ID/R	13	Cisplatin	50 mg/m²	90	40
Raspagliesi[85]	2006	Retro	P/R	40**	Cisplatin/MMC or Cisplatin/dox	25/3.3 mg/m²/L 43/15.25 mgL	*	42.5
Rufian[49]	2006	Retro	FL/R	33	Paclitaxel	60 mg/m²	60	41–43
Lentz[50]	2007	Phase I	FL/C	17	Carboplatin	400-1200 mg/m²	90	43–43.5
Helm[86]	2007	Retro	P/R	18	Cisplatin or MMC	100 mg/m² 40 mg	90	42–43
Cotte[87]	2007	Pro	FL/P/R	81	Cisplatin	20 mg/m²/L max 80 mg	90	44–46 inflow
Bae[88]	2007	Retro	P/C	67	Paclitaxel or Carboplatin	175 mg/m² 350 mg/m²	90	43–44
Harrison[89]	2008	Phase I	R	13	Liposomal dox	15-100 mg/m²	90	40
DiGiorgio[51]	2008	Pro	FL/ID/C/R	45	Cisplatin	75 mg/m²	60	41–43
Cavaliere[90]	2009	Pro	P/R	42	Cisplatin or Cisplatin/dox	25 mg/m²/L 50/15 mg/m²	60-90	41.5–42.5
Munoz-Cesares[91]	2009	Retro	R	14	Paclitaxel	60 mg/m²	60	41–43
Fagotti[92]	2009	Pro	R	25	Oxaliplatin	460 mg/m²	30	41–42.5
Carrabin[93]	2010	Retro	P/R	18	Oxaliplatin	460 mg/m²	30	41–43

[E]Some patients received EPIC
*not stated
**some previously reported in reference 80
(**Abbreviation:** R = recurrent, P = persistent, FL = frontline, ID = interval debulking, C = consolidation
Pro = prospective, Retro = retrospective, MMC = mitomycin
dox = doxorubicin

HYPERO report,[53] despite the fact that 85% of the women treated for recurrence had PC and 29% were platinum resistant, the median OS was 23.5 months. It appears that this population was distinctly different from those who were historically treated with CRS for recurrence.

There are now multiple reports of the use of HIPEC for recurrent disease (Table 9).[46,47,49,51,63,77-90] Despite the large numbers, the studies are difficult to compare and interpret due to their heterogeneity. In those studies in which survival data was clearly stated, the median OS were 22.5 months,[51] 28.1 months,[83] 28.4 months[86] and 31 months[85] while the median PFS 10 months,[85,90,91] 15.5 months,[51] 19.2 months[86] and 21.8 months.[79] In the report by Rufian,[49] patients aged less than or equal to 55 years who were reduced to no visible disease had a 5-year survival of 75%. In another study,[88] 14 patients undergoing CRS and HIPEC for recurrent EOC had 3-year and 5-year survivals of 64 and 50% respectively as compared with 57 and 17% in the same order for those of the 12 patients who underwent CRS alone. These outcomes suggest that HIPEC is having a positive influence on

Section 2

outcomes in this setting when compared with the reports from Bristow [69] and Harter[76] discussed above, and its role should be explored further.

Prognostic factors for survival with HIPEC in recurrent EOC have included the interval from initial diagnosis to HIPEC,[79,85] the PCI,[63,79,83,86] the extent of CRS,[49,63,79,82-86,88] age,[49,79] preoperative performance status,[84] presence of lymph node metastasis[49] and initial platinum response.[53]

THE PROBLEM OF FRONT-LINE FAILURE

Patients with particularly poor outcome in EOC are those with disease that persists at the end of front-line platinum-containing therapy; these patients have tumors that are either totally or partially platinum resistant. Certainly for those with large volume disease at the end of front-line therapy, CRS and HIPEC are not warranted. Surgeons at the Instituto Tumori in Milano initiated a study of CRS and HIPEC in this setting but closed it because of a high level of intolerance of the combined treatments and poor study accrual. This was a pioneering investigation which confirmed the difficulty of finding active therapy in this setting. These patients have refractory disease and are unlikely to respond to any currently available therapy. On the other hand, CRS and HIPEC might have a role for small volume persistent disease such as that found in patients with a complete clinical response who undergo a second look surgery if the disease is easily resectable. This is worthy of further study.

Mortality of HIPEC

The mortality rate for CRS and HIPEC is reported to be between 0% and 10% in 19 studies including treatment at all time-points of EOC[92] whilst a review of 13 reports including 256 cases receiving HIPEC for recurrent EOC revealed a mortality rate of 3.9% (10 of 256 cases).[93] For the 141 patients in the HYPERO registry initial report, the mortality rate was 2.1%.[53] Since much of this data is based on cases that included extensive CRS together with the HIPEC, a significant contribution to the mortality would be expected to come from the CRS alone.

A recent systematic review[94] investigated mortality for CRS alone for initial treatment of primary EOC, and included 2,300 patients from 23 studies. The overall mean perioperative mortality (death from any cause within 30 days of surgery) was 2.8% whilst in single center studies, it was 2.5% (range: 0–6.7%) while in population-based studies, it was 3.7% (range: 2.5–4.8%). The mortality rate for CRS alone in recurrent EOC was 1.4% (range: 0–3.4%);[74] however, these patients probably represent less extensive disease as discussed above (Table 10).

Table 10 Studies reporting mortality rates for HIPEC at all time-points

Studies (N)	Patients (N)	Mortality (%)
6	168	0
1	246	0.4
1	56	2
1*	141	2.1
2	111	3
1	104	4
1	19	5
1	18	6
2	39	10

(*Source:* Adapted from Reference 94)
*HYPERO registry[53]

Morbidity of HIPEC

As with mortality, the estimation of morbidity specifically related to HIPEC is complicated by the fact that the major CRS which often immediately precedes HIPEC is itself associated with significant morbidity.

In a systematic review,[92] 19 studies involving 895 patients undergoing HIPEC for EOC performed at all natural history time-points were analyzed. Complications were reported at the following frequencies by grade: (i) Grade I (no intervention required for resolution): 6–70%, (ii) Grade II (medical treatments required for resolution): 3–50%, (iii) Grade III (invasive intervention including radiological required for resolution): 0–40% and (iv) Grade IV (required urgent definitive intervention such as returning to the operating room or intensive care unit for resolution): 0–15%. Severe complications included ileus, anastomotic leakage, bleeding, pleural effusion, wound and other infections, fistula and thrombocytopenia.

Severe complications occurring in 256 patients undergoing CRS and HIPEC for recurrent/persistent disease[93] included hematologic (4.3%), creatinemia (3.9%), wound infection (4.3%), anastomotic leak (1.6%), bowel perforation (2.3%), peritonitis (0.8%) and abscess formation (1.2%). The rate of anastomotic leak in the absence of a diverting stoma remains unknown. Spontaneous intestinal perforations do occur and may reflect the effect of heated chemotherapy on bowel which has been traumatized, particularly during enterolysis. Complications for 141 patients undergoing CRS and

HIPEC at all time-points taken into account in the initial HYPERO report[53] included ileus, delayed return of bowel function and diarrhea while pleural effusions, atelectasis, pneumonia and pulmonary insufficiency constituted the pulmonary complications, and then infection included wound infection, port site infection and urinary infection. In a recent publication, Pomel[95] reported the premature closure of a phase II prospective study of 31 patients—22 with persistent disease and 9 with no macroscopic disease—following front-line therapy treated with HIPEC oxaliplatin because of a 29% severe morbidity rate which was mainly related to intra-abdominal bleeding in 9 patients. Five of them had adhesiolysis only at the time of surgery. Postoperative bleeding with oxaliplatin has previously been noted at a rate of between 5% and 18% after surgery for pseudomyxoma and appendiceal cancer.[96,97]

A review of severe morbidity following CRS alone for recurrent EOC reported a rate of 11% (67/631);[74] however, as mentioned above, it is likely that this population is different historically from that undergoing HIPEC.

SURGICAL CONSIDERATIONS

Patient Selection

While considering a patient for HIPEC, the surgeon should consider the performance status of the patient and their fitness to undergo surgery. In circumstances where the extent of CRS will be limited by medical comorbidities, this should be a clear indication to consider avoiding HIPEC. The Ovarian Consensus Panel of the 5th International Workshop on Peritoneal Surface Malignancy considered the following as relative contraindications for CRS and HIPEC: (i) heart failure (94%), (ii) pulmonary compromise (94%), (iii) previous pulmonary embolus (63%), (iv) previous deep venous thrombosis without pulmonary embolus (26%), (v) body mass index (BMI), BMI greater than 35 (48%), and (iv) 30–34 BMI (26%).[44] This is not a complete or definitive list and ultimately, it is up to the surgeon to make a decision that weighs the balance between the possibilities of increased morbidity and mortality versus the limited survival without aggressive treatment.

Surgical Approach

The surgical aim should be reduction of the tumor burden to no visible disease or at least to less than or equal to 2.5 mm largest lesion size combined with total adhesiolysis. In the presence of extensive adhesions involving small bowel, great care should be taken to avoid serosal injury since spontaneous perforations do occur after CRS and HIPEC, and it may be that these are related. Surgical Oncologists seem to be split on the need for a diverting stoma following HIPEC at the time of large bowel resection rather than immediate reanastomosis. There is no data on indications, and this must remain up to the surgeon's preference.

Prior to any CRS at which HIPEC delivery is contemplated, the necessary surgical skill should be present or available to carry out maximal CRS. The benefits of such an approach have been more than amply demonstrated.[56] Some of the procedures necessary in the resection of EOC are given in Table 11.

HIPEC Technique

The technique of HIPEC delivery has been described in Chapters 2-4. Whilst there are reports of the open technique leading to better distribution of perfusate within the peritoneal cavity,[98] there is no data showing that there is an advantage of this method in terms of survival. In the HYPERO Initial Report, the closed

Table 11 Some of the procedures necessary for CRS of EOC

Diaphragm stripping/resection
Resection of liver metastasis Serosal Parenchymal
Cholecystectomy
Resection of tumor from porta hepatis
Gastrectomy (partial)
Omentectomy
Lymphadenectomy para-aortic (infra and suprarenal) pelvic Inguinal
Bowel resection large including posterior exenteration Small
Stoma formation colostomy – loop, end ileostomy – loop, end
Appendectomy
Salpingo-oophorectomy
Hysterectomy
Ureteric resection (partial) and reimplantation
Bladder resection (partial)
Peritonectomy procedures

method was the most popular among the contributors with 124 of 141(87.9%) patients undergoing a closed method and 17/141 (12.1%) an open method. The closed method has the advantage with regard to compliance with work-place safety rules for the handling of chemotherapy agents. There are many unanswered questions about the drugs to be used and the duration of perfusion and so, HIPEC is best performed within a defined research protocol.

Laparoscopy versus Laparotomy

Although there have been case reports of delivery of HIPEC at the time of laparoscopy,[99,100] there have been no large series of this method of delivery. The use of a hand port would appear to offer an interesting method of combining minimal invasion with optimum perfusate (heat and chemotherapy agent) distribution.[100] A laparoscopic approach would avoid the complications associated with large incisions but could only be used if the same extent of CRS and adhesiolysis are performed.

The Future of HIPEC for EOC

There are strong theoretical reasons why HIPEC should be investigated for a role in improving outcomes for a disease for which current standard treatments fall way short of acceptability. Whilst millions of dollars and other currency denominations are spent on studies of new systemic chemotherapy and biological agents in EOC, little money is available for HIPEC research. Some studies of novel agents are designed to detect improvements in survival of only a few weeks. When novel agents are approved for use in humans, they can be hugely expensive with a six month course of bevacizumab in the USA; for example, costing several tens of thousands of US dollars. The advantage of HIPEC is that it is a single additional treatment that may not only be given at the time of a routine major surgical intervention indicated for the treatment of EOC but also, if used at initial surgery, can be given at the most optimal time for the treatment of EOC—when the disease burden is at its lowest and there are no adhesions.

There is no doubt that research studies are needed for CRS and HIPEC at all the natural history time-points for EOC. One of the leaders is the Netherlands Cancer Institute with its randomized trial of HIPEC at the time of ID (Principal Investigator, Dr Wilhelmien Van Driel, personal communication). Patients undergoing ID following NAC are randomized to receive either HIPEC or no HIPEC at the time of ID. This trial is accruing and the results are eagerly awaited. Randomised controlled trials at other time-points are badly needed.[101] However, an RCT at the time of recurrent disease is particularly problematic to organize because of the difficulties in defining a control group in patients with PC for whom the outcome is so poor with conventional therapy and for whom CRS alone is not indicated. Recognizing these difficulties, and in an attempt to continue to gather and analyze information about the use, indications and outcomes of HIPEC until further studies are developed, the Gynecologic Oncology team at Saint Louis University is bringing together the efforts of collaborators around the world in the HYPOVA Registry. This will allow data from every patient treated with HIPEC for EOC to be incorporated and studied. The "HIPEC in ovarian cancer study" (HOCS) will prospectively investigate the use of HIPEC at all natural history time-points of ovarian cancer. Participants must have EOC and have had a decision made for HIPEC by their medical team. The study attempts to narrow the variables of HIPEC technique (agents, duration of perfusion, temperature of perfusate) whilst allowing surgeons the leeway to make individual decisions about treatment. These studies will allow sufficient numbers of patients to be accrued to provide information on indications, technique, morbidity and outcomes whilst randomized studies are developed.

Judging by the increasing number of publications, attendance at regional therapy meetings and interest in collaborative research efforts, the necessary biomass of centers and surgeons will be available to conduct valuable trials of HIPEC in EOC. The gynecologic oncology specialty has been slow to develop interest in HIPEC for EOC but the author is hopeful that this will improve.

REFERENCES

1. Parkin DM, Bray F, Ferlay J, et al. Global cancer statistics. CA Cancer J Clin. 2005;55(2):74-108.
2. American Cancer Society. (2010). Cancer Facts and Figures 2010. [online] Available from http://www.cancer.org/Research/CancerFactsFigures/CancerFactsFigures/cancer-facts-and-figures-2010. [Accessed, 2010].
3. Altekruse SF, Kosary CL, Krapcho M, et al. (2010). SEER Cancer Statistics Review, 1975-2007. [online] Available from http://seer.cancer.gov/csr/1975_2007/. [Accessed, 2010].
4. Heintz AP, Odicino F, Maisonneuve P, et al. Carcinoma of the ovary. FIGO 6th Annual Report on the Results of Treatment in Gynecological Cancer. Int J Gynaecol Obstet. 2006;95(Suppl 1):S161-92.
5. AJCC. Ovary and primary peritoneal carcinoma. In: Edge SB, Byrd DR, Compton CC, Fritz AG, Greene FL, Trotti A (Eds). AJCC Cancer Staging Handbook, 7th edition. New York: Springer; 2009. pp. 493-506.

Chapter 6

6. Goodman MT, Shvetsov YB. Incidence of ovarian, peritoneal, and fallopian tube carcinomas in the United States, 1995-2004. Cancer Epidemiol Biomarkers Prev. 2009;18(1): 132-9.
7. Blaustein A, Kurman RJ. Surface epithelial tumors of the ovary. In: Kurman RJ. (Ed). Blaustein's Pathology of the Female Genital Tract, 5th edition. New York: Springer; 2002. pp. 791-904.
8. Trimble CL, Kosary C, Trimble EL. Long-term survival and patterns of care in women with ovarian tumors of low malignant potential. Gynecol Oncol. 2002;86(1):34-7.
9. Munnell EW. The changing prognosis and treatment in cancer of the ovary. A report of 235 patients with primary ovarian carcinoma 1952-1961. Am J Obstet Gynecol. 1968; 100(6):790-805.
10. Griffiths CT. Surgical resection of tumor bulk in the primary treatment of ovarian carcinoma. Natl Cancer Inst Monogr. 1975;42:101-4.
11. Hoskins WJ, Bundy BN, Thigpen JT, et al. The influence of cytoreductive surgery on recurrence-free interval and survival in small-volume stage III epithelial ovarian cancer: a Gynecologic Oncology Group study. Gynecol Oncol. 1992;47(2):159-66.
12. Bristow RE, Tomacruz RS, Armstrong DK, et al. Survival effect of maximal cytoreductive surgery for advanced ovarian carcinoma during the platinum era: a meta-analysis. J Clin Oncol. 2002;20(5):1248-59.
13. Eisenkop SM, Spirtos NM. What are the current surgical objectives, strategies, and technical capabilities of gynecologic oncologists treating advanced epithelial ovarian cancer? Gynecol Oncol. 2001;82(3):489-97.
14. Eisenkop SM, Friedman RL, Wang HJ. Complete cytoreductive surgery is feasible and maximizes survival in patients with advanced epithelial ovarian cancer: a prospective study. Gynecol Oncol. 1998;69(2):103-8.
15. Eisenhauer EL, Abu-Rustum NR, Sonoda Y, et al. The addition of extensive upper abdominal surgery to achieve optimal cytoreduction improves survival in patients with stages IIIC-IV epithelial ovarian cancer. Gynecol Oncol. 2006;103(3):1083-90.
16. Rubin SC, Randall TC, Armstrong KA, et al. Ten-year follow-up of ovarian cancer patients after second-look laparotomy with negative findings. Obstet Gynecol. 1999;93(1):21-4.
17. Dedrick RL, Myers CE, Bungay PM, et al. Pharmacokinetic rationale for peritoneal drug administration in the treatment of ovarian cancer. Canc Treat Rep. 1978;62(1):1-11.
18. Markman M. Intraperitoneal chemotherapy in the management of malignant disease. Expert Rev Anticancer Ther. 2001; 1(1):142-8.
19. Hahn GM. Potential for therapy of drugs and hyperthermia. Canc Res. 1979;39(6 Pt 2):2264-8.
20. Meyn RE, Corry PM, Fletcher SE, et al. Thermal enhancement of DNA damage in mammalian cells treated with cis-diamminedichloroplatinum(II). Cancer Res. 1980;40(4): 1136-9.
21. Alberts DS, Peng YM, Chen HS, et al. Therapeutic synergism of hyperthermia-cis-platinum in a mouse tumor model. J Natl Cancer Inst. 1980;65(2):455-61.
22. Akaboshi M, Tanaka Y, Kawai K, et al. Effect of hyperthermia on the number of platinum atoms binding to DNA of HeLa cells treated with 195mPt-radiolabelled cis-diaminedichloroplatinum(II). Int J Radiat Biol. 1994;66(2): 215-20.
23. Barlogie B, Corry PM, Drewinko B. In vitro thermochemotherapy of human colon cancer cells with cis-dichloro-diammineplatinum(II) and mitomycin C. Cancer Res. 1980; 40(4):1165-8.
24. Wang BS, Lumanglas AL, Silva J, et al. Effect of hyperthermia on the sensitivity of human colon carcinoma cells to mitoxantrone. Cancer Treat Rep. 1987;71(9):831-6.
25. Xu MJ, Alberts DS. Potentiation of platinum analogue cytotoxicity by hyperthermia. Cancer Chemother Pharmacol. 1988;21(3):191-6.
26. Los G, van Vugt MJ, Pinedo HM. Response of peritoneal solid tumours after intraperitoneal chemohyperthermia treatment with cisplatin or carboplatin. Br J Cancer. 1994;69(2):235-41.
27. Maymon R, Bar-Shira Maymon B, Holzinger M, et al. Augmentative effects of intracellular chemotherapy penetration combined with hyperthermia in human ovarian cancer cells lines. Gynecol Oncol. 1994;55(2):265-70.
28. Haveman J, Rietbroek RC, Geerdink A, et al. Effect of hyperthermia on the cytotoxicity of 2',2'-difluorodeoxycytidine (gemcitabine) in cultured SW1573 cells. Int J Cancer. 1995; 62(5):627-30.
29. Rietbroek RC, van de Vaart PJ, Haveman J, et al. Hyperthermia enhances the cytotoxicity and platinum-DNA adduct formation of lobaplatin and oxaliplatin in cultured SW 1573 cells. J Cancer Res Clin Oncol. 1997;123(1):6-12.
30. Hermisson M, Weller M. Hyperthermia enhanced chemosensitivity of human malignant glioma cells. Anticancer Res. 2000;20(3A):1819-23.
31. Urano M, Ling CC. Thermal enhancement of melphalan and oxaliplatin cytotoxicity in vitro. Int J Hyperthermia. 2002; 18(4):307-15.
32. Mohamed F, Marchettini P, Stuart OA, et al. Thermal enhancement of new chemotherapeutic agents at moderate hyperthermia. Ann Surg Oncol. 2003;10(4):463-8.
33. Takemoto M, Kuroda M, Urano M, et al. The effect of various chemotherapeutic agents given with mild hyperthermia on different types of tumours. Int J Hyperthermia. 2003;19(2): 193-203.
34. de Bree E, Theodoropoulos PA, Rosing H, et al. Treatment of ovarian cancer using intraperitoneal chemotherapy with taxanes: from laboratory bench to bedside. Cancer Treat Rev. 2006;32(6):471-82.
35. Istomin YP, Zhavrid EA, Alexandrova EN, et al. Dose enhancement effect of anticancer drugs associated with increased temperature in vitro. Exp Oncol. 2008;30(1):56-9.
36. Herman TS, Teicher BA, Cathcart KN, et al. Effect of hyperthermia on cis-diamminedichloroplatinum(II) (rhodamine 123)2[tetrachloroplatinum(II)] in a human squamous cell carcinoma line and a cis-diamminedichloroplatinum(II)-resistant subline. Cancer Res. 1988;48(18):5101-5.
37. van de Vaart PJ, van der Vange N, Zoetmulder FA, et al. Intraperitoneal cisplatin with regional hyperthermia in advanced ovarian cancer: pharmacokinetics and cisplatin-DNA adduct formation in patients and ovarian cancer cell lines. Eur J Cancer. 1998;34(1):148-54.
38. Gore ME, Fryatt I, Wiltshaw E, et al. Treatment of relapsed carcinoma of the ovary with cisplatin or carboplatin following initial treatment with these compounds. Gynecol Oncol. 1990; 36(2):207-11.
39. Markman M, Rothman R, Hakes T, et al. Second-line platinum therapy in patients with ovarian cancer previously treated with cisplatin. J Clin Oncol. 1991;9(3):389-93.

40. Vermorken JB. Second-line randomized trials in epithelial ovarian cancer. Int J Gynecol Cancer. 2008;18(Suppl 1):59-66.
41. Armstrong DK, Bundy B, Wenzel L, et al. Intraperitoneal cisplatin and paclitaxel in ovarian cancer. N Engl J Med. 2006; 354(1):34-43.
42. Jaaback K, Johnson N. Intraperitoneal chemotherapy for the initial management of primary epithelial ovarian cancer. Cochrane Database Syst Rev. 2006;(1): CD005340.
43. Lee CL, Kay N. Inhibition of ovarian cancer growth and implantation by paclitaxel after laparoscopic surgery in a mouse model. Am J Obstet Gynecol. 2006;195(5):1278-81.
44. Helm CW, Bristow RE, Kusamura S, et al. Hyperthermic intraperitoneal chemotherapy with and without cytoreductive surgery for epithelial ovarian cancer. J Surg Oncol. 2008; 98(4):283-90.
45. Steller MA, Egorin MJ, Trimble EL, et al. A pilot phase I trial of continuous hyperthermic peritoneal perfusion with high-dose carboplatin as primary treatment of patients with small-volume residual ovarian cancer. Cancer Chemother Pharmacol. 1999;43(2):106-14.
46. Look M, Chang D, Sugarbaker PH. Long-term results of cytoreductive surgery for advanced and recurrent epithelial ovarian cancers and papillary serous carcinoma of the peritoneum. Int J Gynecol Cancer. 2004;14(1):35-41.
47. Piso P, Dahlke MH, Loss M, et al. Cytoreductive surgery and hyperthermic intraperitoneal chemotherapy in peritoneal carcinomatosis from ovarian cancer. World J Surg Oncol. 2004;2:21-7.
48. Yoshida Y, Sasaki H, Kurokawa T, et al. Efficacy of intraperitoneal continuous hyperthermic chemotherapy as consolidation therapy in patients with advanced epithelial ovarian cancer: a long-term follow-up. Oncol Rep. 2005;13(1): 121-5.
49. Rufián S, Muñoz-Casares FC, Briceño J, et al. Radical surgery-peritonectomy and intraoperative intraperitoneal chemotherapy for the treatment of peritoneal carcinomatosis in recurrent or primary ovarian cancer. J Surg Oncol. 2006; 94(4):316-24.
50. Lentz SS, Miller BE, Kucera GL, et al. Intraperitoneal hyperthermic chemotherapy using carboplatin: a phase I analysis in ovarian carcinoma. Gynecol Oncol. 2007;106(1): 207-10.
51. Di Giorgio A, Naticchioni E, Biacchi D, et al. Cytoreductive surgery (peritonectomy procedures) combined with hyperthermic intraperitoneal chemotherapy (HIPEC) in the treatment of diffuse peritoneal carcinomatosis from ovarian cancer. Cancer. 2008;113(2):315-25.
52. Lim MC, Kang S, Choi J, et al. Hyperthermic intraperitoneal chemotherapy after extensive cytoreductive surgery in patients with primary advanced epithelial ovarian cancer: interim analysis of a phase II study. Ann Surg Oncol. 2009;16(4):993-1000.
53. Helm CW, Richard SD, Pan J, et al. Hyperthermic intraperitoneal chemotherapy in ovarian cancer: first report of the HYPER-O registry. Int J Gynecol Cancer. 2010;20(1): 61-9.
54. Eisenkop SM, Spirtos NM, Friedman RL, et al. Relative influences of tumor volume before surgery and the cytoreductive outcome on survival for patients with advanced ovarian cancer: a prospective study. Gynecol Oncol. 2003;90(2):390-6.
55. Panici PB, Maggioni A, Hacker N, et al. Systematic aortic and pelvic lymphadenectomy versus resection of bulky nodes only in optimally debulked advanced ovarian cancer: a randomized clinical trial. J Natl Cancer Inst. 2005;97(8):560-6.
56. Chi DS, Eisenhauer EL, Zivanovic O, et al. Improved progression-free and overall survival in advanced ovarian cancer as a result of a change in surgical paradigm. Gynecol Oncol. 2009;114(1):26-31.
57. Surwit E, Childers J, Atlas I, et al. Neoadjuvant chemotherapy for advanced ovarian cancer. Int J Gynecol Oncol. 1996;6(5):356-61.
58. Huober J, Meyer A, Wagner U, et al. The role of neoadjuvant chemotherapy and interval laparotomy in advanced ovarian cancer. J Cancer Res Clin Oncol. 2002;128(3):153-60.
59. Kang S, Nam BH. Does neoadjuvant chemotherapy increase optimal cytoreduction rate in advanced ovarian cancer? Meta-analysis of 21 studies. Ann Surg Oncol. 2009;16(8):2315-20.
60. Bristow RE, Eisenhauer EL, Santillan A, et al. Delaying the primary surgical effort for advanced ovarian cancer: a systematic review of neoadjuvant chemotherapy and interval cytoreduction. Gynecol Oncol. 2007;104(2):480-90.
61. Vergote I, Tropé CG, Amant F, et al. Neoadjuvant chemotherapy or primary surgery in stage IIIC or IV ovarian cancer. N Engl J Med. 2010;363(10):943-53.
62. Di Giorgio A, Cardi M, Sammartino P. Peritonectomy and hyperthermic intraperitoneal chemotherapy (HIPEC) for ovarian peritoneal carcinomatosis: an argued role. Gynecol Oncol. 2010;117(1):146-7.
63. Reichman TW, Cracchiolo B, Sama J, et al. Cytoreductive surgery and intraoperative hyperthermic chemoperfusion for advanced ovarian carcinoma. J Surg Oncol. 2005;90(2):51-8.
64. de Bree E, Rosing H, Beijnen JH, et al. Pharmacokinetic study of docetaxel in intraoperative hyperthermic i.p. chemotherapy for ovarian cancer. Anticancer Drugs. 2003;14(2):103-10.
65. Ryu KS, Kim JH, Ko HS, et al. Effects of intraperitoneal hyperthermic chemotherapy in ovarian cancer. Gynecol Oncol. 2004;94(2):325-32.
66. Mutch DG, Orlando M, Goss T, et al. Randomized phase III trial of gemcitabine compared with pegylated liposomal doxorubicin in patients with platinum-resistant ovarian cancer. J Clin Oncol. 2007;25(19):2811-8.
67. Bolis G, Parazzini F, Scarfone G, et al. Paclitaxel vs epidoxorubicin plus paclitaxel as second-line therapy for platinum-refractory and -resistant ovarian cancer. Gynecol Oncol. 1999;72(1):60-4.
68. Bolis G, Scarfone G, Giardina G, et al. Carboplatin alone vs carboplatin plus epidoxorubicin as second-line therapy for cisplatin- or carboplatin-sensitive ovarian cancer. Gynecol Oncol. 2001;81(1):3-9.
69. Bristow RE, Puri I, Chi DS. Cytoreductive surgery for recurrent ovarian cancer: a meta-analysis. Gynecol Oncol. 2009;112(1):265-74.
70. Pfisterer J, Plante M, Vergote I, et al. Gemcitabine plus carboplatin compared with carboplatin in patients with platinum-sensitive recurrent ovarian cancer: an intergroup trial of the AGO-OVAR, the NCIC CTG, and the EORTC GCG. J Clin Oncol. 2006;24(29):4699-4707.
71. Gordon AN, Tonda M, Sun S, et al. Long-term survival advantage for women treated with pegylated liposomal doxorubicin compared with topotecan in a phase 3 randomized study of recurrent and refractory epithelial ovarian cancer. Gynecol Oncol. 2004;95(1):1-8.
72. Cantù MG, Buda A, Parma G, et al. Randomized controlled trial of single-agent paclitaxel versus cyclophosphamide, doxorubicin, and cisplatin in patients with recurrent ovarian

cancer who responded to first-line platinum-based regimens. J Clin Oncol. 2002;20(5):1232-7.
73. Parmar MK, Ledermann JA, Colombo N, et al. Paclitaxel plus platinum-based chemotherapy versus conventional platinum-based chemotherapy in women with relapsed ovarian cancer: the ICON4/AGO-OVAR-2.2 trial. Lancet. 2003;361(9375):2099-2106.
74. Munkarah AR,Coleman RL. Critical evaluation of secondary cytoreduction in recurrent ovarian cancer. Gynecol Oncol. 2004;95(2):273-80.
75. Harter P, Hahmann M, Lueck HJ, et al. Surgery for recurrent ovarian cancer: role of peritoneal carcinomatosis: exploratory analysis of the DESKTOP I Trial about risk factors, surgical implications, and prognostic value of peritoneal carcinomatosis. Ann Surg Oncol. 2009;16(5):1324-30.
76. Ferrandina G, Legge F, Salutari V, et al. Impact of pattern of recurrence on clinical outcome of ovarian cancer patients: clinical considerations. Eur J Cancer. 2006;42(14):2296-2302.
77. van der Vange N, van Goethem AR, Zoetmulder FA, et al. Extensive cytoreductive surgery combined with intra-operative intraperitoneal perfusion with cisplatin under hyperthermic conditions (OVHIPEC) in patients with recurrent ovarian cancer: a feasibility pilot. Eur J Surg Oncol. 2000;26(7):663-8.
78. Cavaliere F, Perri P, Di Filippo F, et al. Treatment of peritoneal carcinomatosis with intent to cure. J Surg Oncol. 2000;74(1):41-4.
79. Deraco M, Rossi CR, Pennacchioli E, et al. Cytoreductive surgery followed by intraperitoneal hyperthermic perfusion in the treatment of recurrent epithelial ovarian cancer: a phase II clinical study. Tumori. 2001;87(3):120-6.
80. Panteix G, Beaujard A, Garbit F, et al. Population pharmacokinetics of cisplatin in patients with advanced ovarian cancer during intraperitoneal hyperthermia chemotherapy. Anticancer Res. 2002;22(2B):1329-36.
81. de Bree E, Romanos J, Michalakis J, et al. Intraoperative hyperthermic intraperitoneal chemotherapy with docetaxel as second-line treatment for peritoneal carcinomatosis of gynaecological origin. Anticancer Res. 2003;23(3C):3019-27.
82. Chatzigeorgiou K, Economou S, Chrysafis G, et al. Treatment of recurrent epithelial ovarian cancer with secondary cytoreduction and continuous intraoperative intraperitoneal hyperthermic chemoperfusion (CIIPHCP). Zentralbl Gynakol. 2003;125(10):424-9.
83. Zanon C, Clara R, Chiappino I, et al. Cytoreductive surgery and intraperitoneal chemohyperthermia for recurrent peritoneal carcinomatosis from ovarian cancer. World J Surg. 2004;28(10):1040-5.
84. Raspagliesi F, Kusamura S, Campos Torres JC, et al. Cytoreduction combined with intraperitoneal hyperthermic perfusion chemotherapy in advanced/recurrent ovarian cancer patients: the experience of National Cancer Institute of Milan. Eur J Surg Oncol. 2006;32(6):671-5.
85. Helm CW, Randall-Whitis L, Martin RS 3rd, et al. Hyperthermic intraperitoneal chemotherapy in conjunction with surgery for the treatment of recurrent ovarian carcinoma. Gynecol Oncol. 2007;105(1):90-6.
86. Cotte E, Glehen O, Mohamed F, et al. Cytoreductive surgery and intraperitoneal chemo-hyperthermia for chemo-resistant and recurrent advanced epithelial ovarian cancer: prospective study of 81 patients. World J Surg. 2007;31(9): 1813-20.
87. Harrison LE, Bryan M, Pliner L, et al. Phase I trial of pegylated liposomal doxorubicin with hyperthermic intraperitoneal chemotherapy in patients undergoing cytoreduction for advanced intra-abdominal malignancy. Ann Surg Oncol. 2008;15(5):1407-13.
88. Muñoz-Casares FC, Rufián S, Rubio MJ, et al. The role of hyperthermic intraoperative intraperitoneal chemotherapy (HIPEC) in the treatment of peritoneal carcinomatosis in recurrent ovarian cancer. Clin Transl Oncol. 2009;11(11): 753-9.
89. Cavaliere F, Giannarelli D, Valle M, et al. Peritoneal carcinomatosis from ovarian epithelial primary: combined aggressive treatment. In Vivo. 2009;23(3):441-6.
90. Carrabin N, Mithieux F, Meeus P, et al. Hyperthermic intraperitoneal chemotherapy with oxaliplatin and without adjuvant chemotherapy in stage IIIC ovarian cancer. Bull Cancer. 2010;97(4):E23-32.
91. Fagotti A, Paris I, Grimolizzi F, et al. Secondary cytoreduction plus oxaliplatin-based HIPEC in platinum-sensitive recurrent ovarian cancer patients: a pilot study. Gynecol Oncol. 2009; 113(3):335-40.
92. Chua TC, Robertson G, Liauw W, et al. Intraoperative hyperthermic intraperitoneal chemotherapy after cytoreductive surgery in ovarian cancer peritoneal carcinomatosis: systematic review of current results. J Cancer Res Clin Oncol. 2009; 135(12):1637-45.
93. Helm CW. The role of hyperthermic intraperitoneal chemotherapy (HIPEC) in ovarian cancer. Oncologist. 2009;14(7): 683-94.
94. Gerestein CG, Damhuis RA, Burger CW, et al. Postoperative mortality after primary cytoreductive surgery for advanced stage epithelial ovarian cancer: a systematic review. Gynecol Oncol. 2009;114(3):523-7.
95. Pomel C, Ferron G, Lorimier G, et al. Hyperthermic intraperitoneal chemotherapy using oxaliplatin as consolidation therapy for advanced epithelial ovarian carcinoma. Results of a phase II prospective multicentre trial. CHIPOVAC study. Eur J Surg Oncol. 2010;36(6):589-93.
96. Elias D, Lefevre JH, Chevalier J, et al. Complete cytoreductive surgery plus intraperitoneal chemohyperthermia with oxaliplatin for peritoneal carcinomatosis of colorectal origin. J Clin Oncol. 2009;27(5):681-5.
97. Marcotte E, Sideris L, Drolet P, et al. Hyperthermic intraperitoneal chemotherapy with oxaliplatin for peritoneal carcinomatosis arising from appendix: preliminary results of a survival analysis. Ann Surg Oncol. 2008;15(10):2701-8.
98. Elias D, Antoun S, Goharin A, et al. Research on the best chemohyperthermia technique of treatment of peritoneal carcinomatosis after complete resection. Int J Surg Investig. 2000;1(5):431-9.
99. Chang E, Alexander HR, Libutti SK, et al. Laparoscopic continuous hyperthermic peritoneal perfusion. J Am Coll Surg. 2001;193(2):225-9.
100. Ferron G, Gesson-Paute A, Classe JM, et al. Feasibility of laparoscopic peritonectomy followed by intra-peritoneal chemohyperthermia: an experimental study. Gynecol Oncol. 2005;99(2):358-61.
101. Markman M. Hyperthermic intraperitoneal chemotherapy in the management of ovarian cancer: a critical need for an evidence-based evaluation. Gynecol Oncol. 2009;113(1):4-5.

Section 3

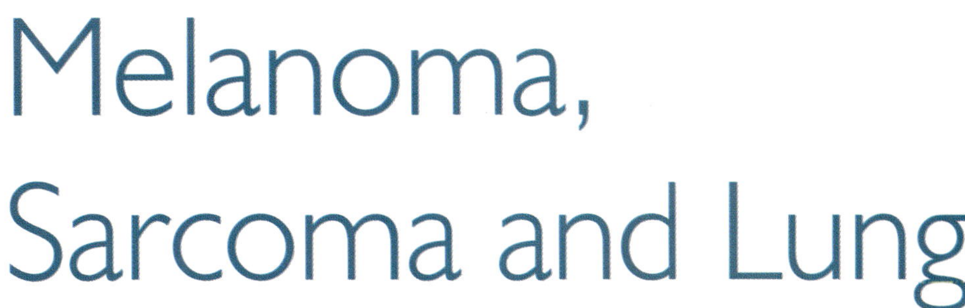

Melanoma, Sarcoma and Lung

7 Isolated Limb Perfusion (ILP) and Isolated Limb Infusion (ILI) for Locally Advanced Malignant Melanoma

Giorgos C. Karakousis, Douglas L. Fraker

BACKGROUND: IN-TRANSIT MELANOMA

There were an estimated 68,130 cases of newly diagnosed malignant melanoma in the United States in 2010 (making it the sixth most common cancer by incidence) with an estimated 8,700 melanoma related deaths.[1] While the majority (nearly 85%) of patients with melanoma present with localized primary disease, a small subset of patients will present with or develop locally advanced melanoma or in-transit disease. In-transit disease is defined by the presence of metastatic melanoma deposits in the dermal or subdermal lymphatic channels beyond 2 cm from the primary melanoma but not beyond the immediate draining regional nodal basin.[2] These lesions typically present as erythematous or pigmented nodules between the site of the primary melanoma and the regional nodal basin. They may occasionally however develop in the direction opposite from the draining regional nodal basin, presumably from obstructed lymphatic flow or the influence of gravity. Patients with in-transit disease are defined as having N2c disease by the current (seventh edition) AJCC staging system and are, therefore, classified as either Stage IIIB or Stage IIIC (the latter stage if nodal metastases or ulceration of the primary tumor are also present).[3] The incidence of in-transit disease in patients with clinical Stages I and II melanoma is estimated to be approximately 2–11%.[4-6] In a large retrospective study by M.D. Anderson of 1,395 patients undergoing sentinel lymph node (SLN) biopsy, the incidence of in-transit recurrence was found to be 6.5%, with the majority (71%) of these recurrences being locoregional without distant disease.[4] Clinical and histopathologic factors that have been associated with development of in-transit disease include female gender, lower extremity anatomic site, thickness, presence of lymphovascular invasion and nodal metastases.[4,7]

When there are a limited number of in-transit lesions, local surgical excision of the metastases with minimal negative margins remains a reasonable approach albeit rendering these patients at appreciable risk of regional relapse. Often, however, the in-transit disease is more extensive making locoregional surgical resection options short of limb amputation unfeasible (Fig. 1). These patients with in-transit disease not

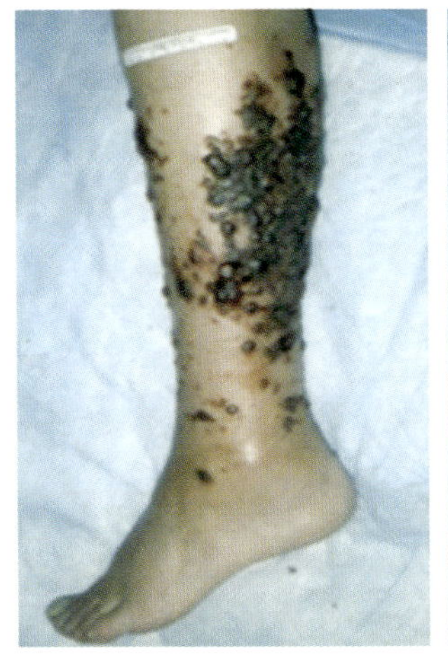

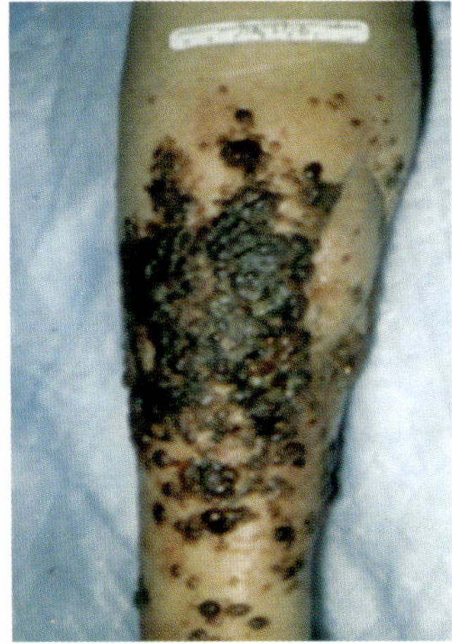

Figure 1 Patient with extensive in-transit melanoma of the distal left leg

amenable to simple local resection would be candidates for isolated limb perfusion (ILP) or isolated limb infusion (ILI). This chapter highlights these regional therapies, discussing the technique of ILP; its efficacy and safety in patients with locally advanced melanoma; factors predicting response and toxicity to ILP, and comparing ILP to the more recently developed ILI technique.

HISTORY AND TECHNIQUE OF ILP

Isolated limb perfusion involves the surgical isolation of the circulation of an extremity and the perfusion of chemotherapeutics at doses much higher than could be safely administered systemically to the affected limb. The technique was first reported by Creech and Krementz in 1958,[8] and has undergone subsequent modifications in the past five decades to improve its efficacy. Mild hyperthermia was introduced in 1969,[9] and the dose of melphalan, an alkylating agent which is the standard chemotherapeutic agent used for perfusion, has been optimized. Other attempted modifications had included the addition of biologic agents to the perfusion circuit including interferon-gamma with tumor necrosis factor-alpha (TNF-α); the effect of which on efficacy has been discussed in more detail below.

The ILP procedure involves surgical access to the inflow and outflow vessels to the limb; typically, the external iliac vessels for the lower extremity and the axillary vessels for the upper extremity. Occasionally, the femoral vessels or popliteal vessels are cannulated if the disease is limited to a more distal location in the lower extremity. Small side branches off the cannulated main vessels are often ligated to prevent systemic leakage, and a tourniquet is placed proximal to the tip of the catheters. Systemic heparin is administered to the patient prior to vessel cannulation, and the catheters are incorporated into an extracorporeal circuit with oxygenating chamber primed with heparinized saline, which is essentially a cardiopulmonary bypass machine (depicted schematically in Figure 2) to complete the limb isolation. The extremity is wrapped with a warming blanket at the onset of the procedure, and temperature probes are used in the extremity to continuously monitor deep and superficial tissue temperatures during the procedure with target temperatures being 38.5–40°C. Melphalan is added to the perfusate at a dose typically calculated by limb volume (10 mg/L for the lower extremity and 13 mg/L

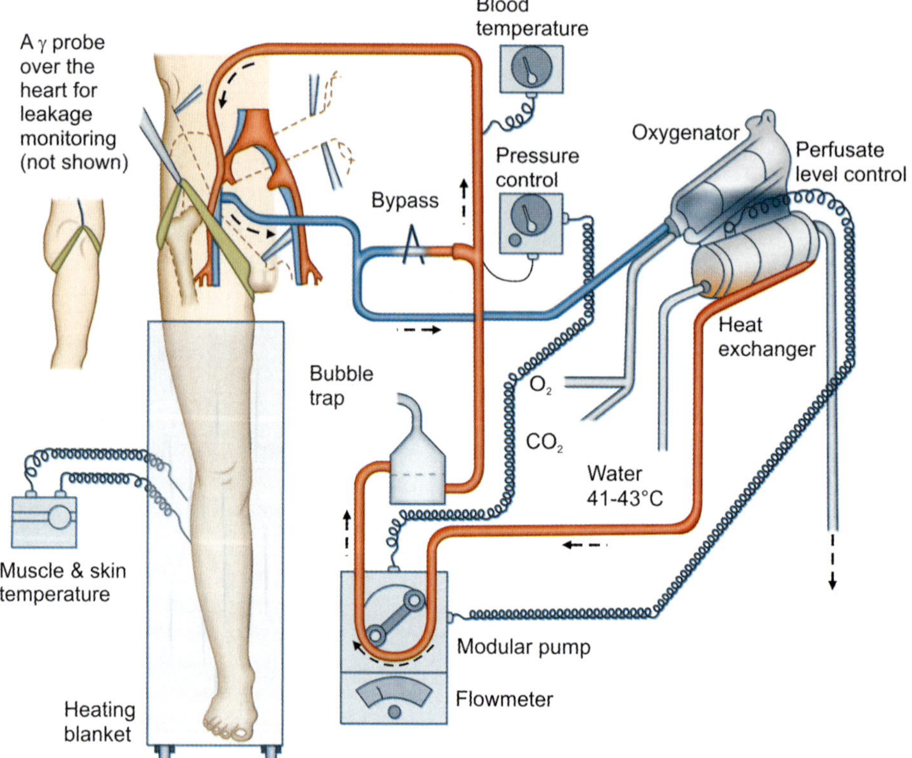

Figure 2 Schematic depiction of ILP circuit
(*Source*: LeJeune FJ, Liénard D, Matter M, et al. Efficiency of recombinant human TNF in human cancer therapy. Cancer Immun. 2006;6:6.)

Section 3

for the upper extremity). Occasionally, dactinomycin and cisplatin are used in conjunction with melphalan. The chemotherapeutic agent is circulated under mild hyperthermia for 60–90 minutes (when TNF added) at flow rates ranging between 400–900 mL/min. Technetium-99 labeled red blood cells or 131-I labeled human serum albumin are occasionally used in the perfusate to assess for systemic leakage. The excess high-dose chemotherapy is then flushed out of the limb prior to decannulation and repair of the arteriotomy and venotomy.

EFFICACY OF ILP

Several studies have investigated the effectiveness of ILP on locoregional (in-field) disease, disease-free and overall survival in patients with in-transit melanoma. There has been one randomized study evaluating the benefit of this modality in the adjuvant or prophylactic setting for high-risk patients.[10] In this multicenter international study, 832 patients with localized melanoma (melanoma thickness > 1.5 mm) were randomized to undergo wide excision of their primary versus wide excision with melphalan ILP. While there was a slight decrease in locoregional recurrences in the group that received the combined therapy, there was no difference in time with regard to distant metastases or overall survival between the two groups, with a higher morbidity in the combined therapy group. Therefore, the use of ILP has not been recommended in the adjuvant setting after wide excision of high-risk primary melanomas.

In a recent review examining the efficacy of ILP for melanoma in 20 studies with 1,587 ILP cases, the median complete response (CR) rate was 58.2% (range, 25–89%) and the median overall response (OR) rate was 90.4% (range, 64.0–100%).[11] In many of these studies, TNF-α was used in combination with melphalan in the perfusate, and in the review of the 562 perfusions with melphalan alone, the CR rate was found to be slightly lower (46.5%; range, 25.0–76.0%) with an OR rate 68.9% (range, 26.0–89.0%). An example of a CR in a patient who underwent ILP with melphalan and TNF is shown in Figure 3.

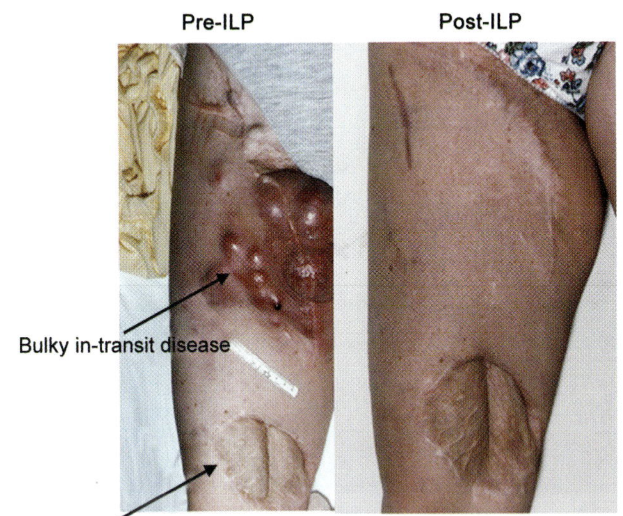

Figure 3 A complete response (CR) after ILP therapy with melphalan and TNF in a patient with in-transit melanoma

While there appears to be a trend with improved efficacy for regional response with the addition of TNF to melphalan in the perfusate compared to melphalan alone, a randomized multicenter trial sponsored by the American College of Surgeons Oncology Group (ACOSOG, Z0020 trial) of 133 enrolled patients with locally advanced melanoma found no statistically significant difference in the CR or OR rates between patients undergoing ILP with TNF and melphalan versus with melphalan alone.[12] At the third month, the CR rates in the combined treatment group versus the melphalan alone group were 25% and 26% respectively; the OR rates of the combined versus melphalan alone groups were 69% and 64% respectively. Moreover, there were 2 patients with treatment related toxicity in the melphalan with TNF group (and only one amputation in the melphalan alone group secondary to disease progression). The conclusion of the trial was that there was no significant short-term response benefit with the addition of TNF to melphalan, but that the combination therapy was associated with a higher morbidity, and therefore TNF is no longer used in ILP therapy in North America. Critics of the trial point to the lack of long-term follow-up from the trial and to the low CR rates identified compared to other studies, and suggest this to be a consequence of the methodology used in the study.[13] Pigmented lesions (even if flat) were likely measured as residual disease, when they may in fact have represented melanosis without viable tumor cells thereby potentially underestimating the response to therapy. TNF continues to be used in the ILP perfusate for in-transit melanoma in European countries, although there has not been data to support a benefit to disease-specific survival.

Generally speaking, disease-specific survival in patients with locally advanced melanoma is felt to be influenced more by disease biology factors, and less by regional treatment approach. In a review evaluating eight studies,[11] the median OS of patients with locally advanced melanoma undergoing ILP was 36.7 months with a 5-year median OS rate of 36.5% (range, 19.0–50.0%). This, of course, considers a heterogeneous group of patients with varying disease burden and stage. Evaluation of the secondary endpoint of local or in-field recurrence by this systematic review in studies reporting on this outcome identified a median local recurrence rate of 40.5% with a median time to recurrence of 10.5 months. Again, these local relapse rates reflect a heterogeneity in treatment (perfusate agents, degree of hyperthermia, etc.) and disease parameters.

Repeat ILP for locally recurrent or progressive disease is feasible, and generally considered to have similar efficacy to initial ILP with acceptable toxicity. In one recent large institutional experience of 25 repeat ILPs with TNF and melphalan in 21 patients, a CR rate of 76% was reported. This was not significantly different when compared to the CR rate (68%) after first ILP from 100 ILP cases in the same institution. Repeat ILP is generally reserved for patients with increased number of recurrent lesions in the extremity not amenable to simple excision, or with increased rapidity of in-field recurrence. ILI post-ILP provides another alternative for this group of patients and is discussed in more detail below.

CLINICAL AND PATHOLOGIC FACTORS PREDICTING RESPONSE AFTER ILP

Several studies have investigated factors with prognostic significance for in-field progression-free survival and overall survival following ILP therapy for in-transit melanoma. The results from such studies are variable; likely in part, secondary to the relatively small study populations and heterogeneity of methodology. Greater tumor burden (size and number of lesion), gender (male), advanced age and advanced stage (presence of nodal metastases) have all been associated with poorer in-field progression-free survival by multivariate analyses in patients undergoing ILP with melphalan and TNF.[13-15] Male gender has also been shown by more recent studies to be a negative prognostic indicator for overall survival post-ILP, along with advanced stage and lack of clinical CR.[13,14] Advanced age was shown in one study to be independently associated with poor overall survival,[16] although this finding has not been uniformly reported,[13,14] and even its impact on locoregional recurrence has been variably reported.[14,17] In a small study comparing patients undergoing TNF based ILP with adjuvant interferon to historical control patients who underwent TNF based ILP therapy alone, the use of adjuvant interferon was associated with improved overall survival by multivariate analysis.[18]

SAFETY AND TOXICITY

Isolated limb perfusion is generally considered a safe procedure with acceptable morbidity in selected patients. Because of the nature of the procedure, the majority of the toxicity is limited to the perfused extremity, although systemic toxicity has been reported. The Wieberdink grading system[19] (Table 1) characterizes the locoregional toxicity of the procedure, ranging from no subjective or objective skin reaction post-procedure (Grade I) to extensive tissue damage of the limb requiring amputation (Grade V). Patients will frequently (30–92%) demonstrate mild erythema or edema (Grade II toxicity), but Grade V toxicity is uncommon (0–3%).[12,15,18,20] Grade IV toxicity involving extensive epidermolysis or deep tissue damage requiring fasciotomy is similarly infrequently reported (0–5%).[15,20,21] Long-term neuropathy (≥ 3 months) in the form of paresthesias, anesthesia or paresis of digits was reported in one study to be 4%, with an apparently higher incidence after perfusions of the upper extremity.[22] Systemic morbidity is very low following ILP, with the ACOSOG Z0020 trial reporting a 6% incidence of Grade III hematologic toxicity, and 8% and 12% rates of Grade III cardiovascular morbidity for patients undergoing perfusion with melphalan and melphalan with TNF respectively.[12] In general, the reported Grade III or Grade IV systemic morbidity for the procedure is less than 5%.

Treatment and patient factors impacting on toxicity have also been investigated. In one retrospective study of 668 ILP procedures for melanoma, the addition of TNF to melphalan perfusate under hyperthermic conditions was found to be independently associated with increased Grades III–V locoregional toxicity.[23] The rate of Grade

Table 1 Wieberdink classification system[19] for grading regional toxicity to the extremity following isolated limb perfusion (ILP) or isolated limb infusion (ILI)

Grade	Reaction
I	No visible reaction
II	Mild erythema or edema
III	Considerable erythema/edema with some skin blistering
IV	Extensive epidermolysis with deep tissue damage and functional disturbance and threatened or actual compartment syndrome
V	Reaction necessitating amputation

III or higher toxicity in the hyperthermic ILP group receiving melphalan with TNF was 36%, and significantly higher when compared to the 16% rate in the group of patients receiving melphalan-only-ILP under normothermic or mild hyperthermic conditions albeit temperatures in the combined therapy group were notably higher than in the melphalan-only-hyperthermic group. Notably, there were no Grade-IV or Grade-V toxicities in the melphalan and TNF group. In the ACOSOG randomized trial Z0020, the incidence of Grade III or higher toxicity was 48% in the melphalan with TNF arm versus 38% in the group undergoing ILP with melphalan alone, with two treatment amputations in the combined treatment arm. Additional factors which have been associated with increased toxicity to the ILP procedure include female gender, and hyperthermia in excess of 40°C.[23,24] Other procedure-related treatment variables (e.g. length of perfusion, perfusate volume required) may likely contribute to toxicity but have not been systematically studied. Post-procedurely, elevated creatine kinase (CK) levels (> 1,000 IU/L) and WBC level have been shown in one study to serve as predictors for increased locoregional toxicity or impending compartment syndrome.[25]

Repeat ILP after progression of disease or recurrent disease can generally be performed, as indicated with acceptable morbidity. In one study of 21 patients undergoing repeat ILP with melphalan and TNF, Grades I/II and III/IV locoregional toxicities were reported to be 67% and 33% respectively and were not found to be statistically different from rates after first ILP.[21] Notably, there was no reported limb-threatening toxicity requiring amputation after repeat ILP.

ISOLATED LIMB INFUSION

Isolated limb infusion is a technique that was developed in the early 1990s at the Sydney Melanoma Unit (SMU) by Dr. Thompson and colleagues as a lesser surgically morbid and low cost procedure to ILP.[26,27] Conceptually, the procedure is similar to ILP and involves the isolation of the vasculature of the extremity and the infusion of high-dose chemotherapy (typically melphalan 7.5 mg/L ± dactinomycin 75 mg/L) into the diseased limb, thereby minimizing systemic toxicity. Unlike ILP, vascular access is achieved percutaneously (usually from the contralateral groin for the lower extremity) under fluoroscopic guidance, typically by interventional radiologists or vascular surgeons. The limb is isolated by a pneumatic compression tourniquet which is positioned proximal to the catheter tips, and the chemotherapeutic is then circulated manually in the limb (lower pressure system) by a syringe with stop flow technique under progressively hypoxic conditions (Fig. 4). This thereby eliminates the need for a cardiopulmonary bypass machine or perfusion team. Because of the progressive hypoxia and resulting acidosis, the duration of limb isolation in ILI is typically 30 minutes compared to 1 hour or greater with ILP, and overall operative times with ILI are considerably shorter (~ 1 hour) compared to ILP (~ 4–6 hours). Because of the percutaneous nature of the procedure, ILI therapy is generally more amenable to repeat treatments in patients with recurrent or progressive disease. Unlike with ILP, however, limb temperatures above 40°C are seldom achieved with ILI. Also, given the location of the tourniquet in the proximal thigh for ILI, the most proximal thigh is not included in the infused field, and therefore treatment of this area is not achieved with ILI, and represents an area potentially at risk for locoregional relapse. Moreover, ILP, unlike ILI, affords exposure to and the possibility of removal of clinically suspicious lymph nodes at the time of limb treatment. A summary comparison of the ILP and ILI techniques is summarized in Table 2.

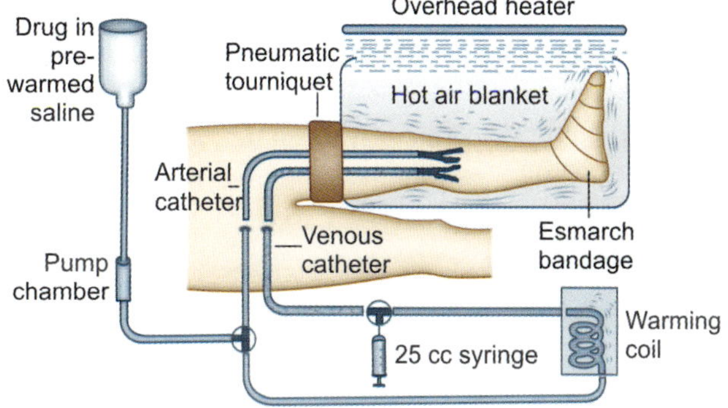

Figure 4 Schematic depiction of ILI circuit
(*Source*: Thompson JF, Kam PC. Isolated limb infusion for melanoma: a simple but effective alternative to isolated limb perfusion. J Surg Oncol. 2004;88(1): 1-3.)

Table 2 Comparison of ILP and ILI techniques for locally advanced melanoma

	ILP	*ILI*
Access of vessels to the extremity	surgical	percutaneous
Need for perfusionist	yes	no
Perfusion/Infusion time	~30 min	~60–90 min
Cost	>	<
Response rates[29] CR OR	 33% 64%	 50.4% 79.4%
Regional toxicity	≈	≈

(**Abbreviations:** CR = complete response; OR = overall response)

Chapter 7

There has been no randomized controlled trial directly comparing ILP to ILI in the treatment of patients with in-transit melanoma. In a retrospective study of 185 patients undergoing ILI at the SMU for locally advanced melanoma (the majority with MD Anderson Stage III disease), the CR and PR rates were 38 and 46% respectively with a median response duration of 13 months, and a median overall survival of 38 months.[28] A multicenter study of a more contemporary cohort of 128 patients treated with ILI for in-transit melanoma in eight US centers identified lower clinical response rates, with CR and PR rates of 31 and 33% respectively.[29] When combined with other clinical experience from Duke University and the SMU data, the CR and PR rates of melanoma patients treated by ILI from this pooled data was 33 and 31% respectively (64% OR rate) compared to CR and PR rates of 50.4 and 29% respectively (79.4% OR rate) for melanoma patients treated by ILP from these same institutions.[29] More severe regional toxicity (Grade III or higher) was similar between treatment modalities in this pooled analysis, although Grade V toxicity (requiring amputation) was lower in the group of patients under ILI (0.3%) versus ILP (2%).[29]

Patient and treatment related factors predictive of response to ILI and outcomes have been evaluated by several studies, and share similarities to those found with ILP. In one recent study of 74 patients undergoing ILI, limb volume greater than 8 L and maximum limb temperature greater than 38.5 were found to be independent predictors of CR; moreover, CR and absence of lymph node metastases were independent predictors of melanoma-specific survival.[30] The multi-center retrospective study actually identified smaller limb volumes along with the use of papaverine (associated with increased toxicity) to be independently associated with improved CR rates.[29] Grades III–IV limb toxicity has been strongly associated with regional response rates in ILI treatment.[31] Independent factors predictive of regional toxicity for ILI identifiable preoperatively or intraoperatively have included female gender, use of the vasodilator papaverine, and higher melphalan concentrations.[32,33] Longer tourniquet time was associated with decreased regional toxicity in ILI in one study, suggesting that perhaps tourniquet times in excess of 30 minutes for ILI may still be safe.[33] Elevated CK levels postoperatively have been associated with increased regional toxicity in ILI, and younger age, unadjusted melphalan dose, and low PO_2 levels at 30 minutes have all been associated with postoperative elevated CK levels by multivariate analysis.

Systemic toxicity, as with ILP, has been reported to be very low with ILI. In patients undergoing ILI at the SMU, melphalan was detected in the systemic circulation in only 6% of patients and typically, at concentrations less than 1% of the administered dose.[32] These low circulating levels of chemotherapeutic are likely in part secondary to the decreased circulation pressures generated through the ILI treatment.

Repeat ILI is technically quite feasible and is considered safe with reasonably favorable clinical outcomes. In a study of 48 patients undergoing repeat ILI, CR rates and OR rates were 23 and 83% respectively, which were not significantly different from response rates after initial ILI (35% and 75%; CR and OR rates respectively). Grade III and higher toxicity was however significantly higher following repeat ILI (42%) compared to after initial ILI (29%), although, it was noted that melphalan concentrations were also significantly higher after repeat ILI compared to after initial ILI. There were no amputations secondary to regional toxicity from repeat ILI. ILI may also be a viable option following regional failure after treatment with ILP.

CONCLUSION

Isolated limb perfusion and the more recently developed ILI remain effective and safe regional limb-sparing treatment approaches for patients with locally advanced extremity melanoma. While ILP and ILI have been performed with melphalan as the main drug of choice, these techniques with limited systemic toxicity, lend themselves to the investigation of other chemotherapeutic agents and targeted therapies, and in fact preclinical studies with temozolomide and systemic O^6-benzylguanine [a suppressor of O^6-alkylguanine DNA alkyltransferase (AGT) activity] have already been reported.[34,35] Recently, the results of a multicenter phase II trial combining melphalan ILI with systemic ADH (a cyclic pentapeptide disrupting N-cadherin) administration were also reported.[36] While regional response rates did not appear to be augmented using this combined therapy, the study offered a novel approach to using a targeted therapy with a regional treatment. With the advent of new systemic therapies for the treatment of metastatic melanoma, further opportunities arise for combining these regional modalities with systemic approaches to potentially impact on disease specific outcome. A clinical trial at Memorial Sloan-Kettering Cancer Center is currently in accrual, studying the use of adjuvant ipilimumab (anti-CTLA4) in the treatment of patients with in-transit melanoma following ILI. Conceptually, while ILP or ILI is regional therapy, it may yield non-regional effect by release or exposure of tumor antigens which can be further modulated by systemic therapies—a paradigm which remains to be further studied.

REFERENCES

1. Surveillance, Epidemiology and End Results Program (www.seer.cancer.gov) Public-Use Data (1975-2007), National Cancer Institute, DCCPS, Surveillance Research Program, Cancer Statistics Branch.
2. Melanoma of the skin. AJCC Staging manual, 7th edition. Springer; 2010. pp. 325.
3. Balch CM, Gershenwald JE, Soong SJ, et al. Final version of 2009 AJCC melanoma staging and classification. J Clin Oncol. 2009;27(36):6199-6206.
4. Pawlik TM, Ross MI, Johnson MM, et al. Predictors and natural history of in-transit melanoma after sentinel lymphadenectomy. Ann Surg Oncol. 2005;12(8):587-96.
5. Veronesi U, Adamus J, Bandiera DC, et al. Inefficacy of immediate node dissection in stage 1 melanoma of the limbs. N Engl J Med. 1977;297(12):627-30.
6. Cascinelli N, Bufalino R, Marolda R, et al. Regional non-nodal metastases of cutaneous melanoma. Eur J Surg Oncol. 1986;12(2):175-80.
7. Borgstein PJ, Meijer S, van Diest PJ. Are locoregional cutaneous metastases in melanoma predictable? Ann Surg Oncol. 1999;6(3):315-21.
8. Creech O Jr, Krementz ET, Ryan RF, et al. Chemotherapy of cancer: regional perfusion utilizing an extracorporeal circuit. Ann Surg. 1958;148(4):616-32.
9. Stehlin JS Jr. Hyperthermic perfusion with chemotherapy for cancers of the extremities. Surg Gynecol Obstet. 1969; 129(2):305-8.
10. Koops HS, Vaglini M, Suciu S, et al. Prophylactic isolated limb perfusion for localized, high-risk limb melanoma: results of a multicenter randomized phase III trial. European Organization for Research and Treatment of Cancer Malignant Melanoma Cooperative Group Protocol 18832, the World Health Organization Melanoma Program Trial 15, and the North American Perfusion Group Southwest Oncology Group-8593. J Clin Oncol. 1998;16(9):2906-12.
11. Moreno-Ramirez D, de la Cruz-Merino L, Ferrandiz L, et al. Isolated limb perfusion for malignant melanoma: systematic review on effectiveness and safety. Oncologist. 2010;15(4):416-27.
12. Cornett WR, McCall LM, Petersen RP, et al. Randomized multicenter trial of hyperthermic isolated limb perfusion with melphalan alone compared with melphalan plus tumor necrosis factor: American College of Surgeons Oncology Group Trial Z0020. J Clin Oncol. 2006;24(25):4196-4201.
13. Alexander HR Jr, Fraker DL, Bartlett DL, et al. Analysis of factors influencing outcome in patients with in-transit malignant melanoma undergoing isolated limb perfusion using modern treatment parameters. J Clin Oncol. 2010;28(1):114-8.
14. Di Filippo F, Giacomini P, Rossi CR, et al. Prognostic factors influencing tumor response, locoregional control and survival, in melanoma patients with multiple limb in-transit metastases treated with TNFalpha-based isolated limb perfusion. In Vivo. 2009;23(2):347-52.
15. Grünhagen DJ, Brunstein F, Graveland WJ, et al. One hundred consecutive isolated limb perfusions with TNF-alpha and melphalan in melanoma patients with multiple in-transit metastases. Ann Surg. 2004;240(6):939-47.
16. Brobeil A, Berman C, Cruse CW, et al. Efficacy of hyperthermic isolated limb perfusion for extremity-confined recurrent melanoma. Ann Surg Oncol. 1998;5(4):376-83.
17. Noorda EM, Vrouenraets BC, Nieweg OE, et al. Safety and efficacy of isolated limb perfusion in elderly melanoma patients. Ann Surg Oncol. 2002;9(10):968-74.
18. Rossi CR, Russano F, Mocellin S, et al. TNF-based isolated limb perfusion followed by consolidation biotherapy with systemic low-dose interferon alpha 2b in patients with in-transit melanoma metastases: a pilot trial. Ann Surg Oncol. 2008; 15(4):1218-23.
19. Wieberdink J, Benckhuysen C, Braat RP, et al. Dosimetry in isolation perfusion of the limbs by assessment of perfused tissue volume and grading of toxic tissue reactions. Eur J Cancer Clin Oncol. 1982;18(10):905-10.
20. Rossi CR, Foletto M, Mocellin S, et al. Hyperthermic isolated limb perfusion with low-dose tumor necrosis factor-alpha and melphalan for bulky in-transit melanoma metastases. Ann Surg Oncol. 2004;11(2):173-7.
21. Noorda EM, Vrouenraets BC, Nieweg OE, et al. Repeat isolated limb perfusion with TNF alpha and melphalan for recurrent limb melanoma after failure of previous perfusion. Eur J Surg Oncol. 2006;32(3):318-24.
22. Vrouenraets BC, Eggermont AM, Klaase JM, et al. Long-term neuropathy after regional isolated perfusion with melphalan for melanoma of the limbs. Eur J Surg Oncol. 1994;20(6):681-5.
23. Vrouenraets BC, Eggermont AM, Hart AA, et al. Regional toxicity after isolated limb perfusion with melphalan and tumour necrosis factor-alpha versus toxicity after melphalan alone. Eur J Surg Oncol. 2001;27(4):390-5.
24. Grünhagen DJ, de Wilt JH, van Geel AN, et al. Isolated limb perfusion for melanoma patients—a review of its indications and the role of tumour necrosis factor-alpha. Eur J Surg Oncol. 2006;32(4):371-80.
25. Vrouenraets BC, Kroon BB, Klaase JM, et al. Value of laboratory tests in monitoring acute regional toxicity after isolated limb perfusion. Ann Surg Oncol. 1997;4(1):88-94.
26. Thompson JF. Isolated limb infusion with melphalan for recurrent limb melanoma: a simple alternative to limb perfusion. Reg Cancer Treat. 1994;7:188-92.
27. Thompson JF, Kam PC, Waugh RC, et al. Isolated limb infusion with cytotoxic agents: a simple alternative to isolated limb perfusion. Semin Surg Oncol. 1998;14(3):238-47.
28. Kroon HM, Moncrieff M, Kam PC, et al. Outcomes following isolated limb infusion for melanoma. A 14-year experience. Ann Surg Oncol. 2008;15(11):3003-13.
29. Beasley GM, Caudle A, Petersen RP, et al. A multi-institutional experience of isolated limb infusion: defining response and toxicity in the US. J Am Coll Surg. 2009;208(5):706-15.

30. Barbour AP, Thomas J, Suffolk J, et al. Isolated limb infusion for malignant melanoma: predictors of response and outcome. Ann Surg Oncol. 2009;16(12):3463-72.
31. Kroon HM, Thompson JF. Isolated limb infusion: a review. J Surg Oncol. 2009;100(2):169-77.
32. Santillan AA, Delman KA, Beasley GM, et al. Predictive factors of regional toxicity and serum creatine phosphokinase levels after isolated limb infusion for melanoma: a multi-institutional analysis. Ann Surg Oncol. 2009;16(9):2570-8.
33. Kroon HM, Moncrieff M, Kam PC, et al. Factors predictive of acute regional toxicity after isolated limb infusion with melphalan and actinomycin D in melanoma patients. Ann Surg Oncol. 2009;16(5):1184-92.
34. Ueno T, Ko SH, Grubbs E, et al. Modulation of chemotherapy resistance in regional therapy: a novel therapeutic approach to advanced extremity melanoma using intra-arterial temozolomide in combination with systemic O^6-benzylguanine. Mol Cancer Ther. 2006;5(3):732-8.
35. Yoshimoto Y, Augustine CK, Yoo JS, et al. Defining regional infusion treatment strategies for extremity melanoma: comparative analysis of melphalan and temozolomide as regional chemotherapeutic agents. Mol Cancer Ther. 2007;6(5):1492-500.
36. Beasley GM, Riboh JC, Augustine CK, et al. Prospective multicenter phase II trial of systemic ADH-1 in combination with melphalan via isolated limb infusion in patients with advanced extremity melanoma. J Clin Oncol. 2011;29(9): 1210-5.

8

Isolated Limb Perfusion for Extremity Sarcoma

Tim Pencavel, Andrew Hayes

INTRODUCTION

Soft-tissue sarcomas are rare tumors arising from the embryonic mesoderm.[1] There are approximately 8,680 new sarcomas diagnosed per year in the United States, of which 46% are expected to be in the lower extremity and 14% in the upper limb.[2] The primary treatment modality for any sarcoma is resectional surgery. Formerly, standard therapy for extremity sarcoma was amputation. However, a randomized study showed that amputation confers no survival benefit over resection with radiotherapy at the expense of considerable morbidity.[3] Consequently, the aim of management now is the preservation of limb function whilst ensuring adequate resection of tumors with a margin of normal tissue. Standard treatment is therefore still to attempt resection if at all feasible, followed by postoperative radiotherapy. Estimates of the proportion of patients requiring amputation in the modern era are in the range of 3–5%.[4]

Regional chemotherapy for sarcoma is indicated in the small proportion of patients in whom an extremity sarcoma is not treatable by function-preserving wide surgical resection, where the only operation that is considered technically possible is an amputation. In this chapter, we review the history of this procedure, technical aspects of limb perfusion and outcomes under differing clinical scenarios. We will also discuss the importance of tumor necrosis factor alpha (TNFα) for sarcoma limb perfusions and also future directions for possible new therapeutic agents.

HISTORY OF ISOLATED LIMB PERFUSION

Isolated limb perfusion (ILP) was first described in human malignancy by Oscar Creech and colleagues at the Tulane University School of Medicine, New Orleans, in 1958.[5] In common with many oncologists of the time, Creech was frustrated by the limitations imposed on the use of the new generation of alkylating agents just because of their severe systemic toxicities. These derivatives of mustard gas had begun to be integrated into clinical practice in the preceding 15 years, and in 1954, Bergel, Stock and Haddow, working at the Institute of Cancer Research, had synthesized melphalan (phenylalanine mustard), the compound Creech chose for use in his ILP studies.[6] The hypothesis was simple; if the tumors could be isolated for the duration of treatment, a higher effective dose of the agent could be administered and, therefore, better response rates gained. After what, by today's standards, was a remarkably short preclinical study in dogs, Creech began his treatment of 24 human subjects with malignancies including malignant melanoma, a variety of pathological subtypes of sarcoma and carcinomas. The lesions were variously present in the limbs, lungs and pelvises of his patients. The perfusions were almost universally undertaken in the palliative setting, and perhaps because of this the defined endpoint was technical success of perfusion rather than tumor response. From this standpoint, the treatment was a resounding triumph; only one of the 24 patients had a technical- or procedure-related failure, in a patient perfused through the aorta and vena cava with a high dose of melphalan who succumbed

15 days postoperatively to the complications of severe bone marrow suppression. Indeed, in the 19 patients who survived to meaningful follow-up, 18 responses were seen in the tumors.

Creech's technique was hailed as a breakthrough as researchers rushed to use it on their own patients. When the work was presented at the American Surgical Association in New York, the comments hinted at this interest, with a question on the applicability of the new technique to liver metastases and also a description of a similar system for use in leukemic patients (Dr. Cooley described a system wherein the perfusate reservoir was housed within a Van Graaf electron generator and blood irradiated prior to being returned to the patient).

TECHNICAL ASPECTS OF ISOLATED LIMB PERFUSION

In summary, ILP involves isolation of the limb from the systemic circulation using operative cannulation of the afferent and efferent vessels to the limb. The limb is then perfused with a low-pressure, high-flow, hyperthermic, oxygenated circuit through which the chemotherapeutic agents are delivered (Fig. 1). The limb is warmed to above physiological temperature to enhance the action of the chemotherapeutic agent. For sarcoma, continuous leak monitoring is performed to ensure that any possible leak of drug (particularly TNFα) from the limb to the systemic circulation is identified promptly. After 1 hour's perfusion, the circuit is washed-out with saline and the cannulae withdrawn before vascular repair is performed, and the limb is returned to the systemic circulation.

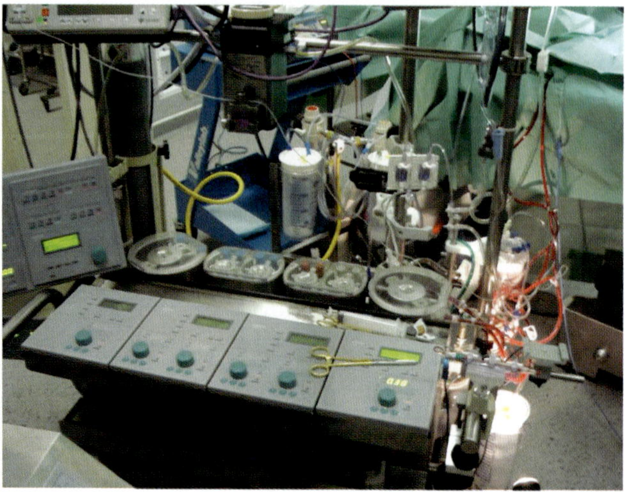

Figure 1 Extracorporeal bypass machine, primed for isolated limb perfusion

Surgical Technique

Isolated limb perfusion can be performed in the upper limb or lower limb at any site in which it is possible to cannulate the supplying vasculature and isolate the limb from the systemic circulation.[7] The majority of perfusions are for lower limb disease, in which cannulation can be at the level of the superficial femoral vessels at the end of Hunter's canal or the external iliac vessels. Upper limb perfusion is via the axillary or brachial vessels. The choice between the sites of perfusion varies according to the site of the primary tumor. For sarcoma, the superficial femoral approach is reserved predominantly for patients with tumors below the distal thigh. For mid and upper thigh tumors, an iliac approach is necessary to ensure inclusion of the whole tumor in the perfusion field. Once the vessels are cannulated, the patient is anticoagulated with a systemic dose of 5,000 IU heparin. Isolation from the systemic circulation is achieved using a tourniquet, either a pneumatic tourniquet inflated to 100 mm Hg above systolic blood pressure in femoral/brachial perfusions or an Esmarch bandage anchored using a Steinmann pin to the iliac crest or scapula for the proximal sites. The higher leak rate seen with iliac perfusions is because of two factors. First the Esmarch bandage, which is necessary for very large tumors impinging close to the inguinal ligament, is less effective than a pneumatic tourniquet, and second, there are many more collateral veins around the hip joint and pelvis that cannot be controlled surgically via the iliac incision.

The vessels are dissected free and cannulated through a small anterior incision on the vessels using appropriately sized standard cardiovascular silastic cannulae. For the duration of the perfusion, they are held in place by vascular 'snuggers', lengths of nylon tape which are able to hold the cannulae without traumatizing the vessel (Figs 2A and B).

For an iliac perfusion cannulation of the iliac vessels mandates an iliac lymph node dissection in order to achieve adequate exposure. At the end of the required perfusion time, usually 60 minutes, a 15-minute washout is performed until the perfusate is clear to remove excess TNFα. The cannulae are withdrawn and the vessels repaired using an appropriate vascular suture. Once adequate hemostasis and distal vessel flow are ensured, the wound can be closed in a standard manner.

Section 3

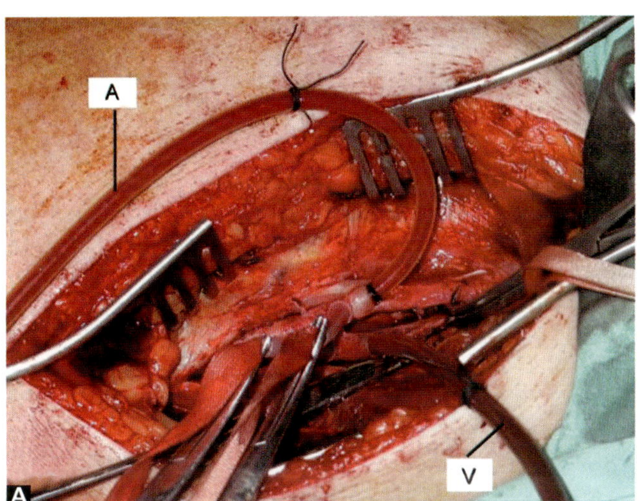

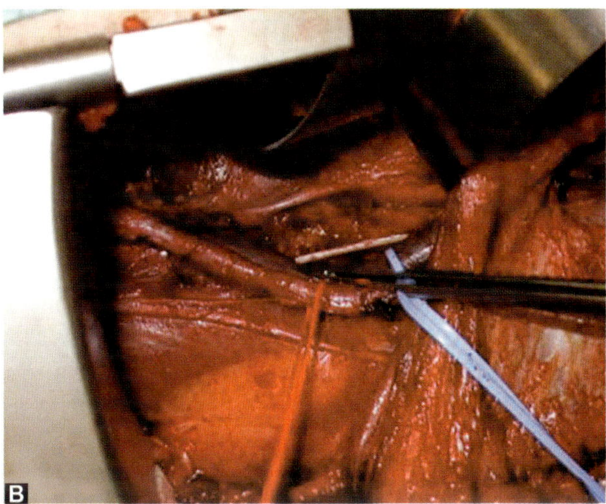

Figures 2A and B (A) Cannulation of the superficial femoral vessels, showing arterial (A) and venous (V) cannulae in position. (B) Exposed external iliac vessels prior to cannulation, showing dissection proximal to the inguinal ligament, artery (red sling) and vein (blue sling). The obturator nerve is visible at the base of dissection

Chemotherapeutic Agents Used in Isolated Limb Perfusion for Sarcoma

Melphalan

Early perfusions were performed with 2–3 mg/kg body weight melphalan.[8] However, this is a relatively high dose of melphalan and, therefore, dose reduction has occurred steadily to the current doses of 1 mg/kg used in modern perfusion. This dose avoids many of the bone marrow side effects and is generally well tolerated.[9] Perhaps the most critical factor in the reduction of dose has been the introduction of TNFα to perfusion regimens, at a dose of 1 mg for upper limb and 2 mg for lower limb perfusions.

Tumor Necrosis Factor Alpha

The strongest indication for the use of TNFα in ILP is for sarcoma. This is because the response rate for melphalan alone perfusion in sarcoma is significantly lower than that for TNFα/melphalan perfusion regimens.[7,10,11] The mechanism underlying this improvement is the effect of TNFα on the tumor vasculature, which increases the amount of cytotoxic agent within the tumor.[7,11-13] The net effect is a synergistic interaction between TNFα and melphalan, despite TNFα having minimal cytotoxicity as a single agent *in vitro*.[13] In malignant melanoma, similar results are seen with bulky, 'sarcoma-like' in-transit deposits, but the effect on smaller volume disease may not be as pronounced.[14,15]

TNFα is a vasoactive cytokine first identified in the mid 1970s as an agent produced in the serum of mice infected with the BCG strain of tuberculosis.[16] When the serum of these animals was purified and reinjected into animals bearing melanoma xenografts, spontaneous regression of the tumors occurred.[17] The name 'Tumor Necrosis Factor' is itself somewhat of a misnomer, as in many tumor lines, including melanoma, TNFα acts at a molecular level as a prosurvival factor for cells exposed to cytotoxic agents.[18] Furthermore, its role in activating immune responses, such as occur in the systemic inflammatory response syndrome (SIRS), is of far greater significance clinically.[19] In ILP, its immunological and molecular effects are sidelined by the reaction it provokes in tumor-associated vasculature. TNFα causes the immature vascular endothelium within the vessels to dilate, and the intracellular gaps to widen, effectively making the tumor vasculature many times more permeable to chemotherapeutic agents (similar to the vascular response in SIRS, which is of the same etiology).[13] The secondary effect, some 12–24 hours after perfusion, is to cause a localized coagulation of the vessels, rendering regions of the tumor ischemic and promoting the 'lock-in' of melphalan.[7]

The levels of TNFα necessary to produce a significant antitumor effect *in vivo* cannot be administered systemically without some form of targeting due to its deleterious side effects.[20] In the 1980s, Lejeune and colleagues recognized that the administration of sufficiently high levels of TNFα to tumors was possible using the isolation-perfusion system and began to incorporate TNFα into clinical perfusion systems.[21] Initially, on the basis of preclinical studies, administration was combined with interferon-gamma (IFNγ), which had shown synergy with TNFα due to the upregulation of TNF receptors and induction of apoptosis on vascular endothelial cells. However, an open-label Phase 2 study designed to compare perfusion with and without IFNγ showed a small but insignificant advantage to its inclusion that did not warrant ongoing use of IFNγ, given the greater rate of side effects.[22] The same study also showed a significant increase in total response rate (defined as partial response rates + complete response rates) for the use of TNFα in perfusion compared with historical melphalan alone controls.

Other Cytotoxic Agents

The newer systemic anti-sarcoma agents, such as doxorubicin (DXR), have also been trialed in ILP. Wray and colleagues have recently reported the results of two trials of ILP, one with TNFα and melphalan and one with DXR alone.[23] The DXR study showed only two minor responses, with no complete responses. However, it is worth noting that, in this trial, TNFα was not administered with the DXR. Rossi and colleagues, in their series of 2005, report one complete clinical response and a further four complete histological responses out of 21 patients.[24] In van der Veen and colleagues' animal study, DXR was poorly active as a single agent.[12] Combination with TNFα resulted in increased concentrations of DXR in tumor tissue (2–3 fold increases), which they felt explained the synergistic results of the combination therapy. This experience adds to the growing evidence that TNFα is a vital part of ILP for sarcoma, which is further bolstered by the reports of increase tumor response rates when cytotoxic alone perfusion is compared to cytotoxic perfusion and TNFα perfusion. The dose of TNFα required has also been steadily reduced as efficacy is maintained to a dose of 0.5–1 mg.[25,26] Such a reduction results in a decrease in systemic side effects.

Leakage Monitoring

Creech's early experiments delineated leak 'after the fact', by adding Evans blue to the perfusion circuit and examining the systemic circulation for the dye. Addition of TNFα mandates real-time leak monitoring because the systemic side effects of the cytokine are potentially fatal. In practical terms, this function is achieved by the use of radioisotopes. A dose of a gamma-emitting isotope, usually ^{99m}Tc-labelled human albumin, is administered systemically and radioactivity recorded using a scintillation counter placed precordially (Fig. 3).

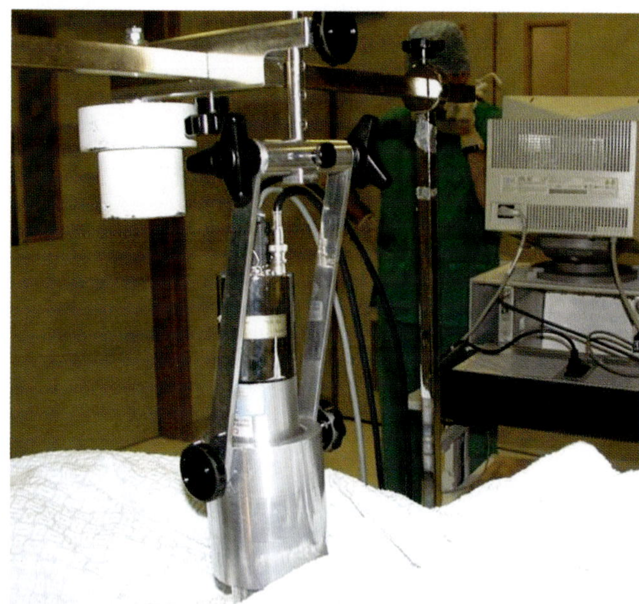

Figure 3 The scintillation counter in position over the precordium of a patient undergoing isolated limb perfusion

A ten-fold higher dose of the same isotope is administered to the perfusion circuit. TNFα is not administered until the absence of leak is confirmed, and monitoring continues throughout bypass, terminating 20 minutes after the end of the washout period. A leak is therefore present, when the level of radiation detected precordially, is above the baseline level recorded in the time preceding bypass. Generally, leak rates of up to 10% are tolerable,[27] but, above this level, action must be taken either to halt the leak or abandon the procedure. It is rare that TNFα leak above this level occurs, partly because, it is not administered if a leak is noted on radioisotope monitoring, but also because a significant leak is accompanied by an almost instantaneous drop in the oxygenation vessel fluid level. In practice, the perfusionist is often aware of a leak a few seconds before it is confirmed by the radiation trace due to a drop in perfusate reservoir level. Figures 4A and B show intraoperative traces from two patients, one of whom developed a leak unexpectedly mid-perfusion.

Hyperthermia

The use of hyperthermia may influence the response rates to perfusion.[28] Hyperthermia in the experimental and clinical settings has been shown to increase the efficacy of melphalan, as well as providing another potentially vasodilatory stimulus to increase tumor uptake of cytotoxic agents.[29] In clinical perfusion, the aim is to achieve hyperthermia of 39°C. Temperature is monitored using

Section 3

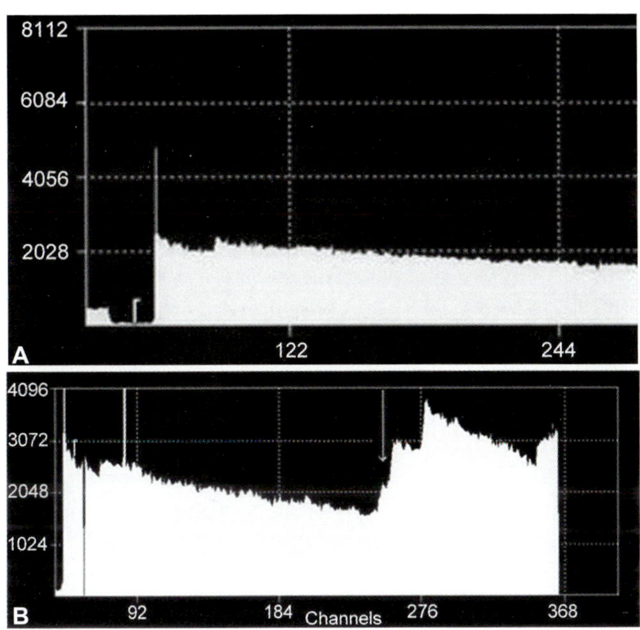

Figures 4A and B Intraoperative radioisotope leak monitoring traces for two patients. (A) A normal trace, with no intraoperative leak. (B) A trace showing the development of a major mid-perfusion circuit-to-systemic leak. The perfusion was immediately terminated and washout commenced

needle thermistors embedded in the musculature of the limb. In practice, temperatures much above 38.5°C are difficult to achieve and rarely employed. Hyperthermia above 40°C significantly increases the procedure related morbidity and is therefore not advisable.[30] Hyperthermia is achieved by warming of the perfusion circuit, keeping the patient and operating room temperatures as high as possible, and the use of extracorporeal heating devices on the limb such as forced warm air heating blankets.

ISOLATED LIMB PERFUSION IN CLINICAL PRACTICE FOR SARCOMA

Currently, there are two major indications for the use of ILP in patients with sarcoma.

1. As a regional chemotherapy for advanced irresectable sarcoma with the aim of avoiding an amputation.[31] Under these circumstances no further surgery on the tumor is undertaken unless the tumor progresses, when an amputation may be necessary. Such tumors often lie in the distal extremity.
2. As induction chemotherapy for a very large tumor that may be considered irresectable in an oncological sense because of its size or juxtaposition to vital neurovascular structures. Such tumors often lie in the proximal extremity. Under these circumstances the aim is to downsize the tumor to allow a subsequent marginal resection at 4–6 weeks after the perfusion.[32]

In many ways, these two indications are very different. The first is essentially a procedure to palliate a tumor that is only treatable by an amputation in the attempt to avoid that procedure. The second is an induction treatment followed by a surgical resection that is a definitive curative approach to a very large, surgically challenging tumor. Many of the series of ILP for sarcoma include patients who undergo the ILP for both of these indications. In the following sections, we will attempt to define the indications and outcomes for both indications, accepting the limitations of the existing data.

Indication 1: ILP and No Subsequent Surgery

Sarcomas can be considered irresectable for a number of reasons including multifocality, spread across compartments or complete encasement of critical structures (particularly nerves). An example is shown in Figures 5A and B, which show an MRI scan and clinical photograph of a large sarcoma arising in the foot that is irresectable because of the extent of involvement of the structures of the foot. The only alternative to an ILP, in this case, was amputation, but the patient was not keen to undergo amputation because of the effect on his quality of life. His prognosis was limited by the presence of synchronous pulmonary metastases.

Figure 6 shows an angiosarcoma arising in the limb in the context of Stewart-Treves syndrome. The tumor was multifocal and had progressed through systemic chemotherapy. The extent of the lymphedema lay above the level of a hindquarter amputation. As can be seen, the patient had a complete response to ILP in the primary tumor and thus was able to keep the limb with excellent local control.

As well as multifocality and locally advanced distal disease, tumors which would require a transcompartmental resection (and therefore significant postoperative functional deficit) and tumors which require excision that would leave large, problematic soft-tissue defects are suitable for palliative ILP. This is especially true in the context of poor-prognosis (high-grade or very large) tumors, concomitant metastatic disease, or the very elderly, in whom amputation carries a significant risk of inhospital mortality or prolonged rehabilitation.

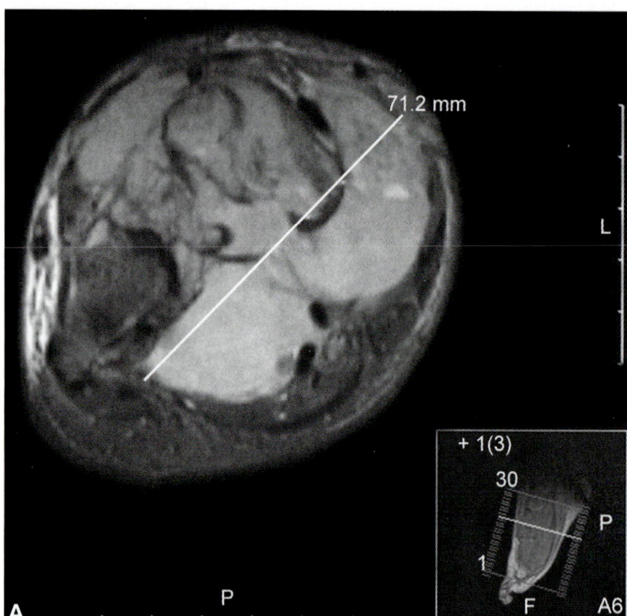

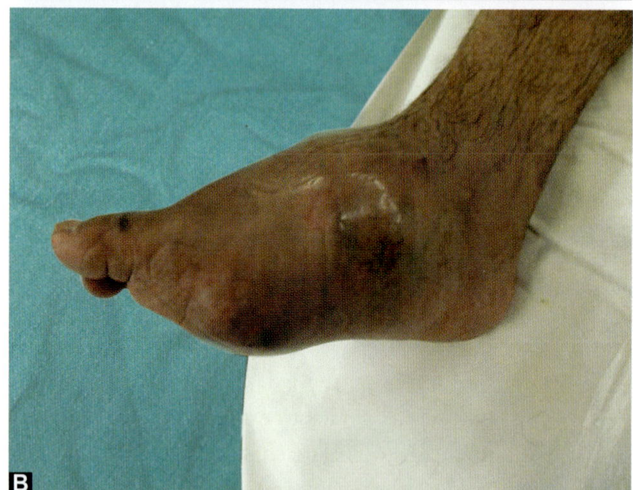

Figures 5A and B An advanced foot sarcoma, treated by isolated limb perfusion

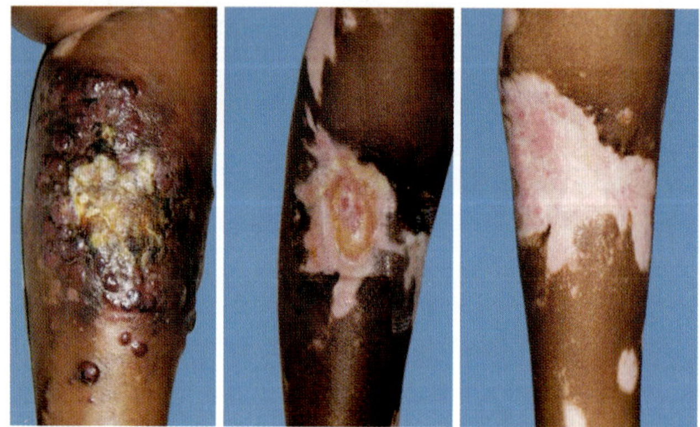

Figure 6 Sequential clinical images of an angiosarcoma, which responded to tumor necrosis factor/melphalan isolated limb perfusion, from presentation to complete response at 12 months

Indication 2: Induction Chemotherapy Prior to an Intended Marginal Excision

There are a large number of series from mainland Europe in which a significant proportion of patients underwent ILP as induction chemotherapy with the aim of down-sizing the tumor to allow a subsequent marginal resection. These tumors were considered irresectable because either their size meant that a resection with a sufficient margin of normal tissue surrounding the tumor was impossible, or because of proximity to neurovascular structures.[32-34] In recent years, this definition has become more relaxed and includes tumors where resection is considered challenging. Post-ILP resection entails a marginal excision,[32] and normally occurs between 4 weeks and 24 weeks post-ILP, depending on the clinical response of the lesion.

Eggermont and colleagues multicentre European trial of 186 patients with advanced extremity sarcoma[32] included 143 patients who had a single large tumor (median size 16 cm) that was considered irresectable by a panel of sarcoma surgeons. Most of the large sarcomas were rendered resectable due to a major response to ILP (82%).

The definition of irresectable in this series was that 'local wide resections (margins of 2–4 cm of normal tissue) were not possible.' However, particularly in the thigh, large tumors may be excised, and patients given postoperative radiotherapy. This may involve resection of encased vascular structures and reconstruction (Figs 7A to C) or resection along a single positive margin, predicted by the extent of the tumor on preoperative imaging investigations. The latter strategy does not appear to worsen local control rates.[35] In our own series of 150 patients with large proximal tumors (median size 17 cm), excision followed by postoperative radiotherapy achieved a 10% local recurrence rate (Fig. 8) and an overall limb salvage rate of 98%. The majority (62%) of patients in the series had grade 2 or 3 lesions. Tumor biology (assessed by tumor grade and pathological subtype) was the significant predictor of outcome in this group.

Hence for large sarcomas, particular in the thigh or upper arm, there are two potential treatment strategies. The first is the more standard approach of attempting a radical resection but accepting focally close margins of certain irresectable structures (e.g. major nerves), with vascular and soft tissue reconstruction if necessary. The second is to employ an ILP as induction chemotherapy and then marginally excise or 'shell out', the tumor remnant, relying upon the success of the ILP to allow such a procedure.

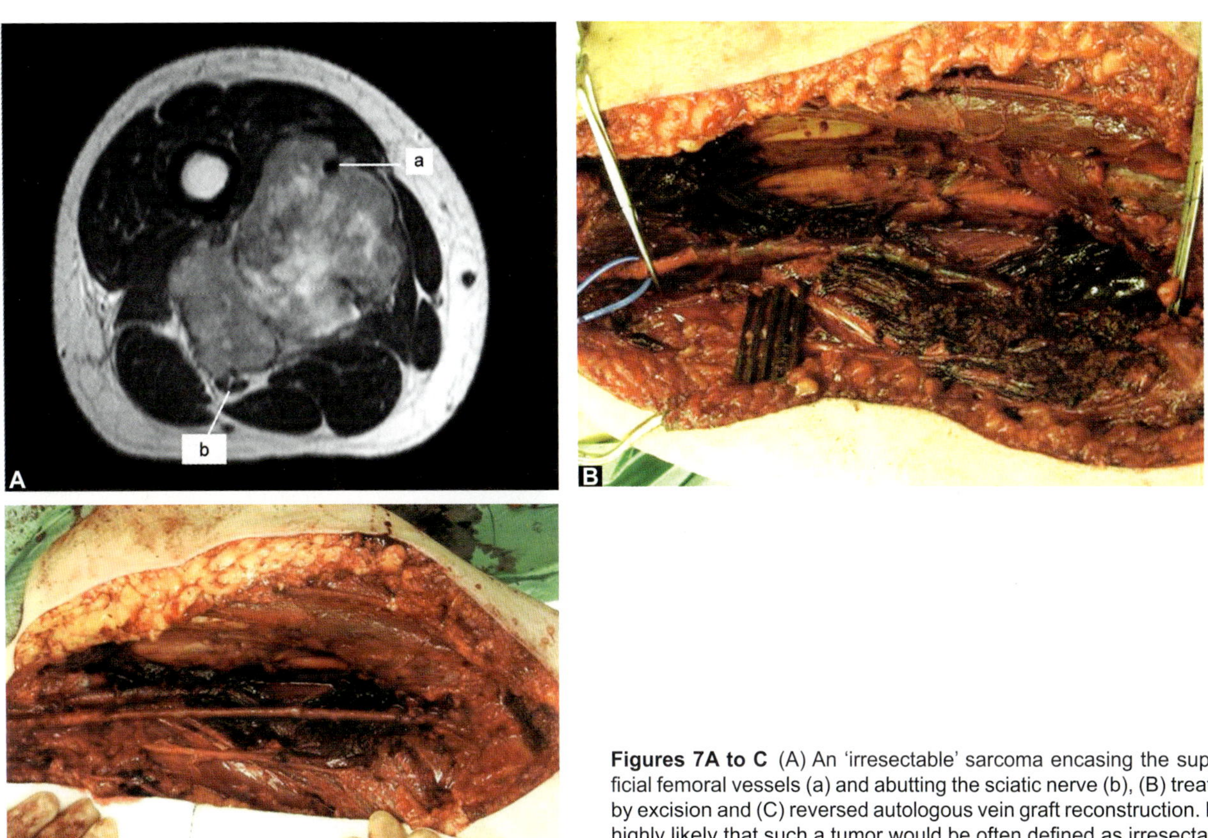

Figures 7A to C (A) An 'irresectable' sarcoma encasing the superficial femoral vessels (a) and abutting the sciatic nerve (b), (B) treated by excision and (C) reversed autologous vein graft reconstruction. It is highly likely that such a tumor would be often defined as irresectable by a surgeon and under such circumstances an isolated limb perfusion and a subsequent marginal resection might be employed as an alternative treatment strategy

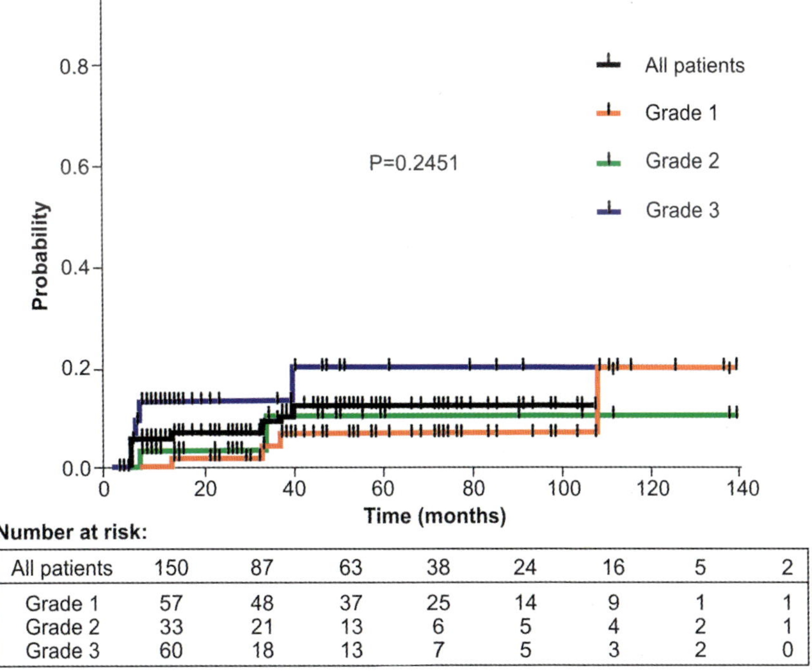

Number at risk:

All patients	150	87	63	38	24	16	5	2
Grade 1	57	48	37	25	14	9	1	1
Grade 2	33	21	13	6	5	4	2	1
Grade 3	60	18	13	7	5	3	2	0

Crude cumulative incidence of local recurrence

Figure 8 Crude cumulative incidence curve for local recurrence in a series of 150 patients with large, proximal extremity sarcomas treated by excision and postoperative radiotherapy

Table 1 Regimen, response rates and response assessment method for published series of isolated limb perfusion in sarcoma

Series (year)	Regimen	Number of ILP	CR	PR	NC/PD	Response assessment	Limb salvage rate
Hill (1993)[36]	TNF + Melphalan	9	100%	0%	0%	Clinical	64%
Santinami (1996)[37]	TNF + Melphalan	10	70%	20%	10%	Clinical	89%
Eggermont (1999)[33]	TNF + Melphalan	196	17%	48%	35%	Clinical	71%, R
Lejeune (2000)[34]	TNF ± IFN + Melphalan	22	18%	64%	18%	Clinical	77%, R
Hohenberger (2001)[38]	TNF ± IFN + Melphalan	55	NR	NR	NR	Clinical	84%, R
Bonvalot (2005)[*,25]	TNF + Melphalan	72	35%	22%	43%	Clinical	84%, R
Van Ginkel (2007)[39]	TNF ± IFN + Melphalan	73	25%	69%	6%	Clinical	61%, R
Pennachioli (2007)[40]	TNF + Doxorubicin/TNF + Melphalan	51	41%	55%	4%	Clinical	82%
Hayes (2007)[41]	TNF + Melphalan	15	20%	33%	47%	Clinical	73%
Cherix (2008)[42]	TNF + Melphalan	57	25%	42%	28%	Clinical	76%, R
Wray (2011)[23]	TNF + Melphalan	17	12%	58%	30%	Clinical	41%
	Doxorubicin	12	0%	0%	100%	Clinical	66%[†]
Eggermont (1996)[43]	TNF + IFN + Melphalan	55	36%	51%	13%	Pathological	84%, R
Eggermont (1996)[32]	TNF ± IFN + Melphalan	246	28%	48%	24%	Pathological	76%, R
Rossi (1999)[44]	TNF + Doxorubicin	20	26%	64%	10%	Pathological	85%, R
Grunhagen (2005)[*,45]	TNF ± IFN + Melphalan	48	38%	31%	29%	Pathological	85%
Grunhagen (2006)[46]	TNF ± IFN + Melphalan	217	18%	51%	31%	Pathological	75%
Nachmany (2009)[*,26]	TNF + Melphalan - HD	26	22%	44%	34%	Pathological	76%, R
	TNF + Melphalan - LD	17	8%	23%	69%	Pathological	53%, R
Grabellus (2011)[47]	TNF + Melphalan	53	17%	83%	0%	Pathological	89%, R
Deroose (2011)[48]	TNF + Melphalan	122	4%	66%	30%	Pathological	89%, R
Noorda (2003)[49]	TNF ± IFN + Melphalan	49	8%	55%	37%	Combined	58%, R
Rossi (2005)[24]	TNF + Doxorubicin	21	5%	57%	38%	Combined	71%, R
Totals/Averages	**All patients**	**1,463**	**26%**	**45%**	**29%**	–	**75%**
	TNF + Melphalan	**1,359**	**28%**	**45%**	**27%**	–	**74%**

[*] TNFα dose reduction studies
[†] Only three patients alive at end of follow-up
Abbreviations: IFN, interferon; ILP, isolated limb perfusion; LD, low dose; NC, no change; PD, progressive disease; PR, partial response; R, also underwent postperfusion resection where possible; TNF, tumor necrosis factor; NR, not reported; CR, complete response; HD, high dose

In the next section we will try to quantify response rates for these two separate indications.

RESPONSE RATES TO ISOLATED LIMB PERFUSION FOR SARCOMA

The response rate to ILP from the major published series are summarized in Table 1. As noted above, many of these series include patients who underwent ILP for indication 1 (ILP alone) and indication 2 (ILP as induction chemotherapy then resection) and accordingly it is difficult to dissect out the response rates and durations of response for these two different indications. Furthermore, the means of assessment of response differs from series to series. Some series used purely radiological and clinical criteria to assess response, even if the patients underwent a resection. Others used the extent of necrosis in the histopathological specimen to assess response, (with 50% or more necrosis qualifying as partial response and > 99% qualifying as a complete response). Two series used both criteria. Despite these difficulties, we will attempt to define response rates for these two separate indications.

Response Rates and Outcome after Isolated Limb Perfusion as Sole Treatment for Irresectable Sarcoma

Response rates to systemic chemotherapy for extremity sarcoma range from 10 to 30%, depending on the type of regimen used,[50] and does not carry a benefit in terms of the time to development of distant metastatic disease.[51] Therefore, an ILP for palliative reasons, which would not be expected to affect time to distant progression, can be justified by its higher response rates.

In our series of ILP for extremity sarcoma,[41] all of which were performed in the setting of advanced, poor-prognosis disease, the response rate was 53% (20% CR, 33% PR). This level of response is clearly superior to that offered by systemic therapy. However, 71% of patients went on to develop local disease progression at a median time of 5 months, and 30% proceeded to amputation. Similarly, Lev-Chelouche and colleagues reported a small series of 13 patients with multifocal, recurrent tumors treated by ILP with the aim of palliation.[52] They report a 92% response rate (38% CR, 54% PR), and a 23% amputation rate. The median time to local recurrence was 9 months, and death occurred for all patients between 4 months and 35 months postperfusion.

For reasons already alluded to, establishing comparable data for other studies is complex. In the large European multicentre trial,[32] 23% of patients had multiple extremity tumors, and 13% presented with metastatic disease at the time of ILP. In the group of patients who already had distant meta-stases, the limb salvage rate was 92 and 80% died at a median time of 9 months. Seventeen percent (31/186) patients underwent amputation for nonresponse to the ILP or local recurrence.

In summary, ILP for the primary palliative treatment of soft-tissue sarcoma, with no intended resection, is a useful strategy with significantly improved response rates over systemic therapy. However, although there are some patients with significant and prolonged responses, in the majority of cases time to local relapse is less than 9 months, and amputation rates of the order of 20–30%. Should patients progress locally without developing further distant disease, the options are repeat ILP or amputation.

Response Rates and Outcome after Isolated Limb Perfusion as Induction Chemotherapy Followed by Resection

The majority of European series on ILP present overall limb salvage rates based on using ILP as a neoadjuvant strategy to allow resection (Table 1, indicated by 'R' next to limb salvage rate). The aim of further surgery after ILP is to provide improved local control rates above those achieved by ILP. Patients who have achieved more than 50% tumor necrosis post-ILP have a better prognosis than those in whom lower rates of necrosis are achieved. As with ILP alone, however, resectional surgery post-ILP is intended for local tumor control and does not confer an overall survival advantage, due to the risk of distant disease progression.

Eggermont and colleague's multicentre European trial of 186 patients with advanced extremity sarcoma[32] included 143 patients who had a single large tumor (median size 16 cm) that was considered irresectable by a panel of sarcoma surgeons. Fourteen of these patients subsequently developed local recurrence between 3 months and 24 months after resection, an overall local recurrence rate of 11%. It is also of note that, of the total series, 60/186 (32%) could not undergo further resection, because of multiple tumors (likely to be included under indication 1, above), the development of systemic metastases or the refusal of an amputation. Of this group, 45% developed local recurrence. Taking these latter two findings together suggests that ILP followed by resection is useful in patients who exhibit a good response to the perfusion, but in patients in whom resection cannot be undertaken subsequently, it exposes the patient to the morbidity of an ILP without necessarily resulting in limb salvage or durable local control. The authors do not suggest a mechanism for predicting patients likely to respond preoperatively, and it could be argued that the group without systemic metastases at presentation who could not undergo subsequent resection would be better served by a curative amputation rather than attempted limb salvage by ILP. As discussed above, in our study of patients with large proximal tumors, resection followed by postoperative radiotherapy resulted in identical rates of local recurrence.

In conclusion, therefore, induction ILP followed by resection is a good treatment, with excellent local control rates. However, the implication for the patient is that they will undergo two operations to obtain local control. If local control rates for large tumors are similar whether the treatment is by ILP and resection or resection followed by radiotherapy, a single operation may be the preferred option. A randomized controlled trial would be the best method of establishing this equivalency. However, given the similarity of patient selection and outcome between our series and the multicentre European series, such a trial would be logistically complex to recruit the large number of patients needed to demonstrate a clear difference, and is unlikely to be done.

SIDE EFFECTS AND TOLERABILITY

Isolated limb perfusion with TNFα and melphalan carries associated risks of both systemic [bone marrow suppression (melphalan); SIRS (TNFα)] and local effects (skin reaction, necrosis, limb ischemia). The local effects are classified according to the suggested schema

Table 2 Grades of local toxicity of isolated limb perfusion

Wieberdink grade	Interpretation
Grade 1	No reaction
Grade 2	Slight erythema/edema
Grade 3	Considerable erythema/edema with blistering
Grade 4	Extensive epidermiolysis or deep tissue damage with functional deficit +/- threatened/incipient compartment syndrome
Grade 5	Reaction necessitating amputation

of Wieberdink and colleagues[53] summarized in Table 2. In general, however, ILP is a well-tolerated treatment modality, with quoted Wieberdink grade III/IV toxicity rates of around 25%.

Despite the potentially severe consequences of leakage of both TNFα and melphalan, ILP is extremely well tolerated. Stam and colleagues reviewed their own series of 10 patients with an average systemic leak rate of 23.9%, and found that, despite an increase in circulating levels of various proinflammatory cytokines (specifically, TNFα and interleukins-6 and -8), the majority of complications observed were WHO grade 0–II.[27] A total of nine grade III/IV toxicities were seen; two patients who developed lymphopenia (one with concomitant thrombocytopenia) due to melphalan leakage, four patients with hyperbilirubinemia and four patients with hypotension requiring inotropic (dopamine) support. However, all patients exhibited signs of a systemic inflammatory response, with fever and nausea the predominant features. A functioning tourniquet and active, real-time leak monitoring is therefore mandatory for all perfusions with TNFα, and a leak must be treated promptly by cessation of the perfusion, immediate washout and involvement of critical care facilities.

The treatment of a TNFα leak is supportive. Even the most severe post-ILP SIRS-type reactions tend to be self-limiting, and treatment is predominantly aimed at correcting hypotension and coagulopathy. Anti-TNFα antibodies, such as infliximab, are not currently recommended for use in the acute phase. In the majority of patients with significant leak of TNFα systemically, intravenous fluid administration was sufficient; in the Rotterdam paper, such patients required 8 liters in the first 16 hours postprocedure as opposed to the 5 liters required routinely in non-leakage ILP. Pulmonary and nephrological sequelae are rare.

TNFα may also increase local toxicity of ILP. In a multivariate analysis evaluating local toxicity after ILP with and without TNFα, Vrouenraets and colleagues found sex, ILP schedule and ILP duration to be the most significant factors in local toxicity.[30] However, the authors suggest that other factors, particularly higher temperatures during TNFα-Melphalan perfusions, may have contributed to this finding. Furthermore, more recent prospective dose-reduction studies have not found a correlation between the dose of TNFα used and the severity or frequency of local tissue toxicity as might be expected if TNFα was the sole agent responsible for the increased toxicity observed after TNFα-based ILP.[25,26]

Further evidence that ILP is well-tolerated can be drawn from a study evaluating the palliative use of ILP, admittedly in melanoma patients.[31] In this study, patients who had undergone ILP reported better health-related quality of life, as assessed by the short-form-36 questionnaire, than healthy control subjects. This was despite the finding that many patients reported chronic symptoms within the limb. Therefore, although local toxicity is more common than systemic toxicity, its effects tend to be short-lived and, even if present in the longer term, sufficiently manageable as to not have a deleterious effect on the patient.

TREATMENT AFTER ISOLATED LIMB PERFUSION

Further Treatment to the Primary Tumor

One area of controversy that has arisen is whether post-ILP and resection, particularly for patients with R1 resections, further radiotherapy should be administered. Evaluation of patients with R0 resections has suggested that there is no additional benefit in such patients to radiotherapy.[48] In an accompanying editorial, Bonvalot and Gronchi point out that a study of ILP +/- resection +/- radiotherapy is unlikely ever to be done.[54] Therefore, current treatment strategies vary. Intuitively, many sarcoma surgeons would feel that a marginal resection of a primary lesion should be followed by radiotherapy to enhance local control; however, it may be that large, poor-prognosis lesions, which are generally treated by ILP, have such unfavorable tumor biology that the development of distant metastatic disease prior to failure of local control is almost inevitable. In that situation, further radiotherapy could not be justified.

Further Treatment for Local Recurrence

Isolated limb perfusion does not preclude the administration of further adjuvant or neoadjuvant therapy. For chemosensitive tumor types, such as synovial sarcoma, ILP can play a role as an induction chemotherapy strategy along with systemic therapy.[55] Similarly, radiotherapy to the primary tumor site or to distant irresectable disease can also be considered. A cautionary note must be attached in the context of radiotherapy, in that acute toxicity may be aggravated by recent ILP. However, functional outcomes are not worse.

ISOLATED LIMB INFUSION

Isolated limb infusion (ILI) is a related procedure to ILP which entails the radiological placement of cannulae in the supplying limb followed by perfusion with cytostatic agents alone. The major difference in the procedure is that the cannulas placed radiologically are much smaller caliber and, accordingly, the flow rate is very much lower. The circuit is not perfused on an oxygenated cardiac bypass circuit but is a much simpler low flow system involving a 50 mL syringe and a three way tap, in which the surgeon manually circulates the perfusate. In practical terms, this means that TNFα cannot be administered through this circuit, because it is not possible to adequately wash out the limb at the end of the procedure, giving a risk of a major postperfusion leak of TNF.

Moncrieff and colleagues presented their experience with ILI for locally advanced sarcoma in 21 patients[56] and found a total response rate of 90% (57% CR, 33% PR) and a limb salvage rate of 76%. These results are comparable to those of ILP and, certainly, warrant further investigation. However, this is a relatively small study in which a significant proportion of patients were amenable to resection at study recruitment, and therefore direct comparison with large ILP studies in patients considered irresectable is problematic.

FUTURE APPROACHES FOR ISOLATED LIMB PERFUSION

As an experimental model for the treatment of locally advanced cancer, ILP is of considerable interest. ILP in any but the smallest rodents is achievable, reproducible and reliable; the site of the tumors renders noninvasive measurement techniques (direct calliper measurement and *in vivo* imaging such as computed tomography or bioluminescent imaging) feasible and the findings from limb perfusion, which is technically easier and less time-consuming to perform, can be used to inform later *in vivo* work on other organs such as the liver, kidneys or lungs.[7,57] Previously, this work had been considered of experimental interest only, but with the advent of lower-dose perfusion and mechanisms for the control of more complex venous anatomy, human clinical series have recently been published evaluating perfusion of pelvic, hepatic and even pulmonary disease. There is also an extending role for peritoneal perfusion in the treatment of advanced gynecological and peritoneal malignancy.[58,59]

Advances in ILP will need to focus on two areas, given the currently very acceptable limb salvage rate: improving the number of complete responses within the limb, and extending benefit to patients in whom systemic disease is either already apparent or biologically inevitable. With this in mind, interest is focusing on broadening the spectrum of chemotherapeutic agents used in ILP, and introducing the use of biotherapeutics such as viral vectors and oncolytic viruses in perfusion systems.

Much has been written about the molecular personalization of cancer therapy. Such an approach should be possible in extremity sarcoma, where a preoperative biopsy is sufficient for molecular characterization by modern high-throughput, high-sensitivity systems. Whether this approach will inevitably lead to an increase in response rates for ILP is uncertain since targeted agents, provided they have sufficient bioavailability and acceptable side effect profiles, will most likely continue to be administered by the simpler intravenous or oral routes.

In many ways, this defines the use of ILP with viral vectors. In particular, oncolytic viruses have shown good preclinical efficacy but the response rates in clinical trials have not yet achieved their potential because of the effects of the reticuloendothelial and immune systems on systemic abrogation prior to tumor infection.[60] ILP provides a mechanism whereby these 'first-pass' effects can be limited. Evidence is mounting that both therapeutic genes and oncolytic agents can be delivered using this approach.[61,62] In addition, in the light of work suggesting priming of immune response in murine models resulting in destruction of distant metastases beyond the site of administration, the prospect of a local therapy with distant results has been raised.[63] Further work is continuing to refine and characterize these processes. We look forward to the integration of novel agents to increase the role of this well tolerated, effective treatment in the armamentarium of the surgical oncologist.

CONCLUSION

Isolated limb perfusion with melphalan and TNF is an important treatment for a small number of patients with limb threatening sarcomas affecting the extremities. For patients in whom no local treatment other than an amputation is possible, and if the patient wishes to avoid this procedure, it is an extremely valuable palliative approach. Clinically useful response rates under these circumstances amount to between 50 and 60%, although many of these responses are short lived. There are, however, some durable ongoing clinical responses.

Isolated limb perfusion is also an effective modality when used as induction chemotherapy to downsize a large primary tumor in the proximal extremity prior to a planned marginal resection. Whether this approach is superior to undertaking primary radical, function preserving operation and adjuvant radiotherapy remains to be clarified.

REFERENCES

1. Pisters PWT. Soft tissue sarcoma. In: Norton JA, Barie PS, Bollinger RR, Chang AE, Lowry S, Mulvihill SJ, Pass HI, Thompson RW (Eds). Surgery: Basic Science and Clinical Evidence, 2nd edition. Philadelphia: Springer LLC; 2008. pp. 2061-208.
2. Howlader N, Noone AM, Krapcho M, et al. (2011). SEER Cancer Statistics Review, 1975-2008, National Cancer Institute. [online] SEER website. Available from http://seer.cancer.gov/csr/1975_2008/ [Accessed June 2011].
3. Rosenberg SA, Tepper J, Glatstein E, et al. The treatment of soft-tissue sarcomas of the extremities: prospective randomized evaluations of (1) limb-sparing surgery plus radiation therapy compared with amputation and (2) the role of adjuvant chemotherapy. Ann Surg. 1982;196(3):305-15.
4. Collin C, Godbold J, Hajdu S, et al. Localized extremity soft tissue sarcoma: an analysis of factors affecting survival. J Clin Oncol. 1987;5(4):601-12.
5. Creech O Jr, Krementz ET, Ryan RF, et al. Chemotherapy of cancer: regional perfusion utilizing an extracorporeal circuit. Ann Surg. 1958;148(4):616-32.
6. Bergel F, Stock JA. Cyto-active Amino-acid and Peptide Derivatives. Part I. Substituted Phenylalanines. J Chem Soc. 1954;2409-17.
7. Eggermont AM, de Wilt JH, ten Hagen TL. Current uses of isolated limb perfusion in the clinic and a model system for new strategies. Lancet Oncol. 2003;4(7):429-37.
8. Kroon BB. Regional isolation perfusion in melanoma of the limbs; accomplishments, unsolved problems, future. Eur J Surg Oncol. 1988;14(2):101-10.
9. Stam TC, Jongen-Lavrencic M, Eggermont AM, et al. Effects of isolated limb perfusion with tumour necrosis factor-alpha on the function of monocytes and T lymphocytes in patients with cancer. Eur J Clin Invest. 1996;26(12):1085-91.
10. Klop WM, Vrouenraets BC, van Geel BN, et al. Repeat isolated limb perfusion with melphalan for recurrent melanoma of the limbs. J Am Coll Surg. 1996;182(6):467-72.
11. Grunhagen DJ, de Wilt JH, ten Hagen TL, et al. Technology insight: Utility of TNF-alpha-based isolated limb perfusion to avoid amputation of irresectable tumors of the extremities. Nat Clin Pract Oncol. 2006;3(2):94-103.
12. van der Veen AH, de Wilt JH, Eggermont AM, et al. TNF-alpha augments intratumoural concentrations of doxorubicin in TNF-alpha-based isolated limb perfusion in rat sarcoma models and enhances anti-tumour effects. Br J Cancer. 2000;82(4):973-80.
13. de Wilt JH, ten Hagen TL, de Boeck G, et al. Tumour necrosis factor alpha increases melphalan concentration in tumour tissue after isolated limb perfusion. Br J Cancer. 2000;82(5):1000-03.
14. Cornett WR, McCall LM, Petersen RP, et al. Randomized multicenter trial of hyperthermic isolated limb perfusion with melphalan alone compared with melphalan plus tumor necrosis factor: American College of Surgeons Oncology Group Trial Z0020. J Clin Oncol. 2006;24(25):4196-4201.
15. Lejeune FJ, Eggermont AM. Hyperthermic isolated limb perfusion with tumor necrosis factor is a useful therapy for advanced melanoma of the limbs. J Clin Oncol. 2007; 25(11):1449-50.
16. Clark IA. How TNF was recognized as a key mechanism of disease. Cytokine Growth Factor Rev. 2007;18(3-4):335-43.
17. Carswell EA, Old LJ, Kassel RL, et al. An endotoxin-induced serum factor that causes necrosis of tumors. Proc Natl Acad Sci USA. 1975;72(9):3666-70.
18. Gray-Schopfer VC, Karasarides M, Hayward R, et al. Tumor necrosis factor-alpha blocks apoptosis in melanoma cells when BRAF signaling is inhibited. Cancer Res. 2007;67(1):122-9.
19. Tjardes T, Neugebauer E. Sepsis research in the next millennium: concentrate on the software rather than the hardware. Shock. 2002;17(1):1-8.
20. Borsi L, Balza E, Carnemolla B, et al. Selective targeted delivery of TNFalpha to tumor blood vessels. Blood. 2003; 102(13):4384-92.
21. Lejeune FJ, Lienard D, Ewalenko P. Hyperthermic isolation perfusion of the limbs with cytostatics after surgical excision of sarcomas. World J Surg. 1988;12(3):345-8.
22. Lienard D, Eggermont AM, Koops HS, et al. Isolated limb perfusion with tumour necrosis factor-alpha and melphalan with or without interferon-gamma for the treatment of in-transit melanoma metastases: a multicentre randomized phase II study. Melanoma Res. 1999;9(5):491-502.
23. Wray CJ, Benjamin RS, Hunt KK, et al. Isolated limb perfusion for unresectable extremity sarcoma: results of 2 single-institution phase 2 trials. Cancer. 2011;117(14):3235-41.
24. Rossi CR, Mocellin S, Pilati P, et al. Hyperthermic isolated perfusion with low-dose tumor necrosis factor alpha and doxorubicin for the treatment of limb-threatening soft tissue sarcomas. Ann Surg Oncol. 2005;12(5):398-405.
25. Bonvalot S, Laplanche A, Lejeune F, et al. Limb salvage with isolated perfusion for soft tissue sarcoma: could less TNF-alpha be better? Ann Oncol. 2005;16(7):1061-8.
26. Nachmany I, Subhi A, Meller I, et al. Efficacy of high vs low dose TNF-isolated limb perfusion for locally advanced soft tissue sarcoma. Eur J Surg Oncol. 2009;35(2):209-14.
27. Stam TC, Swaak AJ, de Vries MR, et al. Systemic toxicity and cytokine/acute phase protein levels in patients after isolated

limb perfusion with tumor necrosis factor-alpha complicated by high leakage. Ann Surg Oncol. 2000;7(4):268-75.
28. Omlor G, Gross G, Ecker KW, et al. Optimization of isolated hyperthermic limb perfusion. World J Surg. 1992;16(6): 1117-9.
29. Chang E, Chalikonda S, Friedl J, et al. Targeting vaccinia to solid tumors with local hyperthermia. Hum Gene Ther. 2005; 16(4):435-44.
30. Vrouenraets BC, Eggermont AM, Hart AA, et al. Regional toxicity after isolated limb perfusion with melphalan and tumour necrosis factor- alpha versus toxicity after melphalan alone. Eur J Surg Oncol. 2001;27(4):390-5.
31. Noorda EM, van Kreij RH, Vrouenraets BC, et al. The health-related quality of life of long-term survivors of melanoma treated with isolated limb perfusion. Eur J Surg Oncol. 2007; 33(6):776-82.
32. Eggermont AM, Schraffordt Koops H, Klausner JM, et al. Isolated limb perfusion with tumor necrosis factor and melphalan for limb salvage in 186 patients with locally advanced soft tissue extremity sarcomas. The cumulative multicenter European experience. Ann Surg. 1996;224(6): 756-64.
33. Eggermont AMM, Schraffordt Koops H, Schlag PM, et al. Limb salvage by isolated limb perfusion (ILP) with TNF and melphalan in patients with locally advanced soft tissue sarcomas: outcome of 270 ILPs in 246 patients. Proc Annu Meet Am Soc Clin Oncol. 1999;18:2067.
34. Lejeune FJ, Pujol N, Lienard D, et al. Limb salvage by neoadjuvant isolated perfusion with TNF alpha and melphalan for non-resectable soft tissue sarcoma of the extremities. Eur J Surg Oncol. 2000;26(7):669-78.
35. Gerrand CH, Wunder JS, Kandel RA, et al. Classification of positive margins after resection of soft-tissue sarcoma of the limb predicts the risk of local recurrence. J Bone Joint Surg Br. 2001;83(8):1149-55.
36. Hill S, Fawcett WJ, Sheldon J, et al. Low-dose tumour necrosis factor alpha and melphalan in hyperthermic isolated limb perfusion. Br J Surg. 1993;80(8):995-7.
37. Santinami M, Deraco M, Azzarelli A, et al. Treatment of recurrent sarcoma of the extremities by isolated limb perfusion using tumor necrosis factor alpha and melphalan. Tumori. 1996;82(6):579-84.
38. Hohenberger P, Kettelhack C, Hermann A, et al. Functional outcome after preoperative isolated limb perfusion with rhTNFalpha/melphalan for high-grade extremity sarcoma. Eur J Cancer. 2001;37:S34-S35.
39. van Ginkel RJ, Thijssens KM, Pras E, et al. Isolated limb perfusion with tumor necrosis factor alpha and melphalan for locally advanced soft tissue sarcoma: three time periods at risk for amputation. Ann Surg Oncol. 2007;14(4):1499-1506.
40. Pennacchioli E, Deraco M, Mariani L, et al. Advanced extremity soft tissue sarcoma: prognostic effect of isolated limb perfusion in a series of 88 patients treated at a single institution. Ann Surg Oncol. 2007;14(2):553-9.
41. Hayes AJ, Neuhaus SJ, Clark MA, et al. Isolated limb perfusion with melphalan and tumor necrosis factor alpha for advanced melanoma and soft-tissue sarcoma. Ann Surg Oncol. 2007;14(1):230-8.
42. Cherix S, Speiser M, Matter M, et al. Isolated limb perfusion with tumor necrosis factor and melphalan for non-resectable soft tissue sarcomas: long-term results on efficacy and limb salvage in a selected group of patients. J Surg Oncol. 2008; 98(3):148-55.
43. Eggermont AM, Schraffordt Koops H, Lienard D, et al. Isolated limb perfusion with high-dose tumor necrosis factor-alpha in combination with interferon-gamma and melphalan for nonresectable extremity soft tissue sarcomas: a multicenter trial. J Clin Oncol. 1996;14(10):2653-65.
44. Rossi CR, Foletto M, Di Filippo F, et al. Soft tissue limb sarcomas: Italian clinical trials with hyperthermic antiblastic perfusion. Cancer. 1999;86(9):1742-9.
45. Grunhagen DJ, de Wilt JH, van Geel AN, et al. TNF dose reduction in isolated limb perfusion. Eur J Surg Oncol. 2005; 31(9):1011-9.
46. Grunhagen DJ, de Wilt JH, Graveland WJ, et al. Outcome and prognostic factor analysis of 217 consecutive isolated limb perfusions with tumor necrosis factor-alpha and melphalan for limb-threatening soft tissue sarcoma. Cancer. 2006;106(8):1776-84.
47. Grabellus F, Kraft C, Sheu-Grabellus SY, et al. Tumor vascularization and histopathologic regression of soft tissue sarcomas treated with isolated limb perfusion with TNF-alpha and melphalan. J Surg Oncol. 2011;103(5):371-9.
48. Deroose JP, Burger JW, van Geel AN, et al. Radiotherapy for soft tissue sarcomas after isolated limb perfusion and surgical resection: essential for local control in all patients? Ann Surg Oncol. 2011;18(2):321-7.
49. Noorda EM, Vrouenraets BC, Nieweg OE, et al. Isolated limb perfusion with tumor necrosis factor-alpha and melphalan for patients with unresectable soft tissue sarcoma of the extremities. Cancer. 2003;98(7):1483-90.
50. Wall N, Starkhammar H. Chemotherapy of soft tissue sarcoma—a clinical evaluation of treatment over ten years. Acta Oncol. 2003;42(1):55-61.
51. Bramwell V, Rouesse J, Steward W, et al. Adjuvant CYVADIC chemotherapy for adult soft tissue sarcoma--reduced local recurrence but no improvement in survival: a study of the European Organization for Research and Treatment of Cancer Soft Tissue and Bone Sarcoma Group. J Clin Oncol. 1994;12(6):1137-49.
52. Lev-Chelouche D, Abu-Abeid S, Kollander Y, et al. Multifocal soft tissue sarcoma: limb salvage following hyperthermic isolated limb perfusion with high-dose tumor necrosis factor and melphalan. J Surg Oncol. 1999;70(3):185-9.
53. Wieberdink J, Benckhuysen C, Braat RP, et al. Dosimetry in isolation perfusion of the limbs by assessment of perfused tissue volume and grading of toxic tissue reactions. Eur J Cancer Clin Oncol. 1982;18(10):905-10.
54. Bonvalot S, Gronchi A. ILP and RT: the study that will never be. Ann Surg Oncol. 2011;18(2):303-5.
55. Grimer R, Judson I, Peake D, et al. Guidelines for the management of soft tissue sarcomas. Sarcoma. 2010; 2010:506182.
56. Moncrieff MD, Kroon HM, Kam PC, et al. Isolated limb infusion for advanced soft tissue sarcoma of the extremity. Ann Surg Oncol. 2008;15(10):2749-56.
57. Ten Hagen TL, Eggermont AMM. Isolated limb and organ perfusion laboratory models. In: Schlag PM, Stein U, Eggermont AMM (Eds). Regional Cancer Therapy, Vol 1. Berlin: Humana Press; 2007. pp. 29-44.

58. Chua TC, Yan TD, Saxena A, et al. Should the treatment of peritoneal carcinomatosis by cytoreductive surgery and hyperthermic intraperitoneal chemotherapy still be regarded as a highly morbid procedure?: a systematic review of morbidity and mortality. Ann Surg. 2009;249(6):900-07.
59. Verwaal VJ, van Ruth S, de Bree E, et al. Randomized trial of cytoreduction and hyperthermic intraperitoneal chemotherapy versus systemic chemotherapy and palliative surgery in patients with peritoneal carcinomatosis of colorectal cancer. J Clin Oncol. 2003;21(20):3737-43.
60. Pencavel T, Seth R, Hayes A, et al. Locoregional intravascular viral therapy of cancer: precision guidance for Paris's arrow? Gene Ther. 2010;17(8):949-60.
61. de Wilt JH, Bout A, Eggermont AM, et al. Adenovirus-mediated interleukin 3 beta gene transfer by isolated limb perfusion inhibits growth of limb sarcoma in rats. Hum Gene Ther. 2001;12(5):489-502.
62. Kubo T, Shimose S, Matsuo T, et al. Oncolytic vesicular stomatitis virus administered by isolated limb perfusion suppresses osteosarcoma growth. J Orthop Res. 2011;29(5):795-800.
63. Qiao J, Kottke T, Willmon C, et al. Purging metastases in lymphoid organs using a combination of antigen-nonspecific adoptive T cell therapy, oncolytic virotherapy and immunotherapy. Nat Med. 2008;14(1):37-44.

9

Hyperthermic Intrathoracic Chemotherapy

Neil A. Christie, Daniel C. Wiener

INTRODUCTION

The results of surgical therapy alone and surgery combined with traditional chemotherapy or radiation therapy have been disappointing for patients with malignant pleural mesothelioma (MPM), locally advanced thymic malignancies, and non-small lung cancer with pleural spread.[1-3] The treatment for most of these malignancies continues to evolve.

Cytoreductive surgery followed by hyperthermic intraperitoneal chemotherapy has been discussed in previous chapters. Encouraging results with intra-abdominal cancers have led to applications of this therapy in the chest. The strategy relies on removing all gross disease and following with intracavitary chemoperfusion. This treatment increases exposure of residual microscopic disease to chemotherapy while limiting systemic side effects. Prerequisites for effective intrathoracic chemotherapy are: (i) the absence of extrathoracic disease and (ii) the ability to achieve a complete macroscopic resection.

MALIGNANT PLEURAL MESOTHELIOMA

Overview

Malignant pleural mesothelioma is a fatal disease with an overall poor prognosis. It is a relatively rare and aggressive disease that arises from the pleural mesothelium and has a reported survival of less than 12 months.[1] Asbestos is a major risk factor with a significant latency period between exposure and disease manifestation. As a result, the incidence of MPM in the United States has continued to rise despite the recognition of asbestos as a causative agent and the resultant environmental regulations instituted in the 1980s.[1]

There are two basic histologic subtypes of MPM, epithelioid and sarcomatoid. There is a drastic difference in behavior with pure epithelioid tumors having the most favorable prognosis. While there is no clear consensus on a specific staging system, there is agreement that nodal status is an important prognosticator.

Treatment

Surgery Alone

Surgical treatment for MPM can either be an extrapleural pneumonectomy (EPP) or pleurectomy and decortication (PD). EPP is an en bloc resection of the lung, pleura, pericardium, and diaphragm (Figs 1 and 2). PD is a resection of the parietal and visceral pleura with or

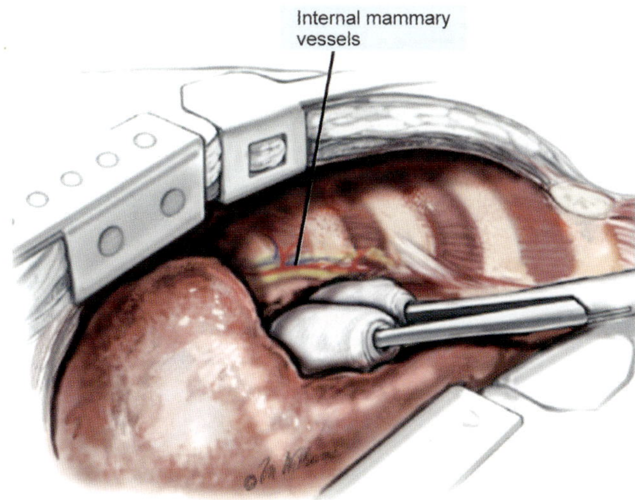

Figure 1 Extrapleural pneumonectomy—exposure via large posterolateral thoracotomy with excision of the sixth rib
(*Source*: Adult Chest Surgery, 1st edition. New York: The McGraw-Hill Companies; 2009)

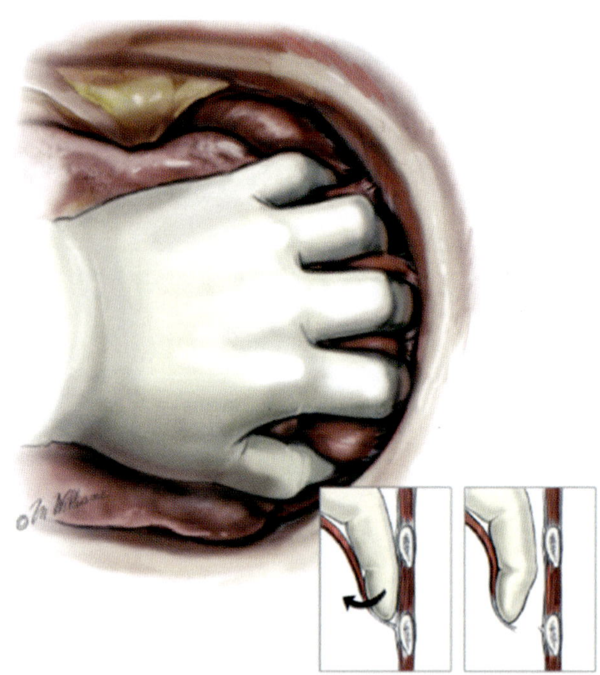

Figure 2 Extrapleural pneumonectomy—diaphragmatic avulsion technique
(*Source*: Adult Chest Surgery, 1st edition. New York: The McGraw-Hill Companies; 2009.)

without the pericardium and diaphragm, with sparing of the lung (Figs 3 and 4). The goal of surgery is to remove all visible disease (R_0 resection). Unfortunately, surgery alone cannot eradicate residual microscopic disease regardless of whether an EPP or PD is performed.[4]

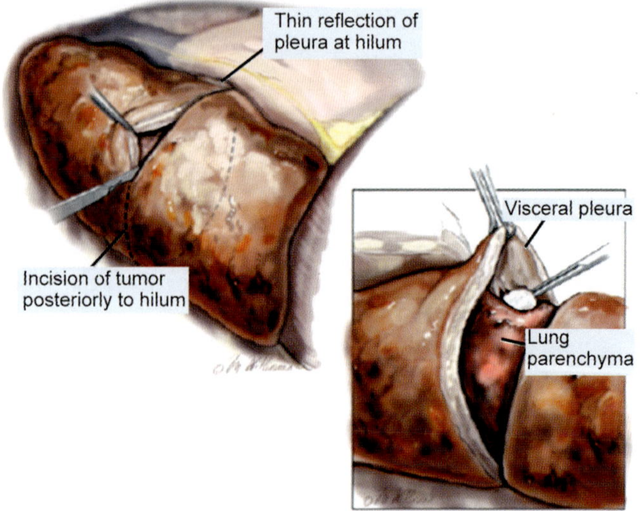

Figure 3 Pleurectomy and decortication
(*Source*: Wolf AS, Daniel J, Sugarbaker DJ. Surgical techniques for multimodality treatment of malignant pleural mesothelioma: extrapleural pneumonectomy and pleurectomy/decortications. Semin Thorac Cardiovasc Surg. 2009;21(2):132-48.)

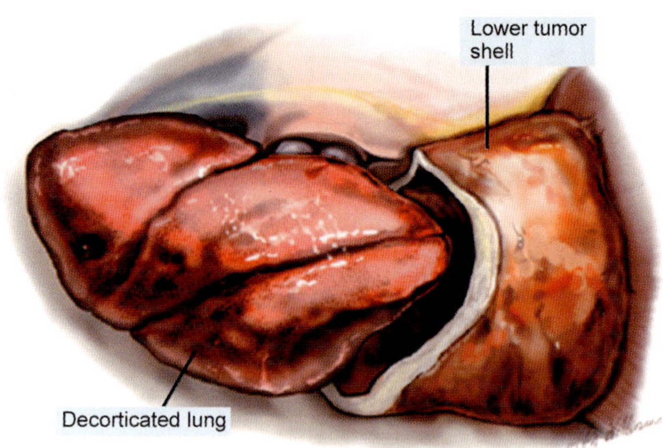

Figure 4 Pleurectomy and decortication
(*Source*: Wolf AS, Daniel J, Sugarbaker DJ. Surgical techniques for multimodality treatment of malignant pleural mesothelioma: extrapleural pneumonectomy and pleurectomy/decortications. Semin Thorac Cardiovasc Surg. 2009;21(2):132-48.)

Outcomes of surgery for MPM have been fairly well documented in the medical literature. One meta-analysis of survival in patients undergoing EPP for MPM reported on 34 studies in 26 institutions for an overall total of 2462 patients.[5] Median disease free survival was 13 months (range: 7–26 months), major morbidity of 33% (range: 13–48%), and a 30-day mortality of 5.5% (range: 0–11%). Median blood loss was 1000 ml (range: 800–2300 ml) and median length of stay was 12 days (range: 8–43 days). N_2 lymph node involvement was found to be a significant prognostic factor on multivariate analysis when grouped with internal thoracic lymph nodes and compared to N_1 and N_0 disease.

Because of the diffuse nature of MPM, there is a high rate of locoregional recurrence with surgery alone which has prompted the development of multimodality therapy.[6]

Multimodality Therapy

Extrapleural Pneumonectomy with Adjuvant Chemoradiation

A number of institutions have combined surgical treatment with chemotherapy and/or radiotherapy. Several studies have shown an improved overall and disease free survival with a multimodality approach compared to historical controls of palliation, chemotherapy, or surgery alone.[7]

The same meta-analysis referenced above describes improved survival with EPP and adjuvant chemoradiation compared to surgical treatment alone with an overall survival ranging from 13–24 months.[5] Studies of EPP and adjuvant chemotherapy and radiotherapy conducted in centers of excellence for mesothelioma demonstrate acceptable morbidity and mortality compared to single modality therapy. In the subset of patients with N_2 node negative, epithelioid histology, and macroscopic complete resection, long-term survival was seen.[7] EPP accompanied by adjuvant conventional chemotherapy and radiation therapy was regarded as offering the best prospect of prolonged survival.[7] The majority of patients however, were still failing locally even with multimodality therapy.

Extrapleural Pneumonectomy versus Pleurectomy and Decortication with Adjuvant Chemoradiation

Surgery is generally recommended for patients with tumor localized to the hemithorax by imaging and who have adequate cardiopulmonary function. Those who favor EPP, argue that the more radical surgery affords a greater chance to achieve a complete macroscopic resection. Furthermore, removing the lung allows for the administration of high-dose postoperative radiation therapy. Significant advances have been made towards decreasing the morbidity and mortality of this surgery over the past decade. Clinicians who favor PD cite lower morbidity and mortality with this less radical resection and equally effective cytoreduction when combined with additional intrapleural therapies.

A large multivariate, multicenter analysis published in 2008 compared the results of EPP with PD.[8] The authors reviewed 663 patients with MPM who underwent either therapy and operated on between 1990 and 2006. Not surprisingly, a survival advantage was seen for epithelioid versus non-epithelioid histology and multimodality therapy versus surgery alone. The median survival was 14 months and the overall 5-year survival was 12%. Median survival was stage dependent (stage I—38 months, stage II—19 months, stage III—11 months, stage IV—7 months).

In terms of EPP versus PD, operative mortality was 7% and 4% respectively and severe complications were more frequent in the EPP group. By univariate analysis, EPP was associated with a significantly worse survival than PD, even when operative deaths were excluded (median survival: 16 months versus 12 months, $p<0.001$). However, as the authors note, there is inherent selection bias with this study design. In their multivariate analysis, PD afforded only a "marginal" benefit with a hazard ratio of only 1.4; and, when analyzed by stage, there was no statistical difference in survival by procedure. Perhaps, the most interesting finding of this study is the pattern of recurrence. Patients undergoing EPP were much more likely to develop distant recurrence (66% versus 35%) whereas local recurrences were higher in patients undergoing PD (33% versus 65%).

Surgery and Radiation

Radiation is a local therapy which can be combined with surgery to help improve local control. EPP, in addition to facilitating complete removal of all gross tumor, also facilitates the administration of postoperative high-dose hemithoracic radiation.[9] Although PD generally provides adequate cytoreduction, especially for patients with earlier stage tumors, and is associated with a lower morbidity and mortality than EPP, it does not facilitate the use of high-dose postoperative radiotherapy. Radiation toxicity to the remaining lung limits the safe application of high ablative doses of radiation.

Patients who undergo EPP and receive adjuvant therapy (particularly high-dose hemithoracic radiotherapy) relapse predominately at distant sites compared to PD alone where local regional recurrence is more common. Local progression after PD leads to death from worsening restrictive lung disease, intractable chest pain, and respiratory failure. Distant progression (usually after EPP) manifests most frequently with dyspnea from contralateral pleural effusion, ascites, or both.[8]

Some challenge the current dogma of the benefit of surgery in MPM. In Europe, the Mesothelioma and Radical Surgery (MARS) trial recently published their feasibility. In this randomized trial comparing multimodality therapy with and without surgery, EPP offered no survival advantage. Proponents of this trial suggest that ultimately our failures are due to a lack of effective systemic therapy and that no matter how effective EPP or PD are in removing gross tumor, the lack of highly effective adjuvant therapy leads to similar survival independent of surgical resection.

It is clear that despite improvements in survival with surgery-based treatments, locoregional recurrence remains problematic. It is felt therefore, that novel strategies are needed to improve local control. Options include intraoperative radiotherapy, brachytherapy, intraoperative photodynamic therapy, and intraoperative chemotherapy with or without hyperthermia.

Intrathoracic Chemotherapy

Intrathoracic administration of chemotherapy can deliver higher doses of drug locally with less toxicity than that which is seen with systemic administration.[10]

Phase I and phase II clinical trials have shown intrathoracic chemotherapy to be relatively safe and feasible. MPM patients appear to be ideal candidates for intrathoracic chemotherapy given that the major mode of failure with conventional treatments is local failure.

Rusch looked at the pharmacokinetics of intrapleural cisplatin (100 mg/m^2) and mitomycin C (8 mg/m^2) after PD with evaluation of pleural fluid and plasma drug levels.[11] Peak plasma levels were observed within 1 hour after intrapleural chemotherapy administration. They were similar to that seen after systemic administration of similar doses of drugs. Mean peak cisplatin and mitomycin C levels in the pleural fluid as well as the mean area under the curve (AUC), were significantly higher than in the plasma samples. Rusch demonstrated a 3.5 fold advantage for pleural administration for both drugs. The type of resection can also affect drug absorption in the pleural space. Systemic drug concentrations have been noted to be higher post PD compared to after EPP, presumably because of the increased absorptive surface area of the remaining lung.

Rusch evaluated a phase II study of PD followed by intrapleural and systemic chemotherapy for MPM.[12] Patients received perioperative hydration with intravenous (IV) fluids at 150 cc/hr for 12 hours. Cisplatin and mitomycin C was administered postoperatively into the pleural space via chest tube for 15 minutes immediately following the operation in the recovery room. Twenty-seven patients were treated; median age 62 years, 41% right hemithorax disease and 70% epithelial histology. Complete resection was obtained in 74% of patients. Mortality was 3.7% and major morbidity was 45%. Two patients developed renal insufficiency, one of whom required dialysis. The authors noted that both patients received less than 100 ml/hr preoperative hydration and that the patient requiring dialysis also received postoperative non-steroidal anti-inflammatory drugs for pain control. Median overall survival was 13.6 months. Local recurrence was the most common mode of failure. The authors concluded that the approach was feasible but there were concerns regarding toxicities.

Rice evaluated resection with PD or EPP followed by intrapleural chemotherapy and systemic chemotherapy.[13] There were 19 patients in the study with 9 PD and 10 EPP. Median age was 62 years with 18 males and 1 female; 53% had epithelial histology, 68% stage I, and 32% stage III. Postoperatively, patients received intrathoracic cisplatin (100 mg/m^2) and mitomycin C (8 mg/m^2) via chest tube in the recovery room for 4 hours. IV hydration was given before, during, and for 24 hours after intrapleural chemotherapy.

For EPP patients, 1–2 weeks following surgery, 100 mg of cisplatin was instilled in the extrapleural space. There were no in-house mortalities and no renal toxicity. Median overall survival was 13 months and median disease free survival was 11 months. The majority (58%) of disease recurrence was local. The authors concluded that their approach offered good palliation of symptoms and was well tolerated, but the local recurrence rate was high.

Lee and coworkers evaluated intrapleural chemotherapy following incompletely resected MPM after PD.[14] Patients received cisplatin (100 mg/m^2) and cytosine arabinoside (1200 mg) via chest tube for 4 hours. IV hydration and mannitol were used to maintain urine output pre and postoperatively. There were 15 patients, 87% were male, 53% had disease in the right hemithorax, and 47% had epithelial histology. There were no mortalities and postoperative morbidity was 13% (one patient with renal insufficiency). The median overall survival was 11 months and all patients developed local recurrences. The authors concluded that, although there was relatively little toxicity, the treatment appeared to offer little beneficial effect on survival.

Sauter looked at intrapleural chemotherapy after subtotal pleurectomy in 13 patients with MPM.[15] Chemotherapy (cisplatin 100 mg/m^2 and cytosine arabinoside 1200 mg) were administered in the operating room at completion of surgery and were left indwelling for 4 hours, after which time the chemotherapy was drained from the chest tubes. The only morbidity was a wound infection and one patient with renal failure. Seven patients also received systemic chemotherapy. There was one mortality. Median overall survival was 9 months. The authors concluded that intrapleural chemotherapy following subtotal pleurectomy resulted in significant toxicity and did not improve overall survival.

Colleoni looked at intrapleural and systemic chemotherapy after PD in 20 patients with MPM.[16] Immediately following surgery, patients received cisplatin (100 mg/m^2) and cytarabine (1000 mg/m^2) instilled via chest tube for 4 hours. Urine output was maintained at 100 ml/hr with 3L IV fluids per day for 48 hours; 40% were stage I, 20% stage II, and 40% stage III. Fifty percent had epithelial histology. Complete macroscopic resection was achieved in only 35% of cases. There were no deaths secondary to treatment. Two patients had severe renal toxicity, one of whom required dialysis. Median overall survival was 11.5 months with median time to progression 7.4 months. Of note, the median survival of the seven patients who underwent complete resection was 24.5 months. The authors concluded that the approach was feasible with encouraging results for those with minimal disease following resection. Overall, although tolerability was established, the survival was still poor.

Hyperthermic Intrathoracic Chemotherapy

The addition of hyperthermia has the advantage of improving the efficacy of intrathoracic chemotherapy by increasing drug absorption and enhancing drug action. Normal tissues are unharmed by temperatures up to 44°C for 1 hour where cancer cells are vulnerable at temperatures above 40°C. The principle mechanism of action is thought to be protein denaturation, which has secondary effects on the cell membrane integrity, cytoskeleton, DNA synthesis, and membrane permeability. Ultimately, hyperthermia tends to increase the rate of tumor cell apoptosis.[17]

Local tissue concentration/perfusate concentration ratio is higher after hyperthermic perfusion compared with normothermic perfusion. It therefore appears to be safe, feasible, and pharmacokinetically advantageous. Furthermore, the addition of hyperthermia to chemotherapy can counteract drug resistance to a variety of agents, including cisplatin.[18]

Yellin evaluated the effectiveness of hyperthermic intrathoracic chemotherapy for malignant pleural disease.[19] Seven patients had MPM, four of who had EPP, one PD, and two cytoreduction only. They were treated with cisplatin 150 mg or 200 mg. One patient died after EPP secondary to gastric herniation. There were no renal toxicities. Three of the four patients who underwent EPP were disease free at 2 years and two patients were alive and disease free at 31 months and 36 months. The authors concluded that the treatment was safe and feasible and offered excellent local control.

Mounese evaluated hyperthermic intrapleural chemotherapy following PD in patients with malignant pleural disease.[20] Sixteen patients underwent PD followed by hyperthermic intrathoracic chemotherapy for 60 minutes. Patients received either mitomycin C alone or mitomycin C and cisplatin. There was one postoperative death, but no renal or hematologic complications. Overall median survival was 18 months. The authors concluded that cytoreductive surgery with hyperthermic intraoperative chemotherapy is safe, feasible, and for a selective group with early disease, may be associated with long-term survival.

Van Ruth looked at 20 patients with stage I MPM.[21] All underwent cytoreductive surgery; 12 via PD and 8 via EPP. Cytoreductive surgery was followed by hyperthermic intrathoracic chemotherapy with cisplatin and doxorubicin for 90 minutes. Nineteen patients were male, with a median age of 57 years and 80% had epithelial histology. Complete macroscopic resection was achieved in 75% of cases. There were no mortalities; however, major morbidity was seen in 65% of cases. There were no significant renal toxicities. Median overall survival was 11 months and most recurrences were local. The author postulated that the lack of effect on survival and recurrence patterns may be due to the low concentrations of the chemotherapeutic agents.

Sugarbaker's group in Boston reported a phase I trial of EPP with hyperthermic 42°C lavage with cisplatin for 1 hour with IV sodium thiosulfate administered during the lavage.[22] Patients were treated with increasing doses of cisplatin to determine the maximum tolerated dose. Mean age was 58 years, 76% of patients were male, 62% were stage III, and 76% had epithelial histology. Operative mortality was 2% with 60% major morbidity.

Maximum tolerated dose was 250 mg/m^2. It was speculated that some of the cisplatin may have been inactivated by the sodium thiosulfate which was administered during the lavage, thus reducing the effectiveness of the cisplatin.

Sugarbaker's group also performed a dose escalation study with hyperthermic intrathoracic chemoperfusion in patients unable to tolerate EPP.[23] Forty-four patients underwent PD immediately followed by a 1-hour lavage with hyperthermic cisplatin. In this study, IV sodium thiosulfate was not administered until after the completion of the lavage. With dose escalation of cisplatin, 225 mg/m^2 was determined to be the maximum tolerated dose. The median length of stay was 11 days (5–71 days). Median age was 71 years and the majority of patients had epithelial histology. Postoperative mortality was 11% with 22% major morbidity. A survival benefit of 18 months versus 6 months was seen in patients receiving higher doses of cisplatin (175–250 mg/m^2) versus those receiving lower doses (50–150 mg/m^2). Renal toxicity was the limiting factor in dose escalation. The authors commented that this study demonstrated not only safety and feasibility but also survival benefit with higher doses of intrathoracic cisplatin.

The sodium thiosulfate might decrease the effectiveness of the cisplatin. Amifostine as a renal protectant administered during hyperthermic chemotherapy lavage, rather than sodium thiosulfate was evaluated.[24] Twenty-nine patients underwent EPP; median age was 57 years, 62% were stage II. Postoperative mortality was 3.4%. One patient had irreversible renal failure and seven other patients had high grade but reversible renal insufficiency. In this study, renal failure was not systematically related to cisplatin dose. Median survival was 29 months.

A further iteration involved EPP followed by hyperthermic intraoperative chemotherapy with cisplatin (225 mg/m^2).[25] The renal protection protocol in this study was IV amifostine before the cisplatin lavage and IV sodium thiosulfate given immediately after as a bolus and infusion. One hundred and twenty-nine patients were enrolled, 25 were unresectable and 96 underwent EPP. Ninety-two received hyperthermic intrathoracic chemotherapy. There was a 1.1% operative mortality rate and postoperative morbidity of 48.9%. Grade III–IV renal toxicity was seen in 9.8% of patients. Overall median survival in the treatment group was 13.1 months with a cancer specific survival of 16.9 months. Recurrences were seen in 47 patients. In this study with high-dose cisplatin and an aggressive combination therapy for renal protection, only 34% recurred in the ipsilateral hemithorax and only two patients recurred solely in the ipsilateral hemithorax. Patients with favorable histology (epithelial) and early-stage disease (stage I or II) had a longer median cancer specific survival (21.4 months) and longer median survival (22 months).

The combination of pemetrexed and cisplatin has emerged as the first-line chemotherapy regimen with a multicenter randomized single blinded study assigning 226 patients to therapies.[26] They saw a significantly longer median survival with combination therapy versus cisplatin alone (12.1 months versus 9.3 months, p=0.02). Consideration for future studies is for the use of multi-drug protocols.

Sandick et al. looked at a comparative study involving 20 patients who underwent surgery with EPP (n=8) or PD (n=12) followed by hyperthermic intrathoracic chemotherapy versus 15 other patients who underwent EPP followed by adjuvant external beam radiation.[27] The median survival was 11 months for the hyperthermic patients versus 29 months for the patients with adjuvant radiation therapy. They found that the group that had hyperthermic chemoperfusion had a longer operating time, longer intensive care unit stay and a shorter time to local recurrence when compared to patients who underwent EPP and postoperative radiotherapy.

Aziz compared 51 patients who underwent EPP with intrapleural chemotherapy followed by postoperative systemic chemotherapy to 13 patients treated with EPP alone.[28] The study found that the median overall survival was significantly improved in the group that received adjuvant intrapleural and systemic chemotherapy (35 months versus 13 months) but it is unclear which form of adjuvant chemotherapy was responsible for the improvement.

In studies of therapy for MPM, outcomes have generally been reported as time to progression and patterns of recurrence. These endpoints are fraught with inaccuracy due to differences in follow-up procedures, definitions of progression of disease and methods of documenting recurrence which vary greatly from institution to institution and study to study. Furthermore, overall survival is primarily dependent on tumor histology and stage. Differing tumor histology and stage, particularly if not well defined, could greatly confound comparisons between different studies. Randomized prospective data is very limited in this arena but slowly growing.[29]

Certainly in patients undergoing PD, one could have a strong rationale for adding hyperthermic intrathoracic chemoperfusion. High doses of cisplatin can be administered safely with aggressive renal protectant protocols. In patients undergoing the more aggressive EPP, where hyperthermic intrathoracic chemoperfusion could potentially increase perioperative morbidity and mortality, and in who postoperative radiotherapy has been proven to be an effective form of local control, the case is more debatable. Ultimately, more effective systemic therapy will need to be developed, as more distant failure is often seen as improved local control is achieved.

THYMIC NEOPLASMS

Both malignant thymomas as well as thymic carcinomas have the potential to spread from the mediastinum to the pleural cavity via direct pleural extension, often in the absence of systemic metastases. All patients with thymoma, with the exception of obviously unresectable tumors, are optimally treated with surgical resection, even when pleural metastases are present. While these pleural deposits can be grossly resected along with the primary mediastinal tumor, as with MPM, it is generally impossible to achieve a microscopic complete resection. Not surprising is the fact that thymoma's with pleural spread carry a higher risk for locoregional recurrence and a poorer outcome with a 5-year survival of 33–48%.[30,31] Outcomes with thymic carcinoma with pleural dissemination are generally even poorer.

Yellin and colleagues reported on the outcomes in 15 patients with stage IV thymic tumors with pleural dissemination treated with hyperthermic chemoperfusion.[2] Ten patients had malignant thymoma and five had thymic carcinoma. The majority of patients were male (11/15) and age was 20–67 years. Nine patients underwent resection without pleurectomy, five had resection with pleurectomy, and one patient underwent resection with an extrapleural pneumonectomy. All the patients underwent intraoperative hyperthermic chemoperfusion with cisplatin at 40°C. Fourteen of the fifteen patients received cisplatin doses of 150 mg or more.

There were no renal complications and no operative mortalities. Two patients required a return to the operating room for bleeding, one patient had a prolonged air leak, and two patients developed delayed respiratory insufficiency secondary to a myasthenic crisis and phrenic nerve palsy.

The median patient follow up was 34 months (range: 7–70 months). Ten patients were alive at 10–70 months after surgery with nine of those ten patients free of any demonstrable disease. Four patients died 7–36 months after surgery; three died secondary to disease progression and one died of unrelated causes.

The authors concluded that macroscopic surgical resection along with intraoperative hyperthermic chemoperfusion for a malignant thymic tumor with pleural dissemination was both safe and feasible. They also noted that it offers excellent local control and survival rates that are superior to surgical controls seen in patients treated with surgery alone.

LUNG CARCINOMA

Lung carcinoma is the most common cause of cancer death in North America. Surgical resection is the main stay of early-stage lung cancers localized to the lung as well as if there are nodal metastases confined to within the visceral pleura. Patients with disseminated cancer are typically treated with systemic chemotherapy with palliative intent. A very controversial approach is aggressive locoregional therapy for lung carcinomas with pleural dissemination restricted to one hemithorax.

Matsuzaki and colleagues compared the outcomes of seven patients with lung cancer and pleural metastases who underwent thoracotomy and resection of the primary tumor along with intraoperative hyperthermic chemoperfusion with the outcomes of seven patients with pleural dissemination who underwent surgical resection of the primary tumor alone.[3] Cisplatin (200 mg/m^2) was infused at 43°C for 2 hours in the study patients. Two patients developed transient pulmonary infiltrates and in no patients was renal insufficiency seen. Control of the pleural effusion was 100% effective in all patients treated with hyperthermic chemoperfusion. Survival time in the hyperthermic chemoperfusion group was 20 months compared to a 6-month survival time in the operative only group in this non-randomized study. Another group of patient underwent hyperthermic chemoperfusion of the pleural cavity without lung resection and survival in this group was only 6 months. The effectiveness of this therapy for non-small cell lung cancer may be more limited by the more extensive systemic metastases that are generally seen, in contradistinction to patients with thymic malignancies and MPM.

REFERENCES

1. Rudd RM. Malignant mesothelioma. Br Med Bull. 2010; 93:105-23.
2. Refaely Y, Simansky DA, Paley M, et al. Resection and perfusion thermochemotherapy: a new approach for the treatment of thymic malignancies with pleural spread. Ann Thorac Surg. 2001;72(2):366-70.
3. Matsuzaki Y, Shibata K, Yoshioka M, et al. Intrapleural perfusion hyperthermo-chemotherapy for malignant pleural dissemination and effusion. Ann Thorac Surg. 1995;59(1): 127-31.
4. Wolf AS, Daniel J, Sugarbaker DJ. Surgical techniques for multimodality treatment of malignant pleural mesothelioma: extrapleural pneumonectomy and pleurectomy/decortications. Semin Thorac Cardiovasc Surg. 2009;21(2):132-48.
5. Cao CQ, Yan TD, Bannon PG, et al. A systematic review of extrapleural pneumonectomy for malignant pleural mesothelioma. J Thorac Oncol. 2010;5(10):1692-703.
6. Baldini EH, Recht A, Strauss GM, et al. Patterns of failure after trimodality therapy for malignant pleural mesothelioma. Ann Thorac Surg. 1997;63(2):334-8.
7. Sugarbaker DJ, Flores RM, Jaklitsch MT, et al. Resection margins, extrapleural nodal status, and cell type determine postoperative long-term survival in trimodality therapy of malignant pleural mesothelioma: results in 183 patients. J Thorac Cardiovasc Surg. 1999;117(1):54-63.
8. Flores RM, Pass HI, Seshan VE, et al. Extrapleural pneumonectomy versus pleurectomy/decortications in the surgical management of malignant pleural mesothelioma: results in 663 patients. J Thorac Cardiovasc Surg. 2008;135(3):620-6.

9. Baldini EH. Radiation therapy options for malignant pleural mesothelioma. Semin Thorac Cardiovasc Surg. 2009;21(2): 159-63.
10. Casper ES, Kelsen DP, Alcock NW, et al. Ip cisplatin in patients with malignant ascites: pharmacokinetic evaluation and comparison with the iv route. Cancer Treat Rep. 1983;67(3):235-8.
11. Rusch VW, Niedzwiecki D, Tao Y, et al. Intrapleural cisplatin and mitomycin for malignant mesothelioma following pleurectomy: pharmacokinetic studies. J Clin Oncol. 1992;10(6): 1001-6.
12. Rusch V, Saltz L, Venkatraman E, et al. A phase II trial of pleurectomy/decortication followed by intrapleural and systemic chemotherapy for malignant pleural mesothelioma. J Clin Oncol. 1994;12(6):1156-63.
13. Rice TW, Adelstein DJ, Kirby TJ, et al. Aggressive multimodality therapy for malignant pleural mesothelioma. Ann Thorac Surg. 1994;58(1):24-9.
14. Lee JD, Perez S, Wang HL, et al. Intrapleural chemotherapy for patients with incompletely resected malignant mesothelioma: the UCLA experience. J Surg Oncol. 1995;60(4):262-7.
15. Sauter ER, Langer C, Coia LR, et al. Optimal management of malignant mesothelioma after subtotal pleurectomy: revisiting the role of intrapleural chemotherapy and postoperative radiation. J Surg Oncol. 1995;60(2):100-5.
16. Colleoni M, Sartori F, Calabro F, et al. Surgery followed by intracavitary plus systemic chemotherapy in malignant pleural mesothelioma. Tumori. 1996;82(1):53-6.
17. Matsuzaki Y, Edagawa M, Shimizu T, et al. Intrapleural hyperthermic perfusion with chemotherapy increases apoptosis in malignant pleuritis. Ann Thorac Surg. 2004;78(5):1769-72.
18. Christophi C, Winkworth A, Muralihdaran V, et al. The treatment of malignancy by hyperthermia. Surg Oncol. 1998; 7(1-2):83-90.
19. Yellin A, Simansky DA, Paley M, et al. Hyperthermic pleural perfusion with cisplatin: early clinical experience. Cancer. 2001;92(8):2197-203.
20. Monneuse O, Beaujard AC, Guibert B, et al. Long-term results of intrathoracic chemohyperthermia (ITCH) for the treatment of pleural malignancies. Br J Cancer. 2003;88(12):1839-43.
21. Van Ruth S, Baas P, Hass RL, et al. Cytoreductive surgery combined with intraoperative hyperthermic intrathoracic chemotherapy for stage I malignant pleural mesothelioma. Ann Surg Oncol. 2003;10(2):176-82.
22. Chang MY, Sugarbaker DJ. Innovative therapies: intraoperative intracavitary chemotherapy. Thorac Surg Clin. 2004; 14(4):549-56.
23. Richards WG, Zellos L, Bueno R, et al. Phase I to II study of pleurectomy/decortication and intraoperative intracavitary hyperthermic cisplatin lavage for mesothelioma. J Clin Oncol. 2006;24(10):1561-7.
24. Zellos L, Richards WG, Capalbo L, et al. A phase I study of extrapleural pneumonectomy and intracavitary intraoperative hyperthermic cisplatin with amifostine cytopretection for malignant pleural mesothelioma. J Thorac Cardiovasc Surg. 2009;137(2):453-8.
25. Tilleman TR, Richards WG, Zellos L, et al. Extrapleural pneumonectomy followed by intracavitary intraoperative hyperthermic cisplatin with pharmacologic cytoprotection for treatment of malignant pleural mesothelioma: a phase II prospective study. J Thorac Cardiovasc Surg. 2009;138(2):405-11.
26. Vogelzang NJ, Rusthoven JJ, Symanowski J, et al. Study of pemetrexed in combination with cysplatin alone in patients with malignant pleural mesothelioma. J Clin Oncol. 2003;21(14):2636-44.
27. van Sandick JW, Kappers I, Baas P, et al. Surgical treatment in the management of malignant pleural mesothelioma: a single institution's experience. Ann Surg Oncol. 2008;15(6):1757-64.
28. Aziz T, Jilaihawi A, Prakash D. The management of malignant pleural mesothelioma; single centre experience in 10 years. Eur J Cardiothorac Surg. 2002;22(2):298-305.
29. Jackman DM. Current options for systemic therapy in mesothelioma. Semin Thorac Cardiovasc Surg. 2009;21(2):154-8.
30. Nakahara K, Ohno K, Hashimoto J, et al. Thymoma: results with complete resection and adjuvant postoperative irradiation in 141 consecutive patients. J Thorac Cardiovasc Surg. 1988; 95(6):1041-7.
31. Pitch A, Chiarle R, Chiusa L, et al. Long-term survival of thymoma patients by histologic patterns and proliferative activity. Am J Surg Pathol. 1995;19(8):918-26.

10

Thermal Ablation of Lung Tumors and Pulmonary Metastases

Chaitan K. Narsule, Benedict D.T. Daly, Hiran C. Fernando

INTRODUCTION

Lung cancer is the most common cause of cancer-related deaths among both men and women in the United States.[1] Pulmonary resection is the treatment of choice for early-stage tumors, offering the best chance of cure for NSCLC. Sadly, many patients have advanced disease at the time of diagnosis, and others with potentially resectable early-stage disease may have medical conditions or poor pulmonary functions which preclude resection. It has been reported that over one-fifth of all patients diagnosed with stage I or stage II NSCLC do not undergo resection.[2] As a result, lung cancer is the number one cause of cancer-related deaths among both men and women in the United States.

The 1995 Lung Cancer Study Group report established lobar resection as the preferred operation for early-stage NSCLC, owing to a three-fold increase in the rate of local recurrence for patients treated with sublobar resection compared to lobectomy in that study.[3] For this reason, most surgeons perform wedge resection or only segmentectomy in those patients who are deemed to be high risk to undergo lobectomy, but are still able to tolerate general anesthesia and limited resection. Local recurrence following resection usually occurs within the first 2 years after surgery and can vary between 17% and 24%.[3,4]

While external beam radiation therapy is an alternative treatment option to surgery for local control in patients with limited disease who are too high risk for resection, survival with this approach has been poor. One study from Duke University on 156 patients treated for stage I NSCLC with radiotherapy alone, reported 2-year and 5-year survival rates of 39% and 13% respectively.[5] Also, a 2003 report by Qiao and associates reviewed 18 studies regarding radiotherapy for stage I NSCLC and suggested a mean 3-year and 5-year overall survival of 34% and 21% respectively.[6]

More recently, percutaneous thermal ablation has been increasingly used for the treatment of lung tumors, and results appear to be superior to standard external beam radiation. Thermal ablation can be performed using either radiofrequency or microwave energy and is commonly reported as radiofrequency ablation (RFA) or microwave ablation (MWA). The evolution of thermal ablation for the treatment of lung tumors has its origins in the initial use of RFA and MWA in managing hepatic tumors.[7,8] RFA and MWA for the treatment of lung tumors were first reported in 2000[9] and 2002[10] respectively.

This review provides an overview of the technique, indications and current results of thermal ablation.

RADIOFREQUENCY ABLATION

Technique

Radiofrequency ablation is the most common thermal ablative technique used for the treatment of tumors, and utilizes an energy source that generates an alternating current with a frequency that is less than 30 MHz (most commercially available generators for medical use function in the 375–500 kHz range). In this technique, a probe is placed within a tumor and it functions as an active electrode. Additionally, grounding pads (i.e. "Bovie" pads) are placed on the patient and function as dispersive electrodes. As the RF energy moves from the active electrode to the dispersive electrode, and then back to the active electrode, ions within the tissue oscillate as they attempt to follow the change in the direction of the alternating current. Frictional heating occurs within the tissue, and as the temperature within the tissue rises beyond 60°C, cell death occurs and a region of coagulation necrosis forms around the active electrode.

The ability to heat lung tissue to a lethal temperature in a specific location with minimal damage to the surrounding tissue is a key advantage of this technique. Radiofrequency energy is effectively applied to the lung tumor because the surrounding alveolar air acts as an insulator, concentrating the thermal energy within the ablation volume. One issue with thermal ablation is that, for tumors being ablated in close proximity to a large blood vessel within the lung, the blood flow within the vessel can act as a heat sink, dissipating heat from the normal lung tissue and limiting the therapeutic ablation margin. This latter effect could be either advantageous or undesirable; while it can protect those blood vessels from injury, a limited therapeutic margin may lead to incomplete ablation and increased local recurrence following ablation.

Available Devices

Currently, three systems approved by Food and Drug Administration (FDA) are available in the United States: (i) Boston Scientific; (ii) Angiodynamics (formerly RITA Medical) and (iii) ValleyLab systems. Figures 1A to D show examples of the different types of probes associated with each system. The Boston Scientific device is an impedance-based device that uses a probe (Fig. 1C) containing multiple tines that are expanded within the tumor being ablated. The tines curve backward toward the main shaft of the device, thus the probe is initially positioned at deep aspect of the nodule and repositioned by withdrawal as necessary. Once activated, the tumor is slowly heated as power is increased at 1-minute intervals. Electrical conduction of the ablated tissue becomes progressively limited as coagulation necrosis sets in, and the resultant significant rise in impedance serves as the endpoint of treatment, signifying that the tumor has been ablated.

The Angiodynamics (RITA) system is a temperature-based device that also uses a probe containing multiple, expandable tines deployed at 1 cm intervals until the target diameter is reached (Fig. 1A). The tines are oriented forward and lateral to the shaft and, for this reason, this probe is deployed near the superficial margin of the tumor. At each deployed size, the tumor is heated to a temperature of 90°C. Thermostats at the end of alternating tines allow for real-time temperature monitoring, and the system continues to heat the tumor until the target temperature is reached.

The ValleyLab system is an impedance-based device that uses a probe (Fig. 1B), consisting of a single needle or a cluster of three parallel needles (without expandable tines) which can also measure the temperature during ablation. Because the probe is infused with cold water to prevent charring around the probe during tumor ablation, it is often referred to as the "cool-tip" probe.

Studies Establishing Safety and Efficacy

Animal models have established the efficacy and feasibility of this technique in lung tissue. In 1996, Goldberg and colleagues[11] reported their experience with RFA in a rabbit model. In their study, VX2 sarcoma cell suspensions were injected into the lungs of eleven rabbits. Subsequently, the tumors of seven rabbits were treated with RFA and the remaining four rabbits were left untreated for control. Computed tomography (CT) imaging performed on the treated subjects demonstrated evidence of coagulation necrosis surrounding the tumor which was manifested by increased opacity enveloping the tumor. This was followed by central tissue attenuation with peripheral hyperattenuation surrounding the treated site. Histologic analysis demonstrated that 95% of the tumor nodules were necrotic, although some rabbits (43%) had residual tumor nests at the periphery of the tumor.

Also, in 2001, Miao et al. reported their experience in which VX2 tumor tissue was implanted in the lungs of 18 rabbits, 12 of which underwent RFA and 6 of which were control subjects.[12] Complete tumor eradication was accomplished with RFA in 33%, and a partial response was seen in 41.6% of rabbits that survived longer than

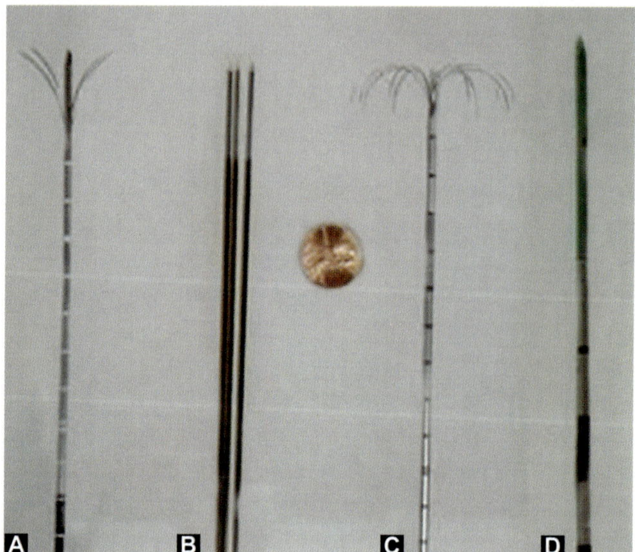

Figures 1A to D Commercially available RFA and MWA probes: (A) RITA Talon RF electrode; (B) ValleyLab Cool-tip cluster RF electrode; (C) Boston Scientific LeVeen RF electrode and (D) ValleyLab MW antenna

(*Source*: Image courtesy of Dr Damian Dupuy)

3 months. On histopathological evaluation, the ablated lesion retained its tissue architecture but had evidence of coagulation necrosis with surrounding edema and inflammation. After 1–3 months of treatment, the ablated tumor became an atrophied nodule of coagulation necrosis within a fibrotic capsule.

In order to evaluate the efficacy of the ablation, some investigators have performed RFA followed by resection. In one such "ablate and resect" study of 15 patients, ablation was possible in 13 cases.[13] The median tumor kill was 70% and, in seven patients, 100% ablation was achieved. Additionally, Nguyen and colleagues reported another study in which supravital staining was used to assess tumor cell viability.[14] In seven tumors, over 80% non-viability was demonstrated. In three tumors which were less than 2 cm in diameter, non-viability was 100%. A factor in this study was that ablations were only performed with 3 cm or 3.5 cm active electrodes, which may have been inadequate for larger tumors. Still, this study demonstrated that, while RFA can effectively destroy tumors, 100% ablation is not guaranteed in every case. For this reason, resection should be performed preferentially whenever possible.

MICROWAVE ABLATION

Technique and Available Devices

Microwave ablation is an even more recent development in the ablative treatment of lung tumors and pulmonary metastases. Commercially available microwave generators for medical use operate in the 900–2,450 MHz range. The mechanism of MWA involves the frictional heating of water molecules in tissue. After probe insertion and activation of the device, polar water molecules in the tissue around the probe spin as a result of their interaction with the rapidly alternating electromagnetic field, generating heat and eventually causing localized cell death and tissue necrosis. MWA may offer advantages over RFA because it does not depend on current flow or thermal conduction and is not limited by charring or boiling of the tissue. Thus, MWA may destroy tumors at higher temperatures than RFA with a potentially larger zone of ablation in a shorter timeframe.

Currently, the ValleyLab evident system is the only device approved by the FDA for MWA that is commercially available in the United States. It uses a 915 MHz generator with a straight antenna that has a 3.7 cm active tip (Fig. 1D). While there are no expandable tines with this device, the ablation volume can be increased by using up to three ablation antennas in parallel to achieve planar ablation. Other systems that have recently received 510(k) premarketing clearance from the FDA include the MicroThermX-100 (BSD Medical, Salt Lake City, UT), the MedWaves system (MedWaves, San Diego, CA), the Certus 140 (Neuwave Medical, Madison, WI), the Acculis Accu2i system (Microsulis Medical Ltd. Denmead, UK) and the Amica system (HS Medical, Boca Raton, FL).

In 2005, Wright and colleagues reported their study comparing MWA to RFA (specifically, the RITA system) in a hepatic porcine model.[15] Nineteen pigs were sacrificed at 0, 2 and 28 days following ablation. In order to assess the influence of vascular convection (the "heat sink" effect) on the efficacy of ablation, the investigators measured the diameters of ablation zones near a blood vessel as well as the diameters of ablation zones at the blood vessel, and determined the percentage difference which was deemed to be the "deflection score". In comparing MWA to RFA, the deflection score (3.6% and 17% respectively) was statistically significant ($P < 0.02$). Additionally, MWA resulted in ablation zones that were significantly larger in the long axis compared with RFA (3.6 cm to 2.2 cm, $P < 0.01$). However, this may have been related to the use of an MWA probe with a longer (3.6 cm) active tip compared to the RFA probe which had a 3 cm active deployment.

Patient Selection

Table 1 outlines the criteria for using thermal ablation for the management of NSCLC or metastases. For

Table 1 Criteria for using thermal ablation in the treatment of NSCLC or pulmonary metastases

Inclusion criteria	*Exclusion criteria*
1. Stage I or II* NSCLC in poor surgical candidate	1. Tumor next to hilum or large pulmonary vessel
2. Stages I-IV NSCLC with solitary pulmonary nodule persisting after standard therapies in poor surgical candidate	2. Malignant effusion
3. Limited pulmonary metastases with controlled or controllable primary cancer in poor surgical candidate	3. Pulmonary hypertension
4. Target lesion 5 cm or less	4. More than three tumors in one lung
	5. Tumor greater than 5 cm

*As N1 nodal disease is not treatable with thermal ablation, additional therapy is required for these patients. Patients with N1 disease have stage II NSCLC.

Chapter 10

NSCLC, thermal ablation should be considered for patients with early-stage disease who are not candidates for lobectomy, and for whom a sublobar resection may be too risky a procedure, or who refuse resection of any type. Traditionally, this same group of patients would have been treated with external beam radiation. Other potential candidates include patients who have previously undergone resection and developed a recurrent ipsilateral tumor which would be more challenging to resect, and patients who have been managed with definitive chemotherapy and/or radiation but have either a persistent isolated focus of cancer or recurrence that is amenable to ablation.

Thermal ablation is also a useful option for patients with limited pulmonary metastases. Appropriate candidates ideally meet the following criteria:[16,17]

- The patient is an unsuitable candidate for resection.
- All tumor lesions are small in diameter.
- Tumor lesions are not abutting mediastinal structures.
- The primary tumor has been controlled or is controllable.
- There are a limited number of metastases.

Preferably, patients should have experienced a long disease-free interval from the primary tumor resection and have disease that is isolated to the chest.[18] As with NSCLC, resection should generally be considered as first-line therapy for the metastases.

Occasionally, there will be cases in which, at the time of operation, it becomes obvious that complete resection of all of the metastases may not be possible. For example, a patient may be found to have a second central nodule identified at the time of a wedge resection for a peripheral metastasis. The use of thermal ablation, in this instance, may avoid the need for a larger resection such as a lobectomy or pneumonectomy. As a general principle, one goal when resecting pulmonary metastases is to spare lung tissue as it is possible that patients will develop further disease and may require repeat resection. This approach differs from that for NSCLC where lobar resection is the standard treatment.

ABLATION TECHNIQUE

Although initial experience with thermal ablation involved an open thoracotomy, the preferred approach for thermal ablation of lung tumors is under computed tomographic guidance. This method is minimally invasive and well-tolerated by the high-risk patients who are considered for this therapy. While procedures can be performed with local anesthesia and moderate sedation, the use of general anesthesia allows for multiple needle deployments, ablations, biopsies, and pleural catheter placements (if needed) with no discomfort to the patient. We have also found this approach to allow for excellent control of the airway, which is particularly helpful in treating patients with severe emphysema who are often unable to lay flat for a prolonged period of time, and are at increased risk should a pneumothorax develop.

Determination of the Treatment Response

Determining whether local control of tumor has been achieved is challenging after thermal ablation. Following treatment, a residual mass remains and it can be difficult to determine whether this represents a post-ablation scar, incomplete tumor ablation or local recurrence. Due to the many factors which can lead to incomplete tumor ablation, it is necessary that all patients treated with thermal ablation also agree in advance to long-term surveillance imaging to detect interval changes.

Immediately after thermal ablation, CT imaging most commonly shows the treated lesion with evidence of wrinkling due to vaporization at its margin, surrounded by concentric rings of variable density which represent a thermal gradient between the lesion and the surrounding normal parenchyma, sometimes referred to as a "cockade phenomenon".[19] Also, it may appear as a rim of ground-glass opacity, and it persists after treatment for 1–3 months. Because of this inflammatory response, the mass initially appears larger and subsequently decreases in size with time (Figs 2A to C). These lesions also sometimes demonstrate

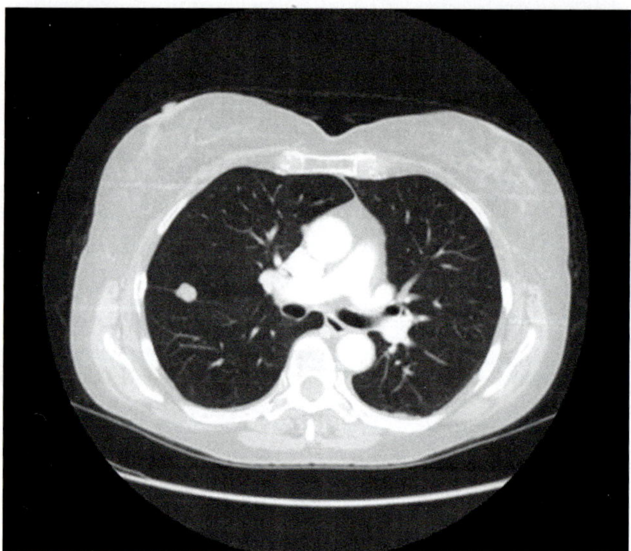

Figure 2A Preoperative image—right lung lesion

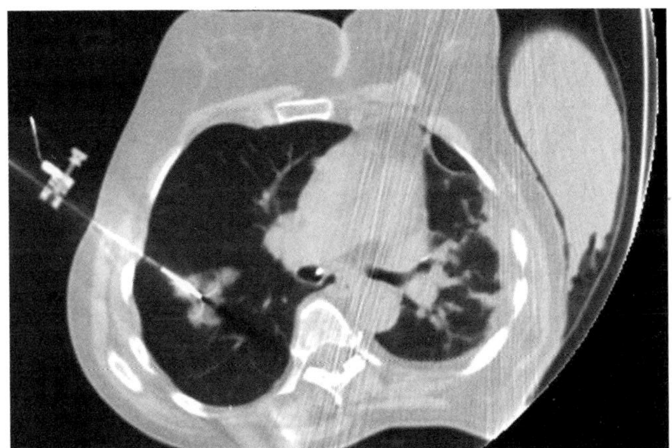

Figure 2B Intraoperative image—LeVeen RFA probe deployed into tumor

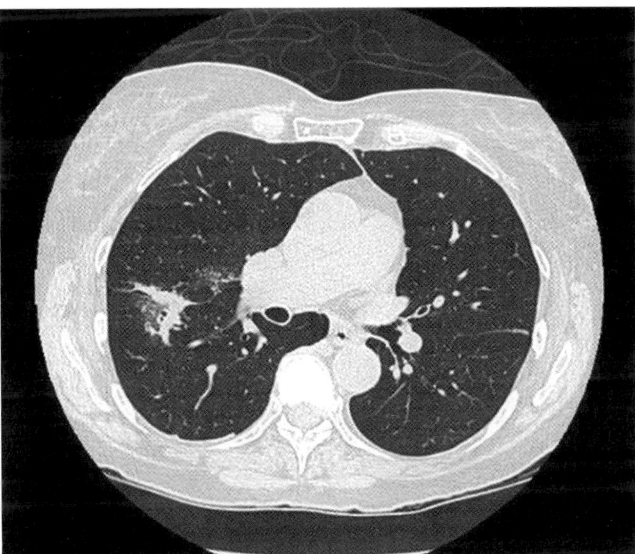

Figure 2C Postoperative changes 24 hours after treatment

central cavitation and develop bubble lucencies, suggesting that the ablation was effective at destroying the lesion. In one report of 32 nodules treated with RFA, 64% of the lesions increased in size, 32% remained unchanged and 4% decreased in size 1 month after treatment.[20] Cavitation was also seen in 31% of lesions within the first 3 months following treatment, and occurred more commonly in larger lesions.

For surveillance, protocols at many centers use CT densitometry to detect local progression, recurrence or persistent disease.[21] This approach is particularly useful for patients with single tumor disease. CT densitometry involves acquiring images of the ablated lesion at 0, 45, 180 and 300 second intervals following the administration of intravenous contrast, and tabulating the change in enhancement of the lesion in terms of Hounsfield units (HU). Intravenous contrast allows the physician to differentiate between non-enhancing ablated tissue and enhancing hypervascular tissue which could represent a viable residual tumor. A lesion that is greater than 9 mm in size, which enhances at greater than or equal to 15 HU over baseline at 1 minute, is considered to be suspicious for cancer. In 2003, Suh and colleagues reported their experience of treating 19 lung tumors with RFA in twelve patients and demonstrated that, at 3-months following treatment, successfully ablated lesions had only minimal contrast enhancement on follow-up CT densitometry which was significantly below the mean pretreatment contrast enhancement levels.[22] It is thought that the decrease in the mean contrast enhancement on follow-up imaging of treated lesions is due to local vascular destruction resulting from the thermal ablation. Therefore, any nodular enhancement that increases on follow-up imaging is very concerning for residual cancer.

Surveillance imaging which involves F-fluorodeoxyglucose positron emission tomography (FDG-PET)[18] is useful; although in practice, FDG-PET is never the only imaging modality used due to its low resolution and the early as well as intense FDG uptake that often occurs because of the inflammatory reaction associated with the newly treated lesion. This is typically seen at the periphery of the treated lesion, and is most prominent within the first month. Akeboshi and colleagues have demonstrated that, following successful ablation of malignant lung lesions, there is disappearance of FDG uptake on follow-up PET imaging.[23] Interestingly, areas of residual or recurrent cancer were observed on the periphery of the zone of ablation, with the focus on FDG uptake corresponding to a punctate or crescentic shape on PET imaging.

Moreover, a modification of the response evaluation criteria in solid tumors (RECIST) is an alternate method for surveillance.[24] In this approach, surveillance CT scans are obtained at 3-month intervals, and whenever possible PET scans are also acquired to determine the response to ablation. The modified RECIST criteria are summarized in Table 2.

Results of Clinical Trials

Radiofrequency Ablation

Table 3 summarizes several reports from the past decade focused on RFA for treating primary lung tumors or pulmonary metastases.

Table 2 Modified RECIST criteria

Response	*CT mass size*	*CT mass quality*	*PET*
Complete (two of the following)	Lesion disappearance (scar) less than 25% of original size	Cyst/cavity formation; low density of entire lesion	SUV < 2.5
Partial (one of the following)	More than 30% decrease in the LD of target lesion	Central necrosis or central cavitation with liquid density	Decreased SUV or area of FDG uptake
Stable lesion (one of the following)	Less than 30% decrease in the LD of the target lesion	Mass solid appearance, no central necrosis or cavitation	Unchanged SUV or area of FDG uptake
Progression (two of the following)	Increase of more than 20% in the LD of target lesion	Solid mass, invasion adjacent structures	Higher SUV or larger area of FDG uptake

(**Abbreviations:** LD = Largest diameter of the lesion; FDG = fluorodeoxyglucose; SUV = standardized uptake value of fluorodeoxyglucose)

For the treatment of NSCLC, many reports in the literature demonstrate the efficacy of RFA in selected patients. A 2007 report by Pennathur et al. described outcomes of RFA in 19 high-risk patients with stage I NSCLC.[29] With a mean follow-up of 29 months, local progression had occurred in 42% of all nodules with a median time to progression at 27 months. The probability of overall survival at 1 year was estimated to be 95%.

In that same year, Simon and colleagues reported their experience with RFA in a subgroup of 116 patients who had primary NSCLC.[30] The overall 1-, 2-, 3-, 4- and 5-year survival rates for stage I NSCLC were 78%, 57%, 36%, 27% and 27% respectively. Also in the following year, Lencioni and associates reported the RAPTURE study—a multicenter, prospective, intention-to-treat, single arm clinical trial of 106 medically inoperable patients (NSCLC, N = 33; colorectal metastases, N = 53; other primary malignancies, N = 20) with 183 lung tumors of 3–5 cm diameter or smaller that were treated by RFA.[31] For those patients with NSCLC, overall survival was 70% at 1 year and 48% at 2 years. Interestingly, for stage I NSCLC patients (N = 13), a 2-year overall survival of 75% and cancer-specific survival of 92% was observed.

For pulmonary metastases, the preliminary results were very encouraging. In 2006 and 2007, Yan and colleagues reported their outcomes of 55 medically inoperable patients with pulmonary metastases from colorectal cancer treated with RFA.[32,33] The local recurrence rate was 38% with a median overall survival of 33 months, and actuarial 1-, 2- and 3-year survival rates of 85%, 64% and 46% respectively were demonstrated. The RAPTURE trial also studied the outcomes of RFA in 53 patients

Table 3 Studies evaluating the clinical outcomes of RFA treatment

Year	*Reference*	*# of pts*	*Pathology*	*Duration (F/U)*	*Outcome results*	
2003	Herrera et al.[26]	18	NSCLC and metastases	Mean: 6 months	Radiographic response in 66% for lesions < 5 cm	
2004	Gadaleta et al.[20]	18	NSCLC and metastases	Median: 8 months	No progression in 94.4% of patients	
2005	Fernando et al.[25]	18	NSCLC	Median: 14 months	Local progression: 38% of lesions. Median PFI: 17.6 Months	
2006	Ambrogi et al.[27]	54	NSCLC and metastases	Mean: 23.7 months	Median local PFI: 24.1 months.	
2006	Hiraki et al.[28]	128	Primary lung and mets	Median: 12 months	Local progression: 27%.	
2007	Pennathur et al.[29]	19	Stage I NSCLC	Mean: 29 months Local progression: 42% Median time to local progression: 27 months	Overall survival at 1 year: 95%. Median survival: NR	
2007	Simon et al.[30]	153	NSCLC and mets	Median: 27.5 months	Overall 1-, 2-, 3-, 4-, 5-year survival for NSCLC: 78%, 57%, 36%, 27% and 27%. For colorectal lung mets: 83%, 64%, 57%, 57% and 57%	
2008	Lencioni et al.[31]	106	Lung cancer and mets	Mean: 15 months	Overall 2-year survival: 48–66%	(Overall 2-year survival for stage I NSCLC: 75%)

with pulmonary metastases from colorectal cancer, and demonstrated overall 1- and 2-year survival rates of 89% and 66% respectively in this subgroup.[31] Moreover, Simon and colleagues reported the outcomes of RFA in 73 patients with pulmonary metastases from colorectal cancer, and they observed overall 1-, 2-, 3-, 4- and 5-year survival rates of 87%, 78%, 57%, 57% and 57% respectively.[30] Interestingly, these results seem to be very similar to those reported after metastasectomy. Thus, in the future, it may be reasonable to consider a study comparing these two approaches for pulmonary metastases.

Microwave Ablation

Compared with RFA, reports of outcomes involving MWA for the treatment of lung tumors and metastases are limited. In 2002, Feng and colleagues published their experience in using MWA for the treatment of 20 patients with lung cancer (N = 8) or metastases (N = 12).[11] After a 24 month follow-up, 80% of the patients were alive. There was an overall response rate of 57.1% and no complications were observed. More recently, Wolf and colleagues reported their experience in treating 82 tumors in 50 patients (NSCLC, N = 27; small cell lung cancer, N = 3; metastases, N = 20).[34] With a mean follow-up of 10 months, 26% had residual disease at the ablation site and an additional 22% had recurrent disease. A 1-year local recurrence rate of 67% was observed, with a mean time to first recurrence at 16.2 months. For this series, actuarial 1-, 2- and 3-year survival rates were 65%, 55% and 45% respectively, and cancer-specific 1-, 2- and 3-year survival rates were 83%, 73% and 61% in the same order. Moreover, cavitation was statistically associated with reduced cancer-specific mortality.

COMPLICATIONS OF LUNG ABLATION

Morbidity after ablation is relatively low, which is important considering that these patients usually have significant baseline comorbidities. Because the lung is the target of intervention, mild fevers and coughs producing brown sputum may occur for up to the first 2 weeks following treatment. Also, small pleural effusions have been known to develop and can be managed without drainage in most cases. Hemoptysis and pulmonary parenchymal hemorrhage are also infrequent, although two cases of massive pulmonary hemorrhage following RFA have been reported.[26,35]

Pneumothorax can occur in 20–35% of the RFA cases, and approximately 6–16% require evacuation with a catheter. It is thought that the higher rate of pneumothorax with RFA as opposed to needle biopsy of the lung is due to the larger size of the electrode (14–17 gauge) as compared to the biopsy needle (20 gauge). Targeting lesions by choosing the shortest path possible between the skin and the lesion while avoiding bulla can help minimize the technical risk. In almost all cases, chest tubes or pigtail catheters can be removed within twenty four hours.

Table 4 Types and frequencies of complication of thermal ablation of the lung

Types	Frequencies
Pneumothorax requiring chest tube or aspiration	0–54% (most < 20%)
Pneumonia	0–22%
Exacerbation of chronic obstructive pulmonary disease	0–6%
Acute respiratory distress syndrome	0–3%
Pulmonary abscess	0–6%
Hemoptysis	0–12%
Hemothorax	0–2%
Pleural effusion requiring drainage	0–4%
Parenchymal hemorrhage	0–1%
Death	4 case reports[36,37]
Bronchopleural fistula	1 case report
Acute renal failure	1 case report
Vocal cord paralysis	1 case report
Atrial fibrillation	1 case report
Pulmonary embolus	1 case report
Third-degree skin burn	1 case report
Stroke	1 case report
Tumor tract seeding	1 case report

(*Source:* This table is adapted from Rose SC, Thistlewaite PA, Sewell PE, et al. Lung cancer and radiofrequency ablation. J Vasc Interv Radiol. 2006;17:927-51)[37]

Other complications include pneumonia, exacerbation of chronic obstructive pulmonary disease, abscess, embolization and skin burns. The frequencies of these complications are listed in Table 4.

CONCLUSION

Thermal ablation is a safe and effective option for the treatment of primary lung cancer and pulmonary metastases. While surgery should always be considered as first-line treatment for local control, RFA and MWA are reasonable alternatives in patients who are considered high-risk for an operation. In these cases, thermal ablation can achieve local control with results that are superior to external beam radiation therapy.

REFERENCES

1. Jemal A, Siegel R, Xu J, et al. Cancer statistics. CA Cancer J Clin. 2010;60(5):277-300.
2. Bach PB, Cramer LD, Warren JL, et al. Racial differences in the treatment of early-stage lung cancer. N Eng J Med. 1999;341(16):1198-1205.
3. Ginsberg RJ, Rubenstein LV. Randomized trial of lobectomy versus limited resection for T1N0 non-small cell lung cancer. Lung Cancer Study Group. Ann Thorac Surg. 1995;60(3): 615-22.
4. Warren WH, Faber LP. Segmentectomy versus lobectomy in patients with stage I pulmonary carcinoma. J Thorac Cardiovasc Surg. 1994;107:1087-94.
5. Landreneau RJ, Sugarbaker DJ, Mack MJ, et al. Wedge resection versus lobectomy for stage I (T1 N0 M0) non-small-cell lung cancer. J Thorac Cardiovasc Surg. 1997;113(4):691-8.
6. Sibley GS, Jamieson TA, Marks LB, et al. Radiotherapy alone for medically inoperable stage I non-small-cell lung cancer: the Duke experience. Int J Radiat Oncol Biol Phys. 1998;40(1):149-54.
7. Qaio X, Tullgren O, Lax I, et al. The role of radiotherapy in the treatment of stage I non-small lung cancer. Lung Cancer. 2003;41(1):1-11.
8. Curley SA, Izzo F, Delrio P, et al. Radiofrequency ablation of unresectable primary and metastatic hepatic malignancies: results in 123 patients. Ann Surg. 1999;230(1):1-8.
9. Lu MD, Chen JW, Xie XY, et al. Hepatocellular carcinoma: US-guided percutaneous microwave coagulation therapy. Radiology. 2001;221(1):167-72.
10. Dupuy DE, Zagoria RJ, Akerley W, et al. Percutaneous radiofrequency ablation of malignancies in the lung. AJR Am J Roentgenol. 2000;174(1):57-9.
11. Feng W, Liu W, Li C, et al. Percutaneous microwave coagulation therapy for lung cancer. Zhonghua Zhong Liu Za Zhi. 2002;24(4):388-90.
12. Goldberg SN, Gazelle GS, Compton CC, et al. Radiofrequency tissue ablation of VX2 tumor nodules in the rabbit lung. Acad Radiol. 1996;3(11):929-35.
13. Miao Y, Ni Y, Bosmans H, et al. Radiofrequency ablation for eradication of pulmonary tumor in rabbits. J Surg Res. 2001;99(2):265-71.
14. Yang S, Whyte R, Askin F, et al. Radiofrequency ablation of primary and metastatic lung tumors: analysis of an ablate and resect study. Presented at the American Association of Thoracic Surgery 82nd Annual Meeting, 2002.
15. Nguyen CL, Scott WJ, Young NA, et al. Radiofrequency ablation of primary lung cancer: results from an ablate and resect pilot study. Chest. 2005;128(5):3507-11.
16. Wright AS, Sampson LA, Warner TF, et al. Radiofrequency versus microwave ablation in a hepatic porcine model. Radiology. 2005;236(1):132-9.
17. Ketchedjian A, Daly B, Luketich J, et al. Minimally invasive techniques for managing pulmonary metastases: video-assisted thoracic surgery and radiofrequency ablation. Thorac Surg Clin. 2006;16(2):157-65.
18. Fernando HC, Ghulam A. Alternatives to surgical resection for non-small cell lung cancer. Pearson's Thoracic and Esophageal Surgery. Philadelphia: Churchill and Livingston; 2008. pp. 796-803.
19. Landreneau RJ, De Giacomo T, Mack MJ, et al. Therapeutic video-assisted thoracoscopic surgical resection of colorectal pulmonary metastases. Eu J Cardiothorac Surg. 2000;18(6): 671-6.
20. Gadaleta C, Mattioli V, Colucci G, et al. Radiofrequency ablation of 40 lung neoplasms: preliminary results. AJR Am J Roentgenol. 2004;183(2):361-8.
21. Bojarski JD, Dupuy DE, Mayo-Smith WW. CT imaging findings of pulmonary neoplasms after treatment with radiofrequency ablation: results in 32 tumors. AJR Am J Roentgenol. 2005;185(2):466-71.
22. Swensen SJ, Viggiano RW, Midthun DE, et al. Lung nodule enhancement at CT: a multicenter study. Radiology. 2000;214(1):73-80.
23. Suh RD, Wallace AB, Sheehan RE, et al. Unresectable pulmonary malignancies: CT-guided percutaneous radiofrequency ablation—preliminary results. Radiology. 2003; 229(3):821-9.
24. Akeboshi M, Yamakado K, Nakatsuka A, et al. Percutaneous radiofrequency ablation of lung neoplasms: initial therapeutic response. J Vasc Interv Radiol. 2004;15(5):463-70.
25. Fernando HC, De Hoyos A, Landreneau RJ, et al. Radiofrequency ablation for the treatment of non-small cell lung cancer in marginal surgical candidates. J Thorac Cardiovasc Surg. 2005;129(3):639-44.
26. Herrera LJ, Fernando HC, Perry Y, et al. Radiofrequency ablation of pulmonary malignant tumors in nonsurgical candidates. J Thorac Cardiovasc Surg. 2003;125(4):929-37.
27. Ambrogi MC, Lucchi M, Dini P, et al. Percutaneous radiofrequency ablation of lung tumours: results in the mid-term. Eur J Cardiothor Surg. 2006;30(1):177-83.
28. Hiraki T, Sakurai J, Tsuda T, et al. Risk factors for local progression after percutaneous radiofrequency ablation of lung tumors. Cancer. 2006;107:2873-80.
29. Pennathur A, Luketich JD, Abbas G, et al. Radiofrequency ablation for the treatment of stage I non-small cell lung cancer in high-risk patients. J Thorac Cardiovasc Surg. 2007;134: 857-64.
30. Simon CJ, Dupuy DE, DiPetrillo TA, et al. Pulmonary radiofrequency ablation: long-term safety and efficacy in 153 patients. Radiology. 2007;243:268-75.
31. Lencioni R, Crocetti L, Cioni R, et al. Response to radiofrequency ablation of pulmonary tumours: a prospective, intention-to-treat, multicentre clinical trial (the RAPTURE study). Lancet Oncol. 2008;9(7):621-8.
32. Yan TD, King J, Sjarif A, et al. Percutaneous radiofrequency ablation of pulmonary metastases from colorectal carcinoma: prognostic determinants for survival. Ann Surg Oncol. 2006; 13(11):1529-37.
33. Yan TD, King J, Sjarif A, et al. Treatment failure after percutaneous radiofrequency ablation for nonsurgical candidates with pulmonary metastases from colorectal carcinoma. Ann Surg Oncol. 2007;14(5):1718-26.
34. Wolf FJ, DiPetrillo TA, Machan JT, et al. Microwave ablation of lung malignancies: effectiveness, CT findings and safety in 50 patients. Radiology. 2008;247:871-9.
35. Vaughn C, Mychaskiw G 2nd, Sewell P. Massive hemorrhage during radiofrequency ablation of a pulmonary neoplasm. Anesth Analg. 2002;94(5):1149-51.
36. Steinke K, Sewell PE, Dupuy DE, et al. Pulmonary radiofrequency ablation—an international study survey. Anticancer Res. 2004;24(1):339-43.
37. Rose SC, Thistlewaite PA, Sewell PE, et al. Lung cancer and radiofrequency ablation. J Vasc Interv Radiol. 2006;17:927-51.

Section 4

Liver

11

Hepatic Arterial Infusion Pumps

Andrea Cercek, Nancy E. Kemeny

INTRODUCTION

In the majority of patients with metastatic colorectal cancer (CRC), treatment is limited to systemic chemotherapy. However, up to 20% of the patients develop liver-only disease. In this subset of patients, locoregional therapy that targets the liver can be pursued. In addition to systemic chemotherapy, possible treatment options in such patients are surgical and regional chemotherapy. A surgical approach is typically pursued in patients with a limited number of lesions, and can incorporate ablative measures such as radiofrequency ablation.[1-5] Despite excellent surgical techniques, the recurrence rates remain high. Hepatic arterial infusion (HAI) therapy refers to the delivery of chemotherapy directly into the liver parenchyma via the hepatic artery (HA). The rationale behind HAI therapy lies in the fact that the blood supply of CRC metastases comes from the HA[1] while the healthy liver parenchyma is supplied by the portal vein. Administration of chemotherapy via the HA therefore enables delivery of the drug to the malignant cells at a higher concentration. Infusion of chemotherapy via the HA has been compared with portal vein infusion in patients with CRC liver metastases. Patients were injected with radioactive 5-Fluoro-2-Deoxyuridine (FUDR) into either the portal vein or the HA. The tumors were removed and subsequently the tumor tissue drug concentration was measured.[6] Arterial administration of FUDR lead to fifteen times higher concentration over portal vein administration.

Hepatic arterial infusion therapy can be used in a presurgical or neoadjuvant approach to decrease tumor volume, and thereby convert some patients with unresectable disease to resectable as well as post-surgical or adjuvant treatment to eliminate microscopic disease, and decrease recurrence rates.

Hepatic arterial infusion therapy was first developed nearly 40 years ago and has evolved from monotherapy to the combination with modern systemic chemotherapeutic regimens to improve response rates and outcomes. This chapter reviews the pharmacological principles behind HAI drug selection, the toxicities associated with therapy and the efficacy of HAI therapy in metastatic CRC.

HEPATIC ARTERIAL INFUSION PUMP PLACEMENT

Evaluation of patients for HAI therapy includes CT arteriography to evaluate the presence of variant hepatic anatomy. The portal vein must be patent to avoid hepatic ischemia. After the placement of the pump, injection of macroaggregated albumin through the side port is done to ensure perfusion of the liver, and not extrahepatic perfusion.

The HAI pump is an implantable biocompatible titanium and silicone rubber disk. It is composed of a hollow cylinder divided into two chambers.[7] The bottom chamber contains fluid with fluorocarbon and is sealed shut. The chemotherapy is inserted into the top chamber which connects to the catheter (Fig. 1). The fluorocarbon is converted to gas when heated to body temperature, thereby creating a constant gaseous pressure leading to a steady flow rate into the catheter at a given temperature. The top drug chamber is refillable via needle through a septum. A cycle of treatment with the pump lasts approximately 4–5 weeks. The chemotherapy infuses over 2 weeks. After 14 days, the pump reservoir is accessed and emptied of all remaining drug, and the pump is filled with heparin and saline which infuses over the next 2 weeks. The flow rate of the chemotherapy into the liver can be accelerated by both increased temperature, above 37°C and altitude, above sea level. If a patient develops fever or lives above sea level, the rate of infusion should

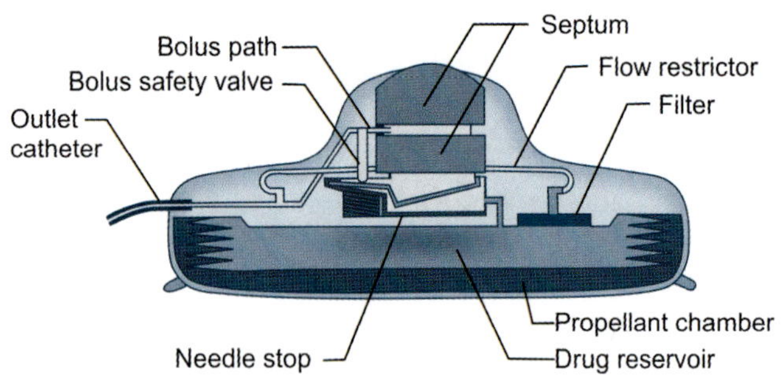

Figure 1 The Codman 3,000 series implantable pump

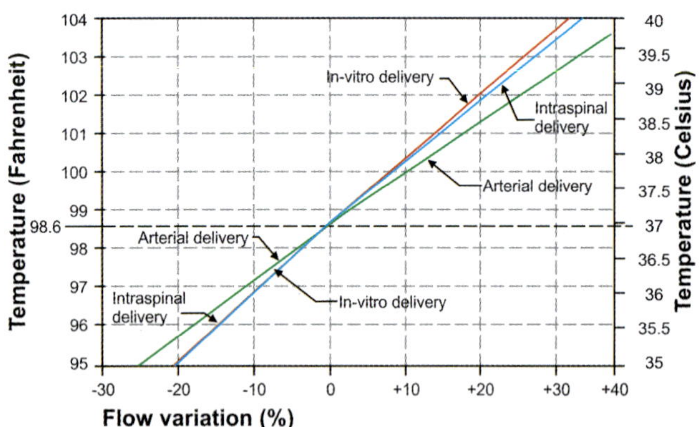

Figure 2 Variation in HAI flow rate as a function of temperature (© Codman pump)

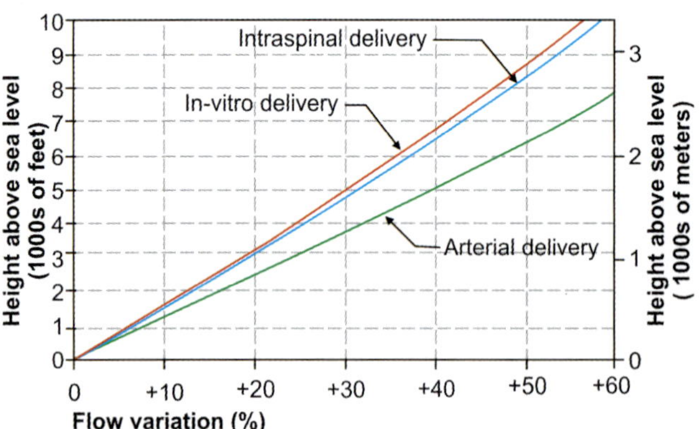

Figure 3 Variation in HAI flow rate as a function of altitude (© Codman pump 3)

be recalculated accordingly (Figs 2 and 3), and the dose should be adjusted.

The pump is placed in a subcutaneous pocket, usually in either the left or right lower quadrant (Fig. 4). The catheter is inserted into the gastroduodenal artery which has a lower rate of thrombosis than the placement directly into the HA.

The surgeon then ligates the right gastric artery and all of the blood vessels supplying the superior border of the stomach and duodenum to prevent perfusion of those structures. If the vessels are not ligated, perfusion with chemotherapy can lead to duodenitis, gastritis and

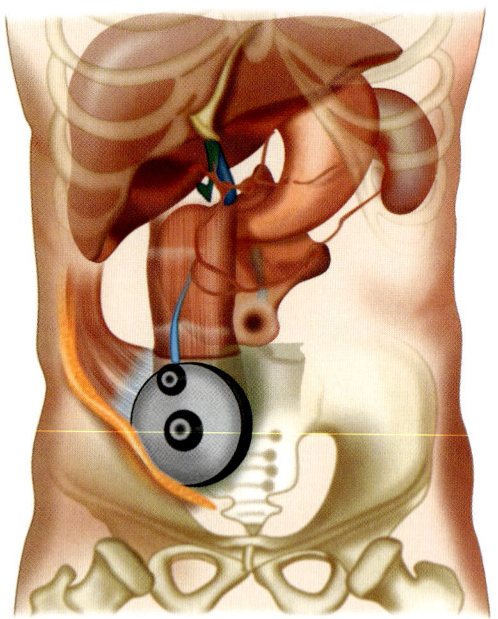

Figure 4 Implantable HAI pump

ulceration. The gallbladder is removed at the time of pump placement because in the early experience with the pump, it led to 30% of the patients getting acalculous cholecystitis if the gallbladder was not removed.

HEPATIC ARTERIAL INFUSION CATHETER RELATED COMPLICATIONS

Catheter related complications of HAI therapy include catheter erosion, displacement or arterial thrombosis or dissection.[7] A retrospective analysis of HAI pump placement reviewed 544 cases; found that the presence of variant anatomy, cannulation of a vessel other than the gastroduodenal artery and lack of an experienced surgeon were significant factors associated with increased risk of complications.[8] In this retrospective review, pump complications were seen in 22% of the patients. However, the majority of the early complications were salvaged in the first 30 days, and the incidence of pump failure was 9% at 1 year and 16% at 2 years (Table 1).

PHARMACOLOGICAL PRINCIPLES FOR DRUG SELECTION

$$\text{Advantage} = \frac{1 + \text{Total body clearance of a drug}}{\text{Hepatic artery flow rate}^*}$$

*(1 = Fraction of drug extracted across the liver)

A number of drug properties are important for selection of therapy for HAI. The overall goal of HAI therapy

Table 1 Catheter related complications

Pump malfunction
Pocket infection
Catheter thrombosis
Catheter displacement/erosion
Arterial thrombosis/dissection
Extrahepatic/incomplete perfusion

Table 2 Ideal drug properties for HAI

High hepatic extraction ratio
Short plasma half-life
High CLTB
First order kinetics
Dose dependant antitumor activity

is to obtain a high concentration of the drug within the liver with a minimal systemic effect.[9] This is achieved by agents that have a high hepatic extraction ratio and a short plasma half-life. The drug needs to be cleared quickly to avoid recirculating and causing systemic toxicity. Ideally, the drugs would have a high hepatic extraction ratio that remains constant at increased doses. This refers to the CL_{TB} which is the total body clearance of the drug, and reflects the rate of elimination relative to its plasma concentration. In drugs that have first order kinetics, the CL_{TB} remains constant regardless of the concentration. Therefore, the ideal drug for HAI exhibits a high CL_{TB} has a high first pass ratio, in addition to first order kinetics and a high hepatic extraction. The Collin's formula describes the advantage of locoregional administration of chemotherapy over systemic chemotherapy for a given drug based on total body clearance, HA flow rate and hepatic extraction[10] (Table 2).

The ideal agent should have dose dependent activity wherein increasing the dose leads to improved response. The advantage of locoregional therapy with HAI is the ability to increase the exposure of tumor cells to higher drug concentration above what is achievable with systemic therapy.

5-FLUORO-2-DEOXYURIDINE

5-Fluoro-2-Deoxyuridine is an antimetabolite which interferes with DNA replication by inhibiting thymidylate synthase (TS). It is a derivative of 5-Fluorouracil. FUDR has been shown to have an excellent first pass metabolism with a 94–99% extraction rate in the liver. The total body clearance is 15–25 mL/min. Intrahepatic FUDR levels have been compared with 5FU, and have been found to have a significant increase in hepatic exposure. Intrahepatic 5FU has a ten-fold increase in levels compared with systemic infusion whereas FUDR has a 100- to 400-fold increase.[11]

Several other agents have been tested for use in HAI. Among these are doxorubicin, mitomycin, cisplatin and BCNU. Although they demonstrated slightly increased response used via HAI, they did not have all of the advantages of FUDR.[12] More recently, oxaliplatin and irinotecan were tested in the regional therapy based on their benefit in the systemic setting. Irinotecan is metabolized in the liver, serum and small intestine to form the active metabolite SN38. Irinotecan lacks first pass metabolism, and pharmacokinetic studies of HA administration failed to show a significant difference in SN38 levels when administered via HA.[13,14] Similar studies of oxaliplatin, however, did show a pharmacokinetic advantage of HA administration.[15] This has led to the evaluation of HA oxaliplatin in a number of phase-II trials.[16-18] Abdominal pain was seen in a significant number of patients treated with HAI oxaliplatin. FUDR remains the single best drug in HAI despite the many studies utilizing other chemotherapeutic agents.

HAI-FUDR TOXICITIES AND MANAGEMENT

5-fluoro-2-deoxyuridine is cleared by the liver and, therefore, very little drug enters systemic circulation. Nausea, diarrhea, mucositis and hematologic toxicity are not seen after HAI-FUDR. Generally the toxicity is limited to hepatic toxicity associated with bile duct injury. Very careful liver function monitoring is required during therapy. Typically, the aspartate transaminase (AST) is the first to rise, and this is followed by a rise in alkaline phosphatase and bilirubin. Approximately 15–25% of the patients receiving HAI-FUDR will develop hyperbilirubinemia.[19] This occurs because of bile duct inflammation; secondary to exposure to high dose of chemotherapy.[20] The rise is usually transient and can be reversed with a short treatment break. In addition to a treatment break, dexamethasone can be added to the pump to decrease the inflammation.[21] In rare cases, this inflammation can lead to biliary sclerosis which mimics sclerosing cholangitis, and may require biliary stent placement. If there is elevation of liver functions or tests, imaging of the liver should be performed to evaluate metastatic lesions as the cause of biliary problems.

Table 3 outlines the recommended FUDR treatment modifications. In the event, FUDR is held due

Table 3 FUDR dose modification table

SGOT (at pump emptying or day of planned retreatment, whichever is higher)	*Reference value**	*FUDR dose (%)*
	0 to < 2 x reference value	100
	2 to < 3 x reference value	80
	3 to < 4 x reference value	50
	> 4 x reference value	Hold
ALK PHOS (at pump emptying or day of planned retreatment, whichever is higher)	0 to 1.2 x reference value	100
	1.2 to < 1.5 x reference value	50
	> 1.5 x reference value	Hold
TOT BILI (at pump emptying or day of planned retreatment, whichever is higher)	0 to 1.2 x reference value	100
	1.2 to < 1.5 x reference value	50
	> 1.5 x reference value	Hold

"Reference value" is the value obtained on the day the patient received last FUDR dose.
If SGOT > 4X reference value, ALK PHOS > 1.5X reference value, total bilirubin > 1.5X reference value, then treatment will be held and will not be reinstituted until values come down to more normal levels, as indicated in section "Resuming Treatment After Temporary Discontinuation".

to increased liver function tests (LFTs), dexamethasone (typically, 25 mg) can be infused to combat the inflammation.

TRIALS EVALUATING HAI-FUDR IN UNRESECTABLE METASTATIC CRC

The development of regional therapy for CRC has focused mainly on the use of FUDR; initially as a single agent and in the last decade, in combination with systemic chemotherapy. The early studies with FUDR in the HAI pump were notable for median response rates of 45%. These results led to several randomized trials comparing HAI-FUDR to systemic 5FU/LV. The results of ten separate randomized trials and three meta-analyses demonstrated an improvement in response rates of liver metastases with HAI-FUDR compared to systemic 5FU/LV. The response rates of HAI therapy ranged 42–64% versus 9–21%.[22-31]

Three randomized trials have been published since 2000. In the German Cooperative Group study, 168 patients with unresectable colorectal liver metastases were evaluated.[29] Fifty-seven patients were assigned to systemic infusional 5FU/LV, 57 to 5FU by HAI, and 54 to HAI-FUDR. The response rates were 19.7%, 45% and 43.2% respectively while the median survival was 17.6 months, 18.7 months and 12.7 months in the same order. The results of this study were disappointing; however, it should be noted that 31% of the patients in the HAI group did not receive HAI therapy as planned. The majority of the patients had HAI therapy administered via a port, and not an implantable pump. Enrollment in the study was terminated because of toxicities including biliary sclerosis; however, dose reductions for FUDR were not incorporated into the protocol and dexamethasone was not administered via HAI.

A second randomized study was performed by the EORTC/MRC group. In this study, 290 patients with unresectable liver metastases were randomized to IV 5FU/LV versus HAI 5FU/LV.[30] In this study, 37% of the patients assigned to HAI therapy did not receive treatment, and all the patients received HAI via a port. There was no improvement in progression-free survival, and the median overall survival was 14.7 months in the HAI group and 14.8 months in the IV group ($p = 0.79$).

In the CALGB study, 135 patients were randomized to HAI-FUDR plus LV and dexamethasone via a pump (not a port) versus systemic bolus 5FU/LV.[31] Cross-over was not permitted, and only 13% of the patients randomized to the HAI arm were not treated. The primary endpoint was survival, and this was achieved [(24.4 months versus 20 months for HAI and systemic 5FU/LV respectively ($p = 0.0034$)]. The systemic arm had an increased incidence of diarrhea, neutropenia and stomatitis ($p < 0.05$). The HAI arm had an increased incidence of biliary toxicity ($p < 0.001$), and 4 patients required biliary stenting. The response rates were 47% for HAI and 24% in the 5FU/LV group ($p = 0.012$).

More recently, a meta-analysis of the 10 randomized trials concluded that the evidence available currently does not support the use of fluoropyrimidine-based HAI alone for the treatment of patients with unresectable CRC liver metastases (at least as first-line therapy).[32] This was based on the conclusion that while there is a statistically significant improvement in response rates with HAI compared with systemic 5FU therapy (42.9% vs 18.4%

Table 4 Trials of HAI in combination with systemic chemotherapy in metastatic CRC

Trial	Number	Trial	Treatment	Response rate	Overall survival
Kemeny et al. 2001	46	Phase I	HAI-FUDR & IV irinotecan	74%	-----
Kemeny et al. 2005	36	Phase I	HAI-FUDR & IV oxaliplatin/5FU or HAI-FUDR & IV oxaliplatin/irinotecan	90% vs 87%	36 vs 22
Fiorentini et al. 2006	76	Randomized	HAI-FUDR vs HAI-FUDR & IV 5FU/LV	47.5 vs 41.7 P = 0.09	20 vs 14 P = 0.0033 (are you sure 20 vs 14 is correct)
Kemeny et al. 2009	49	Phase 1	HAI-FUDR & IV oxaliplatin & irinotecan	92%	50.8 (chemo naïve) 35 (pre-treated with chemo)
Gallagher et al. 2007	39	Retrospective	HAI-FUDR & IV irinotecan	44%	20.1

respectively; $p < 0.001$), there is no statistically significant median overall survival benefit (15.9 months vs 12.4 months in the same order; $p = 0.24$). Although this appears to be true, it should be noted that the majority of the studies were methodically flawed, and crossover was permitted from the HAI to the systemic group limiting the interpretation of the data. There were a number of other confounding factors such as underpowered studies and use of port instead of a pump in many of the studies.

Moreover, as advances have been made in systemic chemotherapy options with improved response rates and outcomes, studies evaluating HAI therapy have moved away from the use of FUDR alone to combination regimes in patients with liver only metastatic disease.

HAI IN COMBINATION WITH SYSTEMIC CHEMOTHERAPY IN UNRESECTABLE METASTATIC CRC

The first studies combining HAI-FUDR with systemic 5FU versus bolus 5FU alone demonstrated a significant improvement in overall survival, time to progression and response rates.[33]

More recently, HAI-FUDR has been studied in combination with modern systemic chemotherapy including oxaliplatin and irinotecan (Table 4). In a phase-I study of 46 previously treated patients with unresectable disease, the combination of HAI-FUDR/dex and systemic irinotecan was notable for a response rate of 74%, and a median overall survival of 20 months.[34] The combination was generally well tolerated, and the most common toxicities were diarrhea and neutropenia. A subsequent phase-I trial evaluated 36 patients with unresectable liver metastases. The patients were treated with HAI-FUDR/dex plus either oxaliplatin and irinotecan (IROX, group A) or FOLFOX (group B).[35] The response rates were 90% in group A and 87% in group B. The median survivals were 36 months and 22 months respectively despite the fact that 89% of the patients were previously treated. The grade-3 or grade-4 toxicities included diarrhea (24% and 20% in groups A and B respectively), neutropenia (10% and 7%), neurotoxicity (24% and 20%) and hyperbilirubinemia (> 3 mg/mL noted in 5% and 7%). With the exception of hyperbilirubinemia, the toxicities were attributable to systemic treatment.

In a third phase-I trial, 49 patients (53% of whom had previously received chemotherapy) were treated with HAI-FUDR/dx and IROX (oxaliplatin plus irinotecan). The results were notable for a response rate of 93% (100% in the treatment naïve group), and 47% of the patients were able to undergo liver resection.[36] It should be noted that the disease was initially unresectable. These patients were clearly unresectable with 98% having bilobar disease and 85% having tumors involving blood vessels. The median overall survival was 35 months in the previously treated patients, and 50.8 months in the chemotherapy naïve group. The most common grade 3/4 toxicities were diarrhea, transaminitis (elevation of ALK PHOS and AST), hyperbilirubinemia and neutropenia. The hepatic toxicities were manageable with appropriate dose reductions.

A phase-II study evaluated the addition of bevacizumab (Bev) to HAI-FUDR/dex plus systemic 5FU/LV with either oxaliplatin or irinotecan. The study was a prospective study to evaluate how many patients can get to resection. The study was closed early because the addition of Bev resulted in statistically significant increase in biliary stenosis. Only 24 patients received HAI plus systemic with Bev. The next 25 received HAI

Table 5 Randomized trials of adjuvant HAI post-resection of liver metastases

Trial	Number of patients	Treatment	Disease-free survival (median or %)	P-value	Overall survival	P-value
Lorenz 1998	226	HAI 5FU vs observation	14.2 vs 13.7	NS	34.5 vs 40.8	P = 0.1519
Kemeny 2002	109	HAI-FUDR & IV 5FU vs observation	46% vs 25% (4-year DFS)	P = 0.04	47 vs 34	P = 0.19
Kemeny 1999	156	HAI-FUDR & IV 5FU vs IV 5FU	31.3 vs 17.2	P = 0.02	68.4 vs 58.8	2-year survival 0.02
Lygidakis 2001	122	HAI Mitomycin C, 5FU, LV, IL2 vs IV mitomycin C, 5FU, LV, IL2	60% vs 35% (5-year DFS)	P = 0.0002	79 vs 66 5 year	P = 0.04
Kemeny 2010	73	HAI-FUDR, 5FU + Bev+oxali or irinotecan + Bev – Bev	31% vs 45% (4-year RFS)	NS	(4-year OS)	P = 0.5

plus systemic without Bev. Overall, 43% (20/47) were converted to complete resection (38% with Bev and 48% without Bev).[37] Seven patients in the Bev arm developed hyperbilirubinemia compared to 1 in the non-Bev arm (p = 0.005). And 10% of the patients versus 0% in the Bev and non-Bev groups respectively required biliary stent placement.[38]

Retrospective analyses have also demonstrated an improvement in response rate and conversion to resection rates with the combination of HAI-FUDR plus systemic chemotherapy. One study reviewed 39 patients with metastatic disease confined to the liver who had progressed on oxaliplatin-based systemic regimens and subsequently received HAI-FUDR/dex with systemic irinotecan. The majority of the patients were heavily pretreated, and had a response rate of 44% and a median overall survival of 20.1 months from the start of HAI treatment. In this group, 18% of the patients proceeded to liver resection.[39]

One of the limitations of these data is that the combination of HAI-FUDR plus modern systemic chemotherapy has not been compared to modern systemic therapy alone in a prospective randomized clinical trial. Such studies are warranted as the response rates of HAI therapy and favorable toxicity profile favor further investigation. The data support further investigation of HAI therapy in patients with metastatic CRC confined to the liver who have progressed on systemic chemotherapy or in patients with extensive liver disease in whom a robust response could convert unresectable disease to resectable disease.

ADJUVANT HAI FOLLOWING LIVER RESECTION

The majority of patients who undergo resection of liver metastases will relapse. Many of these patients relapse in the liver which is likely due to the presence of micrometastatic disease post resection. A pooled analysis of two randomized trials in which patients received adjuvant systemic chemotherapy following resection of liver metastases showed that treatment increases progression-free survival but does not significantly improve overall survival.[40] Adjuvant therapy with HAI is an attractive approach in such patients given that the recurrence is most likely due to the persistence of micrometastatic disease in the liver.

Several studies have addressed this hypothesis (Table 5). A German study randomized 226 patients who underwent liver resection to adjuvant therapy with HAI 5FU/LV via the port versus observation.[41] This study was terminated early because the adjuvant HAI therapy did not demonstrate any benefit over observation. The limitation of the study was that only 84 patients were actually treated in the HAI group, and the HAI therapy was administered via a port and not a pump.

In a cooperative group multicenter study, 109 patients were randomized to postoperative HAI-FUDR combined with intravenous 5FU versus observation.[42] The study met its endpoint, which was recurrence-free survival. The 4-year recurrence-free survival was significantly better in the adjuvant therapy HAI arm at 47.5% and 25.2% respectively. The study was underpowered to evaluate survival.

In a single center study, 156 patients were randomized to either HAI-FUDR plus systemic 5FU/LV or systemic 5FU/LV alone following resection of liver metastases.[43] The results were notable for an overall 2-year survival (endpoint of the study) of 86% versus 72% in the HAI plus chemo and chemo alone groups respectively (p = 0.03). The rates of hepatic disease-free survival (DFS) were 90% versus 60% respectively ($p < 0.001$). Updated results were notable for a significant benefit in progression-free survival for HAI (p = 0.002). The 10-year survival rates were 41% and 27% in the HAI plus systemic and systemic only arms respectively.[44]

In a large meta-analysis of patients who underwent liver resection for metastatic CRC at MSKCC, 1,067

Section 4

patients were identified. In this group, postoperative HAI was associated with improved survival by multivariate analyses.[45] A total of 232 patients who received postoperative pump therapy were compared with 826 who received systemic chemotherapy alone. The median disease specific survival (DSS) was improved in the group that received HAI therapy versus systemic alone; 68 months versus 50 months ($p < 0.001$). In a retrospective analysis of 125 patients who received adjuvant HAI-FUDR in combination with systemic FOLFOX or FOLFIRI compared to matched controls patients who received adjuvant systemic FOLFOX or FOLFIRI alone[46] at a 43 months median follow-up, the DFS was 75% in the HAI plus systemic group versus 52% in the systemic chemotherapy alone group ($p = 0.004$).

More recently, the results of a phase-I trial of systemic oxaliplatin in combination with HAI-FUDR as adjuvant therapy after liver resection resulted in a 4-year survival of 88% and a progression-free survival of 50%.[47] A phase-II study evaluated the addition of Bev to HAI-FUDR/dex and systemic 5FU with either oxaliplatin or irinotecan. The addition of Bev to adjuvant systemic chemotherapy plus HAI did not increase relapse-free survival (RFS) and/or overall survival. With a median follow-up of 30 months, the 4-year survival was 81% and 85% ($P = 0.5$) for the Bev versus no Bev arms respectively. The addition of Bev did, however, correlate with increased biliary toxicity with 4 versus 0 ($p = 0.05$) patients requiring stents in the Bev versus no Bev arms respectively.[48]

These small prospective and retrospective studies support the rationale of HAI-FUDR with systemic chemotherapy as adjuvant therapy in patients with resected liver metastases.

HAI FOR PRIMARY LIVER CANCER

Primary liver cancer, hepatocellular carcinoma (HCC) and intrahepatic cholangiocarcinoma (ICC) derive their blood supply from the HA, thus HAI therapy in these cancers is warranted. Often the tumors present in an advanced or unresectable stage and the efficacy of systemic chemotherapy in terms of response rate is limited.

A phase-II trial evaluating the use of HAI-FUDR in 34 patients (26 ICC and 8 HCC) demonstrated a response rate of 47.1% with a median survival of 29.5 months.[49] Interestingly, a higher response rate was seen in patients with cholangiocarcinoma (53.8% vs 25%), and one patient with cholangiocarcinoma had adequate response to undergo resection and had a complete pathologic response. A second study evaluating the addition of systemic Bev to HAI demonstrated a similar survival of 31 months median survival but increased biliary toxicity with the use of Bev (unpublished results). Although this is a small study, it provides support for further evaluation of HAI therapy in primary liver cancers where the efficacy of systemic chemotherapy is limited and outcomes are poor.

CONCLUSION

Despite the limitation of a number of historical studies utilizing HAI, there is a strong rationale behind its use in patients with metastatic CRC with isolated liver metastases. In such patients, HAI therapy in combination with systemic chemotherapy can be utilized in three different scenarios: (1) as preoperative or neoadjuvant therapy to enable hepatic resection; (2) as second-line therapy to improve response rates and (3) in postoperative or adjuvant therapy to decrease recurrence rates. Improvements in surgical techniques and careful administration of therapy and close monitoring of liver enzyme toxicities are minimal and manageable. Future randomized studies utilizing HAI therapy in combination with systemic chemotherapy in the adjuvant as well as the neoadjuvant setting are needed. These studies must incorporate analysis of molecular markers to provide further insight into the biology of patients with liver-only metastatic disease who would benefit from such therapy.

REFERENCES

1. Scheele J, Stang R, Altendorf-Hofmann A, et al. Resection of colorectal liver metastases. World J Surg. 1995;19:59-71.
2. Fong Y, Fortner J, Sun RL, et al. Clinical score for predicting recurrence after hepatic resection for metastatic colorectal cancer: analysis of 1001 consecutive cases. Ann Surg. 1999;230(3):309-18.
3. Nordlinger B, Guiguet M, Vaillant JC, et al. Surgical resection of colorectal carcinoma metastases to the liver. A prognostic scoring system to improve case selection, based on 1568 patients. Association Francaise de Chirurgie. Cancer. 1996;77(7):1254-62.
4. Curley SA, Izzo F, Delrio P, et al. Radiofrequency ablation of unresectable primary and metastatic hepatic malignancies: results in 123 patients. Ann Surg. 1999;230(1):1-8.
5. Pearson AS, Izzo F, Fleming RY, et al. Intraoperative radiofrequency ablation or cryoablation for hepatic malignancies. Am J Surg. 1999;178(6):592-9.
6. Sigurdson ER, Ridge JA, Kemeny N, et al. Tumor and liver drug uptake following hepatic artery and portal vein infusion. J Clin Oncol. 1987;5(11):1836-40.
7. Skitzki JJ, Chang AE. Hepatic artery chemotherapy for colorectal liver metastases: technical considerations and review of clinical trials. Surg Oncol. 2002;11(3):123-35.

8. Allen PJ, Nissan A, Picon AI, et al. Technical complications and durability of hepatic artery infusion pumps for unresectable colorectal liver metastases: an institutional experience of 544 consecutive cases. J Am Coll Surg. 2005;201(1):57-65.
9. Ensminger WD. Intrahepatic arterial infusion of chemotherapy: pharmacologic principles. Semin Oncol. 2002;29(2):119-25.
10. Collins JM. Pharmacologic rationale for regional drug delivery. J Clin Oncol. 1984;2(5):498-504.
11. Ensminger WD, Rosowsky A, Raso V, et al. A clinical-pharmacological evaluation of hepatic arterial infusions of 5-fluoro-2'-deoxyuridine and 5-fluorouracil. Cancer Res. 1978; 38(11 Pt 1):3784-92.
12. Ensminger WD, Gyves JW. Clinical pharmacology of hepatic arterial chemotherapy. Semin Oncol. 1983;10(2):176-82.
13. De Jong FA, Mathijssen RH, Verweij J. Limited potential of hepatic arterial infusion of irinotecan. J Chemother. 2004; 16(Suppl. 5):48-50.
14. van Riel JM, van Groeningen CJ, Kedde MA, et al. Continuous administration of irinotecan by hepatic arterial infusion: a phase I and pharmacokinetic study. Clin Cancer Res. 2002;8(2): 405-12.
15. Dzodic R, Gomez-Abuin G, Rougier P, et al. Pharmacokinetic advantage of intra-arterial hepatic oxaliplatin administration: comparative results with cisplatin using a rabbit VX2 tumor model. Anticancer Drugs. 2004;15(6):647-50.
16. Boige V, Malaka D, Elias D, et al. Hepatic arterial infusion of oxaliplatin and intravenous LV5FU2 in unresectable liver metastases from colorectal cancer after systemic chemotherapy failure. Ann Surg Oncol. 2008;15(1):219-26.
17. Bouchahda M, Adam R, Giacchetti S, et al. Rescue chemotherapy using multidrug chronomdoulated hepatic arterial infusion for patients with heavily pretreated metastatic colorectal cancer. Cancer. 2009;115(21):4990-9.
18. Goéré D, Deschaies I, de Baere T, et al. Prolonged survival of initially unresectable hepatic arterial infusion of oxaliplatin followed by radical surgery of metastases. Ann Surg. 2010; 251(4):686-91.
19. Koea JB, Kemeny N. Hepatic artery infusion chemotherapy for metastatic colorectal carcinoma. Semin Surgical Oncol. 2000; 19:125-34.
20. Strazzabosco M, Fabris L. Functional anatomy of normal bile ducts. Anat Rec (Hoboken). 2008;291(6):653-60.
21. Kemeny N, Seiter K, Niedzweikei D, et al. A randomized trial of intrahepatic infusion of fluorodeoxyuridine with dexamethasone versus fluorodeoxyuridine alone in the treatment of metastatic colorectal cancer. Cancer. 1992;69(2):327-34.
22. Chang AE, Schneider PD, Sugarbaker PH, et al. A prospective randomized trial of regional versus systemic continuous 5-fluorodeoxyuridine chemotherapy in the treatment of colorectal liver metastases. Ann Surg. 1987;206(6):685-93.
23. Kemeny N, Daly J, Reichman B, et al. Intrahepatic or systemic infusion of fluorodeoxyuridine in patients with liver metastases from colorectal carcinoma. A randomized trial. Ann Intern Med. 1987;107(4):459-65.
24. Hohn DC, Stagg RJ, Friedman MA, et al. A randomized trial of continuous intravenous versus hepatic intraarterial floxuridine in patients with colorectal cancer metastatic to the liver: the Northern California Oncology Group trial. J Clin Oncol. 1989;7(11):1646-54.
25. Martin JK Jr, O›Connell MJ, Wieand HS, et al. Intra-arterial floxuridine vs systemic fluorouracil for hepatic metastases from colorectal cancer. A randomized trial. Arch Surg. 1990; 125(8):1022-7.
26. Wagman LD, Kemeny MM, Leong L, et al. A prospective, randomized evaluation of the treatment of colorectal cancer metastatic to the liver. J Clin Oncol. 1990;8(11):1885-93.
27. Rougier P, Laplanche A, Huguier M, et al. Hepatic arterial infusion of floxuridine in patients with liver metastases from colorectal carcinoma: long-term results of a prospective randomized trial. J Clin Oncol. 1992;10(7):1112-8.
28. Allen-Mersh TG, Earlam S, Fordy C, et al. Quality of life and survival with continuous hepatic-artery floxuridine infusion for colorectal liver metastases. Lancet. 1994;344(8932):1255-60.
29. Lorenz M, Müller HH. Randomized, multicenter trial of fluorouracil plus leucovorin administered either via hepatic arterial or intravenous infusion versus fluorodeoxyuridine administered via hepatic arterial infusion in patients with nonresectable liver metastases from colorectal carcinoma. J Clin Oncol. 2000;18(2):243-54.
30. Kerr DJ, McArdle CS, Ledermann J, et al. Intrahepatic arterial versus intravenous fluorouracil and folinic acid for colorectal cancer liver metastases: a multicentre randomised trial. Lancet. 2003;361(9355):368-73.
31. Kemeny NE, Niedzwiecki D, Hollis DR, et al. Hepatic arterial infusion versus systemic therapy for hepatic metastases from colorectal cancer: a randomized trial of efficacy, quality of life, and molecular markers (CALGB 9481). J Clin Oncol. 2006; 24(9):1395-1403.
32. Mocellin S, Pilati P, Lise M, et al. Meta-analysis of hepatic arterial infusion for unresectable liver metastases from colorectal cancer: the end of an era? J Clin Oncol. 2007;25(35):5649-54.
33. Fiorentini G, Cantore M, Rossi S, et al. Hepatic arterial chemotherapy in combination with systemic chemotherapy compared with hepatic arterial chemotherapy alone for liver metastases from colorectal cancer: results of a multi-centric randomized study. In Vivo. 2006;20(6A):707-9.
34. Kemeny N, Gonen M, Sullivan D, et al. Phase I study of hepatic arterial infusion of floxuridine and dexamethasone with systemic irinotecan for unresectable hepatic metastases from colorectal cancer. J Clin Oncol. 2001;19(10):2687-95.
35 Kemeny N, Jarnagin W, Paty P, et al. Phase I trial of systemic oxaliplatin combination chemotherapy with hepatic arterial infusion in patients with unresectable liver metastases from colorectal cancer. J Clin Oncol. 2005;23(22):4888-96.
36. Kemeny NE, Melendez FD, Capanu M, et al. Conversion to resectability using hepatic artery infusion plus systemic chemotherapy for the treatment of unresectable liver metastases from colorectal carcinoma. J Clin Oncol. 2009;27(21):3465-71.
37. D'Angelica M, Gonen M, Do RK, et al. Prospective phase II trial of hepatic intra-arterial Floxuridine combined with best systemic chemotherapy and Bevacizumab for unresectable liver metastases from colorectal carcinoma: assessing the rate of conversion to complete resection. Submitted ASCO 2011.
38. Power DG, Capanu M, Patel D, et al. Unexpected increased biliary toxicity when systemic bevacizumab is added to hepatic artery infusion. J Clin Oncol. 2010;28:15s.
39. Gallagher DJ, Zheng J, Capanu M, et al. Response to neoadjuvant chemotherapy does not predict overall survival for

Section 4

patients with synchronous colorectal hepatic metastases. Ann Surg Oncol. 2009;16(7):1844-51.
40. Mitry E, Fields AL, Bleiberg H, et al. Adjuvant chemotherapy after potentially curative resection of metastases from colorectal cancer: a pooled analysis of two randomized trials. J Clin Oncol. 2008;26(30);4906-11.
41. Lorenz M, Müller HH, Schramm H, et al. Randomized trial of surgery versus surgery followed by adjuvant hepatic arterial infusion with 5-fluorouracil and folinic acid for liver metastases of colorectal cancer. German Cooperative on Liver Metastases (Arbeitsgruppe Lebermetastasen). Ann Surg. 1998; 228(6):756-62.
42. Kemeny MM, Adak S, Gray B, et al. Combined-modality treatment for resectable metastatic colorectal carcinoma to the liver: surgical resection of hepatic metastases in combination with continuous infusion of chemotherapy—an intergroup study. J Clin Oncol. 2002;20(6):1499-1505.
43. Kemeny N, Huang Y, Cohen AM, et al. Hepatic arterial infusion of chemotherapy after resection of hepatic metastases from colorectal cancer. N Engl J Med. 1999;341:2039-48.
44. Kemeny NE, Gonen M. Hepatic arterial infusion of chemotherapy after resection. N Engl J Med. 2005;352:734-35.
45. Ito H, Are C, Gonen M, et al. Effect of postoperative morbidity on long-term survival after hepatic resection for metastatic colorectal cancer. Ann Surg. 2008;247(6):994-1002.
46. House MG, Jarnagin WR. Comparison of adjuvant systemic chemotherapy with or without hepatic arterial infusional chemotherapy after hepatic resection for metastatic colorectal cancer. American Society of Clinical Oncology Gastrointestinal Cancer Symposium, 2009.
47. Kemeny N, Capanu M, D' Angelica M, et al. Phase I trial of adjuvant hepatic arterial infusion (HAI) with floxuridine (FUDR) and dexamethasone plus systemic oxaliplatin, 5-fluorouracil and leucovorin in patients with resected liver metastases from colorectal cancer. Ann Oncol. 2009;20(7): 1236-41.
48. Kemeny NE, Jarnagin WR, Capanu M, et al. A randomized phase II trial of adjuvant hepatic arterial infusion and systemic chemotherapy with or without bevacizumab in patients with resected hepatic metastases from colorectal cancer. J Clin Oncol. 2010;28(15s):3557.
49. Jarnagin WR, Schwartz LH, Gultekin DH, et al. Regional chemotherapy for unresectable primary liver cancer: results of a phase II clinical trial and assessment of DCE-MRI as a biomarker of survival. Ann Oncol. 2009;20(9):1589-95.

12

Hepatic Arterial Therapies for Colorectal Liver Metastases

Hebat Allah Mohamed Saad El-Din Fouad, Robert C.G. Martin II

INTRODUCTION

Colorectal cancer (CRC) is the third most common malignancy worldwide. CRC metastasizes to various organs, with the lymph nodes being the most frequent followed by the liver and lungs. By the time of diagnosis, about 25% of the patients have liver metastases (synchronous metastases); another 25–30% will present hepatic lesions in the following 2–3 years (metachronous metastases). The overall life expectancy is primarily determined by the progression of metastatic liver disease and not by the primary carcinoma, even in patients with an isolated hepatic tumor. Without treatment, life expectancy is less than 1 year.[1]

Surgery is the only therapy that offers a possibility of cure for the patients with hepatic metastatic diseases. Unfortunately, only 25% of the patients with colorectal liver metastases are candidates for liver resection while the others are not amenable to surgical resection.[2] Several modalities have been developed for local treatment of liver tumors including cryotherapy, radiofrequency ablation, percutaneous ethanol injection, laser and photodynamic therapy.[3] Techniques for regional hepatic therapy for metastatic colon cancer to the liver include hepatic arterial infusion chemotherapy, chemoembolization, infusion radiotherapy with yttrium-90 labeled particles, and isolated hepatic perfusion (Table 1). While these approaches have been available for a long time, their role in the management of metastatic colon cancer continues to evolve.[4]

The first-line treatment for unresectable hepatic metastases from CRC is chemotherapy, which may be administered systemically or with a hepatic arterial infusion. Because the progression of hepatic disease contributes significantly to morbidity and mortality, transarterial therapies may be used for palliative or adjuvant therapy to help stabilize disease, or to reduce the hepatic tumor burden.[5,6] Transarterial therapies take advantage of the dual blood supply of the liver. Approximately 80% of the blood supply to hepatic metastases from CRC arrives via the hepatic artery, whereas three fourth of the blood supply to normal hepatic parenchyma is portal venous. Hence, cytotoxic agents that are infused selectively into the hepatic artery preferentially target tumor cells over normal hepatic tissue.[7]

HEPATIC ARTERIAL INFUSION CHEMOTHERAPY

Traditional transarterial therapies are based on the infusion of chemotherapeutic drugs into the hepatic artery either intermittently or through a surgically implanted hepatic artery pump.[7] The concept of hepatic artery infusion (HAI) dates back to the early 1960s

Table 1 Options for transarterial therapies

Traditional methods
Without embolization:
• Intermittent chemotherapy infusion into the hepatic artery
• Continuous infusion with a hepatic artery pump
With embolization:
• Bland embolization
• TACE (Transarterial chemoembolization)
Recent advances
Embolization with drug-eluting microspheres
Embolization with radiation-emitting microspheres
Experimental methods
Gene therapy

when it was tried in a few patients with gastrointestinal tumors metastatic to the liver, and was associated with favorable outcomes. The rationale for HAI is to expose the metastases to high chemotherapy concentrations while minimizing systemic toxicity. The other rationale is the high first-pass hepatic extraction of the drug used for this approach. Both factors cause high local drug concentrations with reduced systemic toxicity, and allow relatively higher dosages as compared with intravenous treatment.[8] Some studies comparing intra-arterial chemotherapy with conventional systemic chemotherapy have demonstrated consistently higher response rates in patients receiving intra-arterial chemotherapy.[9]

Multiple agents such as 5-fluorouracil (5-FU), mitomycin, cisplatin and doxorubicin have been infused, but 5-fluoro-2′-deoxyuridine (floxuridine, FUDR) has been the chemotherapeutic agent most frequently studied. FUDR has a 95% hepatic extraction when continuously infused in the hepatic artery, resulting in a 16-fold higher concentration in liver metastasis compared with venous administration.[10] It has a high first-pass metabolism/clearance through the liver that minimizes the chances for systemic toxicity.[11] Infusing FUDR in the hepatic artery is achieved through an implantable subcutaneous infusion pump connected to a surgically placed hepatic artery catheter, which delivers the chemotherapeutic agent at a slow fixed rate, usually for 2 weeks.[12]

Incidents related to hepatic artery thrombosis, catheter displacement, hematomas, infections and liver perfusion are all reported as pump-related complications.[12,13] The technical complications are closely associated with surgeon experience and arterial anatomy (37% for inexperienced surgeons vs 7% for experienced surgeons).[14] Treatment-related toxicities include chemical hepatitis, biliary sclerosis and peptic ulceration. Chemical hepatitis, which is the most common (42%), presents with elevation in liver enzymes or bilirubin. Liver function monitoring, dose reduction or treatment cessation are recommended based on the severity of the clinical presentation. Although most cases are reversible, biliary sclerosis can develop in 3–26% of the patients.[15] Kemeny et al.[16] reported a trend toward a lower incidence of increased bilirubin levels in patients receiving dexamethasone plus FUDR when compared to those receiving FUDR alone (9% and 30% respectively, had a two-fold or greater increase in the bilirubin level from baseline). Response rate and survival also improve with the addition of dexamethasone.[17] The most suitable subjects for HAI have disease confined to the liver, have undergone hepatic angiography to define their hepatic arterial anatomy, and are deemed appropriate surgical candidates for the catheter and pump placement. Contraindications include portal vein thrombosis, more than 70% liver replacement by tumor, significant impairment of liver function or a hepatic artery anatomy that would preclude perfusion of the entire liver.[18] The utilization of HAI pump has decreased secondary to a small number institutions seeing benefit, significantly high pump-related complications secondary to both surgeon technique and medical oncologist management as well as three recently failed cooperative trials—NSABP, ACOSOG and SWOG—secondary to accrual limitations.

TRANSARTERIAL CHEMOEMBOLIZATION

Transarterial chemoembolization (TACE) is a catheter-based technique that combines both regional chemotherapy and embolization to increase the dwell time of cytotoxic agents and induce ischemia in the tumor. Conventional TACE therapy, in which arterial inflow is reduced to delay drug washout, enables chemotherapeutic drug concentrations within a tumor that are up to 100 times greater than those achievable with systemic chemotherapy.[19-21] It has been shown that anoxic damage increases vascular permeability, and thereby promotes penetration of chemotherapeutic agents into the tumor[22,23] (Table 2).

Hepatic artery chemoembolization (HACE) was developed to treat unresectable non-disseminated liver tumors.[24,25] Although HACE has not shown any benefit

Table 2 Reported literature of conventional chemoembolization for mCRC

Author	N	Drug	Mort (%)	RR (%)	OS
Hong	21	Cis—100 mg Dox—50 mg Mito—10 mg	5.4	NR	7.7 mon
Morise	4	DSM w/80 mg CPT-11 8 mg Mito	0	80	6.5 mon
Sanz-Altamira	40	5FU—1000 mg Mito C—10 mg Ethiodol—10 cc Stasis	7.5	NR	10 mon
Lang	46	Doxo—50-100 mg Ethiodol—7-10 ml	28	24	12 mon
Tellez	30	Cis—10 mg Dox—3 mg Mito C—3 mg	0	63	8.6 mon
Van Riel	25	5-day infusion CPT-11—20 mg/m^2	0	13.6	PFS 2.8

Chapter 12

on survival, it increased the response rate compared with systemic administration of cytotoxic agents. HACE has been studied mostly in the treatment of hepatocellular carcinoma, and was also used in CRC liver metastases for some clinical trials.[26] Preoperative HACE has been proposed as a possible means of decreasing perioperative tumor dissemination, but only in a small number of patients. Some centers reported that HACE in patients with borderline resectable tumors caused sufficient tumor shrinkage to allow resection.[27,28]

Although conventional TACE implementation is tailored according to the liver function of each patient as well as the extent of the tumor and portal vein involvement, the use of more selective TACE can often result in a better outcome with fewer adverse effects. There is increasing evidence that selective TACE achieves better antitumoral effects, and reduces both the dosage of drugs used for TACE and the number of TACE sessions needed to achieve extensive tumor necrosis as compared to the use of conventional TACE.[29-31] The current limitations of the TACE literature have come from the wide variations in chemotherapeutic agents used, the utilization of non-standard chemotherapy (i.e. doxorubicin), and no established standard embolic and stasis interventional techniques (Table 2).

DRUG-ELUTING BEADS

The use of drug-eluting microspheres in a new variation of the TACE method is designed to improve the precision of drug delivery.[7] Drug-eluting microspheres are made of polyvinyl alcohol hydrogel and are biocompatible, hydrophilic and nonresorbable.[32] The primary advantage of using drug-eluting microspheres for chemotherapy is the sustained release of the chemotherapeutic agent over a long period of time, which contrasts with the more rapid release of agents from the lipiodol solution in standard TACE therapy.[32-34] With a controlled gradual and local release, contact time of the drugs with the tumor is greater, and plasma levels of the drugs are lower than those with standard TACE therapy. Preprocedural planning with cross-sectional imaging and liver function testing is imperative. Accurate staging of disease by assessing the intrahepatic and extrahepatic tumor burden is crucial to exclude the possibilities of surgical therapy, radiofrequency ablation and cryotherapy. Cross-sectional imaging can be extremely useful for assessing the hepatic arterial anatomy and portal vein patency.[32-34]

Patients with unresectable liver metastases are usually treated with systemic chemotherapy based on 5-FU, oxaliplatin and irinotecan. Recently it has been shown that combination regimens, including oxaliplatin or irinotecan and monoclonal anti-EGFR or anti-VEGF antibodies, lead to higher response rates and an improved survival.[35,36]

Pharmacokinetics

Drug loading and elution kinetics are dependent on the particle size. For example, DC Beads (Biocompatibles UK, Surrey, England) are manufactured in various sizes ranging 100–1200 μm. For a specific drug concentration, smaller microspheres require less time for drug loading than larger ones do, with a loading efficiency of 99% up to a maximum concentration of 45 mg/ml. Elution kinetics are similarly affected by microsphere size, with smaller microspheres eluting slightly more quickly than larger ones.[32]

Technique and Administration

Prior to administration via a catheter, the loaded beads are mixed with an equal volume of non-ionic contrast medium to guide the injection. The specific targeting of the drug at the site of the tumor implies enhanced efficacy by a maximized tumor dose and, at the same time, reduced toxicity due to negligible systemic exposure and toxicity.[36] According to the product information, irinotecan-loaded DC Beads™ or drug-eluting bead, irinotecan (DEBIRI) (100 mg irinotecan per 2 ml DC Beads™) are stable over a period of 14 days when stored refrigerated. After mixing with non-ionic contrast media, irinotecan-loaded beads have to be administered immediately. The bead admixture is reported to be stable for a maximum 24 hours at 2–8°C or 4 hours at room temperature.

Baseline angiography of the celiac, superior mesenteric and hepatic arteries, as well as indirect portal venography should be performed to determine the vascular anatomy, and assess tumor vascularity. Administration through the proper hepatic artery is feasible for the treatment of bilobar disease. In patients with variant arterial anatomy, such as a replaced left hepatic artery or a middle hepatic artery, bilobar disease may be treated incrementally by dividing the drug dose and infusing separate portions into the individual hepatic arteries. After the infusion of drug-eluting microspheres, a solution containing bland microspheres (without drugs) may be administered to achieve complete embolization, which is characterized by the cessation of flow in the catheterized vessel.

Table 3 Hepatic intra-arterial injection of drug-eluting bead, irinotecan (DEBIRI) in unresectable colorectal liver metastases refractory to systemic chemotherapy: results of multi-institutional study (response rates for all 55 patients evaluated)

Response (n = 55)	*3 months*	*6 months*	*12 months*
Complete response	7 (12%)	7 (12%)	8 (15%)
Partial response	28 (53%)	21 (38%)	14 (25%)
Stable disease	15 (30%)	19 (34%)	23 (42%)
Progression of disease	3 (5%)	8 (15%)	10 (18%)
Dead of disease	0	5	9
Death of other cause	2	0	0

Follow-up cross-sectional imaging with the same modality that was used at baseline is critical for determining the tumor response. Determinants of tumor response observed at imaging include loss of arterial contrast enhancement which signifies necrosis, and/or reduction of fluorine-18 fluorodeoxyglucose (FDG) uptake at positron emission tomography (PET). In cases of tumor progression or partial necrosis with residual areas of enhancement suggestive of viable tumor cells, therapy with drug-eluting microspheres may be repeated (Table 3).[37]

Recent publications in the literature have demonstrated the safety and efficacy of DEBIRI in patients with unresectable metastatic CRC (mCRC).[38,39] These initial results confirmed the safety of DEBIRI, provided modifications in interventional techniques were utilized. Among the most significant modifications were the addition of pretreatment medications, pretreatment with intra-arterial lidocaine, and the avoidance of overzealously pursuing a hard endpoint of stasis.[40] Lastly, given that these tumors are relatively hypervascular on angiography and are multifocal—thus the reason they are unresectable or not amenable to ablation—the DEBIRI infusion should be performed in a lobar approach (Fig. 1). These results have been further validated to allow for a greater percentage of surgical down-staging as well as to ensure safety of using DEBIRI prior to surgical resection in patients with mCRC to the liver.[41,42] Recent publications have also demonstrated the ability to treat chemo-refractory tumors through the ability to deliver targeted chemotherapy directly to the tumor.[37] However, the dose of 100 mg in the DEBIRI is relatively small compared to normal bimonthly systemic dosing of irinotecan which is 125 mg/m^2. Thus, recent data has demonstrated that one DEBIRI treatment will not be enough and for robust response, at least 2–3 DEBIRI treatments are necessary (Fig. 1).

Yttrium-90 Radioembolization

The therapeutic use of external-beam irradiation of the liver has been limited due to the vulnerability of the normal hepatic parenchyma to damage by radiation. Approximately 50% of the patients who receive a whole-liver radiation dose of 35 Gy (a dose insufficient to induce tumor cell death) develop radiation-induced liver disease.[43-45] Yttrium-90 (^{90}Y) bearing microspheres, however, act as point sources of radiation that, when delivered via the hepatic artery, are deposited predominantly within tumor tissue. ^{90}Y emits beta radiation with a mean energy of 0.94 MeV, and mean penetration of 2.5 mm. ^{90}Y-bearing microspheres can deliver an intratumoral radiation dose of 100–150 Gy, which is highly effective for tumor destruction. In addition, the preferential deposition of the microspheres within the tumor allows selective irradiation of the target rather than normal hepatic parenchyma, and thereby reduces the risk of radiation-induced hepatitis.[46] ^{90}Y-bearing microspheres are commercially available in two formulations (Table 4).

Therapy Planning

The first step in therapy planning is proper staging with the use of cross-sectional imaging and laboratory evaluation of liver function. CT or MR imaging is performed before ^{90}Y therapy to help determine the tumor volume, liver volume, extrahepatic tumor burden, presence of anatomic variants in the hepatic arterial supply and portal vein patency. In addition, PET may be helpful for assessing the intrahepatic and extrahepatic tumor burden; particularly, in colorectal metastatic disease.[47]

Before treatment, the performance status of all patients should be graded according to the Eastern Cooperative Oncology Group scheme (Table 5).[48,49] Patients with a compromised performance status (score of 2–4) may incur an increased risk of treatment-related morbidity. In addition, a total bilirubin level of more than 1.2 is a marker of impaired hepatic function, and a relative contraindication to radioembolization with ^{90}Y-bearing microspheres.[48]

The second step in therapy planning is baseline angiography to assess the anatomy of the celiac, superior mesenteric and hepatic arteries. If multiple hepatic arteries supply the tumor or the diseased lobe, embolization of the smaller accessory arteries should be considered, and the ^{90}Y-bearing microspheres should be injected into the larger artery. If two large vessels

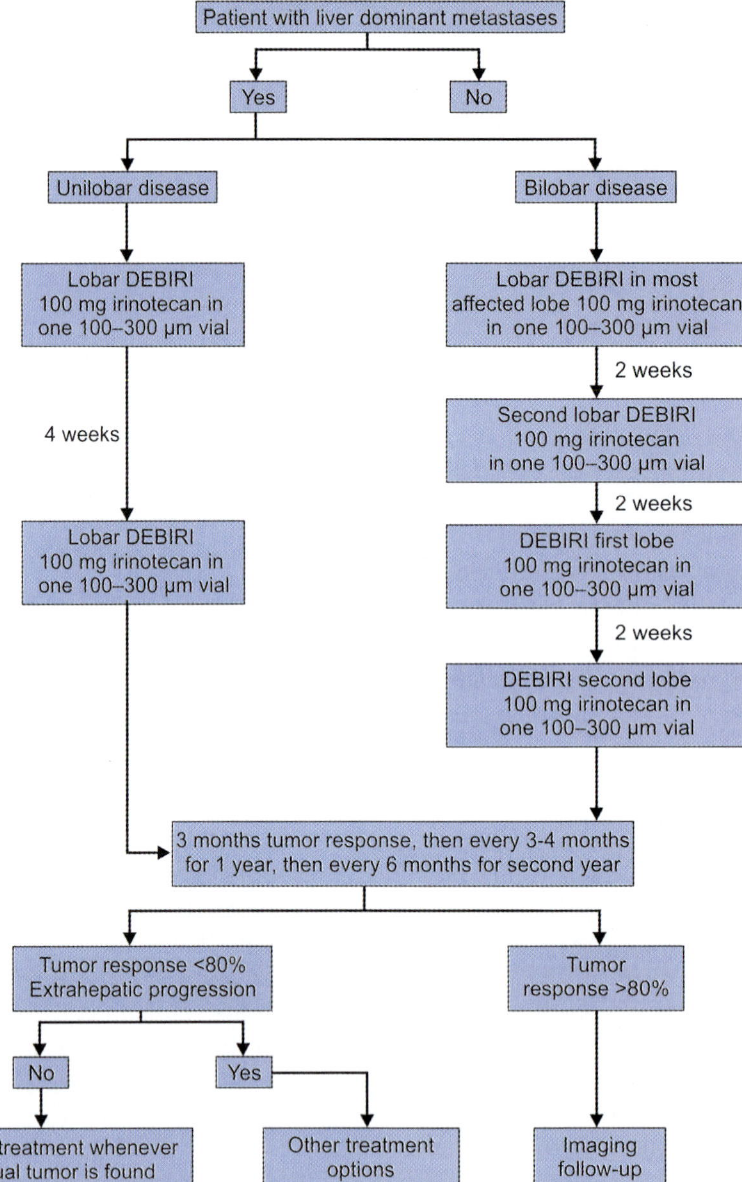

Figure 1 Treatment algorithm most commonly used in the treatment of unresectable liver tumors with DEBIRI

Table 4 Comparison of two ^{90}Y-bearing microsphere formulations

Characteristic	*TheraSphere*[*]	*SIR-Spheres*[†]
Composition	Glass	Resin
Specific activity (Bq per microsphere)	2,500	50
No. of microspheres[‡]	4×10^6	50×10^6
FDA approval category[§]	Humanitarian exemption for use in patients with unresectable hepatocellular carcinoma	Premarket approval for use adjuvant chemotherapy in patients with hepatic metastasis from colorectal carcinoma
Hepatopulmonary shunt limit[‖]	10	20

[*]Manufactured by MDS Nordion, Ottawa, Ontario, Canada.
[†]Manufactured by Sirtex Medical, Sydney, Australia.
[‡]Numbers are the mean per dose.
[§]FDA = U.S. Food and Drug Administration.
[‖]Numbers are the shunt fraction as a percentage.

Table 5 ECOG* system for scoring patient performance status

Score	Characterization
0	Fully active
1	Unable to pursue strenuous physical exercise
2	Symptomatic but able to completely fulfill normal activities of daily living
3	Limited ability to perform activities of daily living, spends more than half the day in bed
4	Completely bedridden

*ECOG = Eastern Cooperative Oncology Group

supply the tumor, two options may be considered: (i) the interventional radiologist may consider catheterizing both vessels and infusing half the dose via each vessel; (ii) alternatively, one artery can be treated during the first session, and the remaining artery treated in a future session with a half to a full dose administered at each session.[47]

The third step in therapy planning is the determination of the degree of hepatopulmonary shunting due to the tumor. Tumor-associated arteriovenous shunting is more common in hepatocellular carcinoma than in metastatic disease.[50]

Delivery

Radioembolization is usually performed as an outpatient procedure. The delivery kit, which is available from the respective manufacturing companies, includes an apparatus that shields the radiation and provides a closed circuit to prevent accidental spills. Whole-liver treatment with ^{90}Y-bearing microspheres can be performed at the level of the common or proper hepatic artery, but segmental or lobar infusions are performed with increasing frequency,[48] with their primary advantage being a reduction in the risk of reflux of microspheres into the gastroduodenal artery or small perforating vessels.[48,49] For whole-liver treatment, Salem and Thurston recommend a "bilobar lobar" infusion in which either the right or the left hepatic artery is catheterized, the microsphere formulation is administered, and then the sequence is repeated with the other hepatic artery.[48]

Follow-up Evaluations

Immediately after the therapeutic procedure is completed, planar scintigraphy or single photon emission computed tomography is performed to detect bremsstrahlung from interactions between beta rays and tissue. Post-procedural scintigraphy provides an opportunity to detect any inadvertent extrahepatic deposition of microspheres.[51]

The oncologic standard for determining tumor response is the tumor size as categorized according to the Response Evaluation Criteria in Solid Tumors (RECIST) parameters and modified Response Evaluation Criteria in Solid Tumors (mRECIST) which are summarized in Table 6.[52,53] However, size alone may not be a reliable criterion for assessing the response of a tumor to regional therapies because necrosis, edema and hemorrhage may cause an initial increase in the size of a tumor that is responding to therapy. Instead, to accurately determine the tumor response, the tumor size should be assessed in conjunction with the presence and extent of tumor necrosis (Tables 7–10).[54]

In addition, early studies with diffusion-weighted MR imaging demonstrated a post-treatment decrease in the apparent diffusion coefficient of tumors—a finding consistent with treatment-induced cell death both after therapeutic embolization with ^{90}Y-bearing microspheres and after standard TACE therapy.[55,56]

Table 6 Definition of disease response according to RECIST and modified RECIST parameters

RECIST	Modified RECIST
CR—Disappearance of all target lesions	CR—Disappearance of any intratumoral arterial enhancement in all target lesions
PR—At least 30% decrease in the sum of diameters of target lesions, taking as reference the baseline sum of the diameters of target lesions	PR—At least 30% decrease in the sum of diameters of viable (enhancement in arterial phase) target lesions, taking as reference the baseline sum of the diameters of target lesions
SD—Any cases that do not qualify for either partial response or progressive disease	SD—Any cases that do not qualify for either partial response or progressive disease
PD—An increase of at least 20% of the sum of the diameters of target lesions, taking as reference the smallest sum of the diameters of the target lesions recorded since treatment started	PD—An increase of at least 20% of the sum of the diameters of viable (enhancing) target lesions, taking as reference the smallest sum of the diameters of viable (enhancing) target lesions recorded since treatment started

CR = complete response; PR = partial response; SD = stable disease; PD = progression of disease

Table 7 Completed prospective clinical studies on Y^{90} microspheres in mCRC

mCRC 1st-line	*Treatment regimen(s)*	*Design*	*n*
Gray et al.	FUDR HAC + SIR-Spheres	Ph III RCT	74
Van Hazel et al.	5FU/LV + SIR-Spheres	Ph II RCT	21
Sharma et al.	FOLFOX + SIR-Spheres	Ph I	20
mCRC 2nd-line			
Lim et al.	5FU/LV + SIR-Spheres	Ph II	30
Van Hazel et al.	Irinotecan + SIR-Spheres	Ph I	25
mCRC salvage therapy			
Cosimelli et al.	SIR-Spheres	Ph II	50

Potential complications of ^{90}Y-bearing microsphere therapy include gastrointestinal ulcers, radiation pneumonitis, radiation hepatitis and radiation cholecystitis. The risk of complications can be minimized with meticulous treatment planning; particularly, on the basis of baseline angiography, which may reveal extrahepatic vessels or a cystic artery at risk from reflux of microspheres. Myelosuppression was a reported complication during early experience with ^{90}Y microsphere therapy in the 1970s; however, the new resin and glass microspheres devised as radiotherapy delivery vehicles have virtually eliminated the leaching of ^{90}Y that presumably led to bone marrow suppression.[57,58]

Table 8 SIR-Spheres microspheres in 1st-line mCRC

Investigator	*n*	*Treatment*	*CR + PR*	*PFS*	*Survival*
Gray	74	SIR-Spheres + FUDR FUDR	44% 18% P = 0.01	15.9 mon 9.7 mon P = 0.001	39% at 2 year, 29% at 2 year, P = 0.06
van Hazel	21	SIR-Spheres + 5FU/LV 5FU/LV	76% 0% P = 0.001	18.6 mon 3.6 mon P = 0.0005	29.4 mon 12.8 mon P = 0.025
Sharma	20	FOLFOX4 + SIR-Spheres	90%	9.2 mon 14.2 mon*	Nr
Published chemotherapy (FOLFOX4) data			27–59%	7.6–9.2 mon	16.2–20.7 mon

Nr: not reported
*In-patients with liver-only disease

Table 9 SIR-Spheres microspheres in 2nd-line mCRC

Investigator	*n*	*Treatment*	*CR + PR*	*PFS*	*Survival*
Lim	30	SIR-Spheres (+ 5FU/LV)	33%	5.3 mon	not reported
van Hazel	25	SIR-Spheres + irinotecan	48%	6.0 mon	12.2 mon
Comparative chemotherapy phase II/III studies					
2nd-line		Irinotecan irinotecan + cetuximab	4–13% 16–27%	2.6–4.3 mon 3.3–4.0 mon	6.4–10 mon 8.6–10.7 mon
3rd-line		Panitumumab	9–14%	2–3.5 mon	6.3–9 mon

Table 10 SIR-Spheres microspheres in chemorefractory mCRC

Investigator	*N*	*Treatment*	*CR + PR*	*SD*	*PFS*	*Survival*
Kennedy	208‡	SIR-Spheres Responders Compare: non-responders/controls	 35.5% Na	 55% Na	 7.2 mon Na	 10.5 mon 4.5 mon P = 0.0001
Jakobs	41‡	SIR-Spheres	17%	61%	5.9 mon	10.5 mon
Cosimelli	50	SIR-Spheres	24%	24%	4 mon	13 mon

‡Retrospective data

Gene Therapy

Other experimental therapies that take advantage of a transarterial approach are in the early stages of development. Gene therapy is based on the transfer of DNA or RNA into host tissues; a procedure that may lead to new protein synthesis or to the deactivation of gene expression with the ultimate goal of inducing tumor lysis, blocking tumor growth, inducing antitumor immunity, activating a prodrug or inhibiting angiogenesis.[59]

REFERENCES

1. McMillan DC, McArdle CS. Epidemiology of colorectal liver metastases. Surg Oncol. 2007;16(1):3-5.
2. Liu LX, Zhang WH, Jiang HC. Current treatment for liver metastases from colorectal cancer. World J Gastroenterol. 2003;9(2):193-200.
3. Rothbarth J, van de Velde CJ. Treatment of liver metastases of colorectal cancer. Ann Oncol. 2005;16(Suppl. 2):ii144-9.
4. Bartlett DL, Berlin J, Lauwers GY, et al. Chemotherapy and regional therapy of hepatic colorectal metastases: expert consensus statement. Ann Surg Oncol. 2006;13(10):1284-92.
5. Gray B, Van Hazel G, Hope M, et al. Randomised trial of SIR-Spheres plus chemotherapy vs chemotherapy alone for treating patients with liver metastases from primary large bowel cancer. Ann Oncol. 2001;12(12):1711-20.
6. Stubbs RS, Cannan RJ, Mitchell AW. Selective internal radiation therapy with 90 yttrium microspheres for extensive colorectal liver metastases. J Gastrointest Surg. 2001;5(3):294-302.
7. Kalva SP, Thabet A, Wicky S. Recent advances in transarterial therapy of primary and secondary liver malignancies. Radiographics. 2008;28(1):101-17.
8. Homsi J, Garrett CR. Hepatic arterial infusion of chemotherapy for hepatic metastases from colorectal cancer. Cancer Control. 2006;13(1):42-7.
9. Lygidakis NJ, Sgourakis G, Dedemadi G, et al. Regional chemoimmunotherapy for nonresectable metastatic liver disease of colorectal origin. A prospective randomized study. Hepatogastroenterology. 2001;48(40):1085-7.
10. Ensminger WD, Gyves JW. Clinical pharmacology of hepatic arterial chemotherapy. Semin Oncol. 1983;10(2):176-82.
11. Cohen AD, Kemeny NE. An update on hepatic arterial infusion chemotherapy for colorectal cancer. Oncologist. 2003;8(6):553-66.
12. Heinrich S, Petrowsky H, Schwinnen I, et al. Technical complications of continuous intra-arterial chemotherapy with 5-fluorodeoxyuridine and 5-fluorouracil for colorectal liver metastases. Surgery. 2003;133(1):40-8.
13. Curley SA, Chase JL, Roh MS, et al. Technical considerations and complications associated with the placement of 180 implantable hepatic arterial infusion devices. Surgery. 1993;114(5):928-35.
14. Campbell KA, Burns RC, Sitzmann JV, et al. Regional chemotherapy devices: effect of experience and anatomy on complications. J Clin Oncol. 1993;11(5):822-6.
15. Skitzki JJ, Chang AE. Hepatic artery chemotherapy for colorectal liver metastases: technical considerations and review of clinical trials. Surg Oncol. 2002;11(3):123-35.
16. Kemeny N, Seiter K, Niedzwiecki D, et al. A randomized trial of intrahepatic infusion of fluorodeoxyuridine with dexamethasone versus fluorodeoxyuridine alone in the treatment of metastatic colorectal cancer. Cancer. 1992;69(2):327-34.
17. Kemeny N, Conti JA, Cohen A, et al. Phase II study of hepatic arterial floxuridine, leucovorin, and dexamethasone for unresectable liver metastases from colorectal carcinoma. J Clin Oncol. 1994;12(11):2288-95.
18. Dizon DS, Kemeny NE. Intrahepatic arterial infusion of chemotherapy: clinical results. Semin Oncol. 2002;29(2):126-35.
19. Ramsey DE, Kernagis LY, Soulen MC, et al. Chemoembolization of hepatocellular carcinoma. J Vasc Interv Radiol. 2002;13(9 Pt 2):S211-21.
20. Konno T. Targeting cancer chemotherapeutic agents by use of lipiodol contrast medium. Cancer. 1990;66(9):1897-903.
21. Nakamura H, Hashimoto T, Oi H, et al. Transcatheter oily chemoembolization of hepatocellular carcinoma. Radiology. 1989;170(3 Pt 1):783-6.
22. Vogl TJ, Mack MG, Balzer JO, et al. Liver metastases: neoadjuvant downsizing with transarterial chemoembolization before laser-induced thermotherapy. Radiology. 2003;229(2):457-64.
23. Wallace S, Carrasco CH, Charnsangavej C, et al. Hepatic artery infusion and chemoembolization in the management of liver metastases. Cardiovasc Intervent Radiol. 1990;13(3):153-60.
24. Chen MS, Li JQ, Zhang YQ, et al. High-dose iodized oil transcatheter arterial chemoembolization for patients with large hepatocellular carcinoma. World J Gastroenterol. 2002;8(1):74-8.
25. Wu ZQ, Fan J, Qiu SJ, et al. The value of postoperative hepatic regional chemotherapy in prevention of recurrence after radical resection of primary liver cancer. World J Gastroenterol. 2000;6(1):131-3.
26. Huang XQ, Huang ZQ, Duan WD, et al. Severe biliary complications after hepatic artery embolization. World J Gastroenterol. 2002;8(1):119-23.
27. Abramson RG, Rosen MP, Perry LJ, et al. Cost-effectiveness of hepatic arterial chemoembolization for colorectal liver metastases refractory to systemic chemotherapy. Radiology. 2000;216(2):485-91.
28. Popov I, Lavrnić S, Jelić S, et al. Chemoembolization for liver metastases from colorectal carcinoma: risk or a benefit. Neoplasma. 2002;49(1):43-8.
29. Ji SK, Cho YK, Ahn YS, et al. Multivariate analysis of the predictors of survival for patients with hepatocellular carcinoma undergoing transarterial chemoembolization: focusing on superselective chemoembolization. Korean J Radiol. 2008;9(6):534-40.
30. Matsui O, Kadoya M, Yoshikawa J, et al. Subsegmental transcatheter arterial embolization for small hepatocellular carcinomas: local therapeutic effect and 5-year survival rate. Cancer Chemother Pharmacol. 1994;33(Suppl):S84-8.
31. Miyayama S, Matsui O, Yamashiro M, et al. Ultraselective transcatheter arterial chemoembolization with a 2-f tip microcatheter for small hepatocellular carcinomas: relationship between local tumor recurrence and visualization of the portal vein with iodized oil. J Vasc Interv Radiol. 2007;18(3):365-76.
32. Lewis AL, Gonzalez MV, Lloyd AW, et al. DC bead: in vitro characterization of a drug-delivery device for transarterial chemoembolization. J Vasc Interv Radiol. 2006;17(2 Pt 1):335-42.

33. Johnson PJ, Kalayci C, Dobbs N, et al. Pharmacokinetics and toxicity of intraarterial adriamycin for hepatocellular carcinoma: effect of coadministration of lipiodol. J Hepatol. 1991;13(1):120-7.
34. Hong K, Khwaja A, Liapi E, et al. New intra-arterial drug delivery system for the treatment of liver cancer: preclinical assessment in a rabbit model of liver cancer. Clin Cancer Res. 2006;12(8):2563-7.
35. Vogl TJ, Zangos S, Eichler K, et al. Colorectal liver metastases: regional chemotherapy via transarterial chemoembolization (TACE) and hepatic chemoperfusion: an update. Eur Radiol. 2007;17(4):1025-34.
36. Taylor RR, Tang Y, Gonzalez MV, et al. Irinotecan drug eluting beads for use in chemoembolization: in vitro and in vivo evaluation of drug release properties. Eur J Pharm Sci. 2007;30(1):7-14.
37. Martin RC, Joshi J, Robbins K, et al. Hepatic intra-arterial injection of drug-eluting bead, irinotecan (DEBIRI) in unresectable colorectal liver metastases refractory to systemic chemotherapy: results of multi-institutional study. Ann Surg Oncol. 2011;18(1):192-8.
38. Martin RC, Joshi J, Robbins K, et al. Transarterial chemoembolization of metastatic colorectal carcinoma with drug-eluting beads, irinotecan (DEBIRI): multi-institutional registry. J of Oncology. 2009;12(5):539-45.
39. Martin RC, Robbins K, Tomalty D, et al. Transarterial chemoembolisation (TACE) using irinotecan-loaded beads for the treatment of unresectable metastases to the liver in patients with colorectal cancer: an interim report. World J Surg Oncol. 2009;7:80.
40. Martin RC, Howard J, Tomalty D, et al. Toxicity of irinotecan-eluting beads in the treatment of hepatic malignancies: results of a multi-institutional registry. Cardiovasc Intervent Radiol. 2010;33(5):960-6.
41. Bower M, Metzger T, Robbins K, et al. Surgical downstaging and neo-adjuvant therapy in metastatic colorectal carcinoma with irinotecan drug-eluting beads: a multi-institutional study. HPB (Oxford). 2010;12(1):31-6.
42. Brown RE, Bower MR, Metzger TL, et al. Hepatectomy after hepatic arterial therapy with either yttrium-90 or drug-eluting bead chemotherapy: is it safe? HPB (Oxford). 2011;13(2): 91-5.
43. Dawson LA, Normolle D, Balter JM, et al. Analysis of radiation-induced liver disease using the Lyman NTCP model. Int J Radiat Oncol Biol Phys. 2002;53(4):810-21.
44. Geschwind JF, Salem R, Carr BI, et al. Yttrium-90 microspheres for the treatment of hepatocellular carcinoma. Gastroenterology. 2004;127(5 Suppl. 1):S194-205.
45. Lewin K, Millis RR. Human radiation hepatitis. A morphologic study with emphasis on the late changes. Arch Pathol. 1973;96(1):21-6.
46. Murthy R, Nunez R, Szklaruk J, et al. Yttrium-90 microsphere therapy for hepatic malignancy: devices, indications, technical considerations, and potential complications. Radiographics. 2005;25(Suppl. 1):S41-55.
47. Miller FH, Keppke AL, Reddy D, et al. Response of liver metastases after treatment with yttrium-90 microspheres: role of size, necrosis, and PET. AJR Am J Roentgenol. 2007; 188(3):776-83.
48. Salem R, Thurston KG. Radioembolization with 90Yttrium microspheres: a state-of-the-art brachytherapy treatment for primary and secondary liver malignancies. Part 1: Technical and methodologic considerations. J Vasc Interv Radiol. 2006;17(8):1251-78.
49. Oken MM, Creech RH, Tormey DC, et al. Toxicity and response criteria of the Eastern Cooperative Oncology Group. Am J Clin Oncol. 1982;5(6):649-55.
50. Ho S, Lau WY, Leung TW, et al. Clinical evaluation of the partition model for estimating radiation doses from yttrium-90 microspheres in the treatment of hepatic cancer. Eur J Nucl Med. 1997;24(3):293-8.
51. Houle S, Yip TK, Shepherd FA, et al. Hepatocellular carcinoma: pilot trial of treatment with Y-90 microspheres. Radiology. 1989;172(3):857-60.
52. Therasse P, Arbuck SG, Eisenhauer EA, et al. New guidelines to evaluate the response to treatment in solid tumors. European Organization for Research and Treatment of Cancer, National Cancer Institute of the United States, National Cancer Institute of Canada. J Natl Cancer Inst. 2000;92(3):205-16.
53. Lencioni R, Llovet JM. Modified RECIST (mRECIST) assessment for hepatocellular carcinoma. Semin Liver Dis. 2010;30(1):52-60.
54. Keppke AL, Salem R, Reddy D, et al. Imaging of hepatocellular carcinoma after treatment with yttrium-90 microspheres. AJR Am J Roentgenol. 2007;188(3):768-75.
55. Deng J, Miller FH, Rhee TK, et al. Diffusion-weighted MR imaging for determination of hepatocellular carcinoma response to yttrium-90 radioembolization. J Vasc Interv Radiol 2006. 2006;17(7):1195-1200.
56. Kamel IR, Reyes DK, Liapi E, et al. Functional MR imaging assessment of tumor response after 90Y microsphere treatment in patients with unresectable hepatocellular carcinoma. J Vasc Interv Radiol. 2007;18(1 Pt 1):49-56.
57. Mantravadi RV, Spigos DG, Tan WS, et al. Intraarterial yttrium 90 in the treatment of hepatic malignancy. Radiology. 1982;142(3):783-6.
58. Herba MJ, Illescas FF, Thirlwell MP, et al. Hepatic malignancies: improved treatment with intraarterial Y-90. Radiology. 1988;169(2):311-4.
59. Avila MA, Berasain C, Sangro B, et al. New therapies for hepatocellular carcinoma. Oncogene. 2006;25(27):3866-84.

13 Ablations RFA vs Microwave vs Other

Lisa Rutstein, Abby Crume

Nearly half of the patients with colorectal cancer will develop liver metastases at some point in their lives.[1] Surgical resection is considered to be the first-line treatment for any patient undergoing intent to cure. Most patients however are deemed unresectable for various reasons. Radiofrequency ablation (RFA) is currently the most popular alternative treatment for colorectal liver metastases.[2] Microwave ablation is a newer technology and is gaining popularity in the treatment of metastatic disease.

RADIOFREQUENCY ABLATION

Methods

Radiofrequency ablation uses an alternating electric current to heat tissue. The high frequency initiates ionic movement which creates frictional heat. RFA heats tissue to at least 60°C.[3] Tissues heated above 60°C undergo coagulation and denaturing of proteins which causes irreversible cell damage while tissue heated above 100°C is vaporized.[3] The goal of RFA is to create a homogeneous heating of the lesion with a surrounding margin of approximately 1 cm. The liver however is not homogeneous, and different tissues conduct heat differently. Impedance is the primary factor that influences current delivery.[3] The liver parenchyma has a higher impedance (and therefore resistance) than surrounding blood vessels and bile ducts. As a result, the current may follow the path of least resistance through the blood vessels and bile ducts leading to incomplete ablation. This is commonly referred to as the electrical-sink or heat-sink effect, and is one reason why the proximity to blood vessels is a factor in determining candidacy for RFA. Although bile ducts can create a heat-sink effect, the more worrisome factor that must be considered is injury to the duct. When a bile duct is injured by RFA, the patient is at increased risk of bile leak, abscess, and biliary strictures. The tissue surrounding the zone of ablation is also affected, and has some degree of thermal injury. Up to 8 mm in diameter of partial tissue, destruction can occur surrounding the ablated area.[2]

Ablation of a lesion 4–7 cm may be possible but the risk of leaving residual disease is increased. Overlapping zones of ablation are frequently used for larger tumors (Fig. 1). This can be done in one setting with multiple probe sites or at different times.

The location of the intended ablation helps determine the approach. For lesions near the periphery close to other organs such as the diaphragm, stomach, duodenum, and colon, an open or laparoscopic procedure is safer due to direct visualization and the ability to recognize iatrogenic injury. Another benefit to laparoscopy and laparotomy is the ability to use intraoperative ultrasound to better localize tumors and potentially detect additional tumors in up to 40% of the patients.[2] The percutaneous approach is favored by many when the tumor is amenable due to the less invasive nature and potential for repeat ablations. This is commonly used for patients who have had a short disease-free interval as the need for repeat ablations is increased.

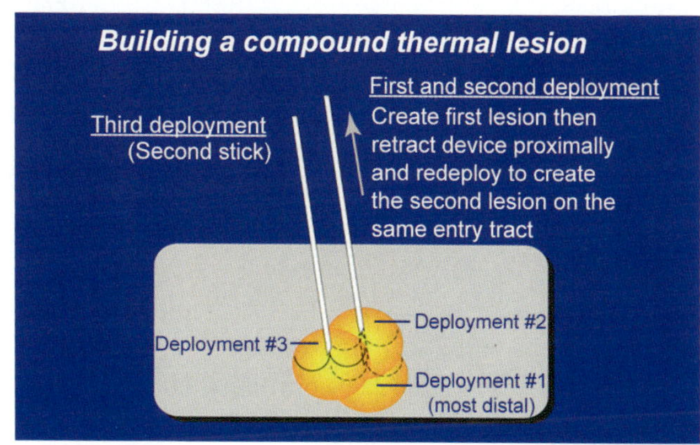

Figure 1 Overlapping zones of ablation

Indications

The common practice has been to use RFA as a second-line treatment if surgical resection is not an option, or in conjunction with resection. Historically resection was limited to tumors less than 5 cm, less than five lesions, single lobe tumors and metastatic disease confined to the liver. Recently the criteria have changed and more centers are expanding their limits of resection. The percentage of functioning residual liver is now the underlying factor in determining resectability. When tumors are deemed not resectable or the patient is not a good operative candidate, RFA can be used either as a primary treatment or as an adjunct to surgery. Cancer is a chronic disease, and RFA is an important tool for providing patients with a disease-free interval. There are factors however that limit the use of RFA. Although marketed as being capable of destroying tumors up to 7 cm in diameter with a single application, there have been numerous studies which advocate the use of a smaller cut-off.[1,4] Ayav and colleagues analyzed 311 tumor ablations and found that there was an increased risk of incomplete ablation and local recurrence when the tumor was greater than 3 cm.[4] Close proximity to large blood vessels is also a relative contraindication due to the heat-sink effect and the possibility for incomplete destruction. As with liver resection, enough healthy liver must be left for the patient to survive. RFA has also been used in less studied metastatic tumors. Patients with neuroendocrine metastases may benefit from RFA because tumor destruction may help diminish their endocrine symptoms.[5] RFA is becoming more popular for treating metastatic breast cancer which has been shown beneficial in selected patients.[6]

Complications

Although complication rates are low for RFA, physicians must be aware of their potential complications. Published complications include hemothorax, pneumothorax, intrahepatic bleeding or abscess, cholecystitis, liver failure, thermal injury to surrounding structures, and bile duct injuries resulting in bilomas or fistulas.[4,7-10] Curley and colleagues studied both the early (within 1 month) and late complications of multiple types of malignant liver tumors treated with RFA. In this series, they looked at 608 patients and 1,225 tumors. Open intraoperative RFA was performed in 62.8% of the patients with 48% of those also having a surgical resection, and percutaneous RFA was performed in 37.2% of the patients. The mortality rate of 0.5% represented three patients. One died of liver failure after both resection and RFA; one of pneumonia, and one of a fatal MI after bleeding into a RFA site. Early complications occurred in 7.1% of the patients and late complications in 2.4% of the patients. The most common early complication was a symptomatic pleural effusion requiring treatment (11 patients), whereas the most common late complication was biloma (6 patients). They concluded that early complications are more likely to occur in patients treated with open RFA and in cirrhotics while there was no difference in late complications.[9] Berber et al. studied 30-day morbidity and mortality rates of 428 patients who underwent a total of 521 RFA procedures; all done laparoscopically. They reported a 30-day mortality rate of 0.4% and morbidity rate of 3.8%. In their study, repeat ablations did not increase morbidity nor did combining RFA with another surgical procedure such as a colon resection or laparoscopic cholecystectomy. It did however show an increased rate of liver abscess formation in patients who had a previous bilio-enteric anastomosis such as a whipple.[10]

RFA versus Resection

Comparisons between surgical resection and RFA are difficult due to the inability to conduct randomized trials. Most studies comparing the two have a bias one way or another. Usually, RFA is reserved for patients excluded from surgery. These patients usually have unfavorable or worse tumor anatomy or are too sick to undergo a major operation. Hur and colleagues compared surgical resection and RFA of solitary colorectal liver metastases, and found that recurrence—intrahepatic and extrahepatic (both local)—was higher in the RFA group than the resection group. Overall survival was higher in the resection group than the RFA group.[1] Table 1 summarizes some recent publications regarding resection and RFA.

Otto and colleagues reported their experience using RFA as a first-line treatment for patients with colorectal liver metastases within 1 year of their initial colon surgery. Their goal was to spare patients the morbidity that comes along with a second large operation after a recent colon resection. The criteria used for RFA included lesions less than 5 cm in diameter, not more than five lesions, and not in proximity to large blood vessels or bile ducts. They were treated percutaneously unless the lesion was felt to be too superficial. The study found that RFA compared to surgical resection showed both the local recurrence and new metastases to be higher in the RFA group. At

Table 1 Recent studies comparing resection versus RFA

Study		*5-year OS*	*Local recurrence free survival*	*Tumors less than 3 cm*
Hyuk				5-year OS
	Resection	50.10%	89.70%	56.10%
	RFA	25.50%	69.70%	55.40%
McKay				
	Resection	43%	93%	
	RFA	23%	40%	
Hur				
	Resection	50.10%	89.70%	56.10%
	RFA	25.50%	69.70%	55.40%
Lee				
	Resection	65.70%	84.60%	
	RFA	48.50%	42.60%	

(**Abbreviation:** OS = Overall survival)
(*Source*: References 1, 11-13)

the third year however overall survival and disease-free survival were the same for both groups.

MICROWAVE ABLATION

Microwave ablation is a newer technology available for the treatment of liver metastatic disease. Microwave ablation has been shown in several studies to have equal effectiveness, safety and survival with shorter ablation times compared with RF ablation of both primary liver cancers and metastatic deposits. To better understand the potential advantages of microwave ablation, the mechanism of action must be understood.

Mechanism of Action

Microwave ablation uses dielectric hysteresis to produce heat. Tissue destruction occurs when tissues are heated to lethal temperatures from an applied electromagnetic field at 900–2,500 MHz. Polar molecules which are primarily H20, realign with the oscillating electric field increasing kinetic energy, and therefore the temperature of the tissue. Solid organs and tumors are most conducive to this type of heating. The microwave energy radiates into the tissue through an antenna that functions to couple energy from the generator power source to tissue. Direct heating occurs in a volume of tissue around the antenna. The ablation zone size and shape produced by an antenna in live tissue depends on the antenna design, tissue type, thermal conduction from the active heating zone, and thermal "sinks" caused by nearby structures such as blood vessels. This mechanism of action provides many theoretical advantages.[14-21]

Advantages

Microwave energy has the potential to produce faster heating over a larger volume of tissue with less susceptibility to heat-sink effect. Microwave can be effective in tissues with high impedance such as lung or charred tissue; capable of generating very high temperatures often in excess of 100°C, is highly conducive to the use of multiple applicators and does not require grounding pads or other ancillary components.[16,22-24] It also has organ specific advantages, particularly when one examines its application in liver tumors. Liver is a highly vascular solid organ with large blood vessels which creates the potential for heat-sink effects. Microwave is more apt to overcome perfusion and large heat sinks. Microwave energy has been shown to ablate tissue up to and around large hepatic vessels as large as 1 cm.[18,23,25-27] From an overall practical standpoint, the speed and effectiveness of microwave ablation allows for the treatment of multiple lesions in fewer sessions.

Hepatic Microwave Trials

The greater effectiveness of microwave ablation has been examined both in liver metastatic lesions and primary liver cancers. Most of the clinical trials have accumulated outcomes for the treatment of both primary and secondary liver cancers. Table 2 lists preclinical hepatic microwave trials, such as the Brace et al. study, which created circular ablation zones with minimal effects related to even large intrahepatic vessels, suggesting that there is minimal heat-sink effect adjacent to vessels.[18,19,27] Table 3 outlines clinical hepatic microwave trials which

Table 2 Preclinical microwave trials

Study	Model	System parameters	Ablation zone size
Brace	In vivo porcine	2.45 GHz, 68W 17-gauge, 2–12 min	Mean diameter: 2 min/2.3 cm, 6 min/2.6 cm, 12 min/2.9 cm
Awad	In vivo porcine	2.45 GHz, 100 W, 5.7 mm antenna, 2–8 min	Mean volume: 2 min/33.5 cm^3, 4 min/37.5 mm^3, 8 min/92 cm^3

(*Source:* References 18 and 27)

Table 3 Clinical microwave ablation trials

Study	No. pts	Mean tumor size (cm)	Mean follow-up (mo)	Local recurrence (%)	Survival
Yin	109	3.9	22	17	Median 30.3 mo
Shiomi	161	perc 2.6, thor 2.6	24.6	perc 15.1 thor 1.1	HCC 3 y perc 89.9% thor 89.9%; CRC 3 y perc 5% thor 6.6%
Ianitti	87	3.6	19	2.70	Survival 47% at 19 mo
Lu	102	2.5	25.1	11.80	Microwave: 1 y 81.6%, 2 y 61.2%, 3 y 50.5%, 4 y 36.8% RFA: 1 y 71.7%, 2 y 47.2%, 3 y 37.6%, 4 y 24.2%
Seki	68	2.0	31	12	1 y 97%, 3 y 90%, 5 y 48%

(**Abbreviations:** Mo = Months, perc = Percutaneous, thor = Thorascopic, HCC = Hepatocellular carcinoma, CRC = Colorectal carcinoma)
(*Source:* References 21, 32, 33, 37 and 38)

collectively demonstrate the proposed advantages of microwave ablation technology.[28–39] Dong et al. described 234 patients who underwent percutaneous microwave ablation, and demonstrated favorable survival without severe complications.[31] Lu et al. retrospectively compared 102 patients who underwent treatment with microwave or RF ablation with no significant difference in survival or complication rates between the two groups.[21] Ianitti et al. treated 87 patients with hepatocellular carcinoma and metastatic disease, and found an overall survival rate of 47% (all tumor types) at 19 months.[33] Preclinical data have suggested that microwaves may be effective in the treatment of larger tumors (> 3 cm), particularly with the use of multiple applicators. In addition, clinical studies have also suggested that microwaves are effective in the treatment of colorectal hepatic metastatic disease which requires a larger ablation margin, and therefore a larger ablation zone. Shibata et al. perspectively randomized 30 patients with multiple metastatic colorectal tumors to undergo microwave ablation or surgical resection and demonstrated no difference in the 1-, 2- and 3-year survival rates.[30] There was also less blood loss in the microwave ablation group. Ogata et al. treated 102 unresectable colorectal metastases with a local control rate of 95% during a median follow-up of 33 months.[40] This group reported a new lesion and extrahepatic recurrence rate of 78% with a median survival of 43 months.

Disadvantages of Microwave

Microwave power is more difficult to generate, and deliver safely and efficiently to the tissue compared with RF ablation. The coaxial cables carrying the microwave energy are larger and more prone to heating. The cable and shaft heating remains an issue when distributing such high power to tissues. There is ongoing effort to create effective cooling systems that limit excessive tissue damage. A clinical study comparing cooled with noncooled antennas in a cohort of 1,136 patients[41] showed that the use of a cooled-shaft antenna led to fewer treatment sessions and fewer complications related to normal tissue destruction such as abscess, necrosis, bile duct injury and vessel thrombosis. To date, there exists technical limitations related to underpowered systems, shaft heating, large diameter probes and long thin ablation zones. There is also some unpredictability as to the size and shape of the ablation zone.

REFERENCES

1. Hur H, Ko YT, Min BS, et al. Comparative study of resection and radiofrequency ablation in the treatment of solitary colorectal liver metastases. Am J Surg. 2009;197(6):728-36.
2. Yamane B, Weber S. Liver-directed treatment modalities for primary and secondary hepatic tumors. Surg Clin North Am. 2009;89(1):97-113.
3. Sindram D, Lau KN, Martinie JB, et al. Hepatic tumor ablation. Surg Clin North Am. 2010;90(4):863-76.
4. Ayav A, Germain A, Marchal F, et al. Radiofrequency ablation of unresectable liver tumors: factors associated with incomplete ablation or local recurrence. Am J Surg. 2010;200(4):435-9.
5. Mazzaglia PJ, Berber E, Milas M, et al. Laparoscopic radiofrequency ablation of neuroendocrine liver metastases: a 10-year experience evaluating predictors of survival. Surgery. 2007;142(1):10-9.

6. Meloni MF, Andreano A, Laeseke PF, et al. Breast cancer liver metastases: US-guided percutaneous radiofrequency ablation—intermediate and long-term survival rates. Radiology. 2009;253(3):861-9.
7. Otto G, Düber C, Hoppe-Lotichius M, et al. Radiofrequency ablation as first-line treatment in patients with early colorectal liver metastases amenable to surgery. Ann Surg. 2010;251(5): 796-803.
8. Amersi FF, McElrath-Garza A, Ahmad A, et al. Long-term survival after radiofrequency ablation of complex unresectable liver tumors. Arch Surg. 2006;141(6):581-7.
9. Curley SA, Marra P, Beaty K, et al. Early and late complications after radiofrequency ablation of malignant liver tumors in 608 patients. Ann Surg. 2004;239(4):450-8.
10. Berber E, Siperstein AE. Perioperative outcome after laparoscopic radiofrequency ablation of liver tumors: an analysis of 521 cases. Surg Endosc. 2007;21(4):613-8.
11. McKay A, Fradette K, Lipschitz J. Long-term outcomes following hepatic resection and radiofrequency ablation of colorectal liver metastases. HPB Surg. 2009.
12. Hur H, Ko YT, Min BS, et al. Comparative study of resection and radiofrequency ablation in the treatment of solitary colorectal liver metastases. Am J Surg. 2009;197(6):728-36.
13. Lee WS, Yun SH, Chun HK, et al. Clinical outcomes of hepatic resection and radiofrequency ablation in patients with solitary colorectal liver metastasis. J Clin Gastroenterol. 2008;42(8):945-9.
14. Brace CL. Microwave ablation technology: what every user should know. Curr Probl Diagn Radiol. 2009;38(2):61-7.
15. Duck FA. Physical properties of tissue: a comprehensive reference book. London: Academic Press; 1990. pp. 176-204.
16. Brace CL. Radiofrequency and microwave ablation of the liver, lung, kidney, and bone: what are the differences? Curr Probl Diagn Radiol. 2009;38(3):135-43.
17. Simon CJ, Dupuy DE, Mayo-Smith WW. Microwave ablation: principles and applications. Radiographics. 2005;25(Suppl. 1): S69-83.
18. Brace CL, Laeseke PF, Sampson LA, et al. Microwave ablation with a single small-gauge triaxial antenna: in vivo porcine liver model. Radiology. 2007;242(2):435-40.
19. Hines-Peralta AU, Pirani N, Clegg P, et al. Microwave ablation: results with a 2.45-GHz applicator in ex vivo bovine and in vivo porcine liver. Radiology. 2006;239(1):94-102.
20. Shock SA, Meredith K, Warner TF, et al. Microwave ablation with loop antenna: in vivo porcine liver model. Radiology. 2004;231(1):143-9.
21. Lu MD, Xu HX, Xie XY, et al. Percutaneous microwave and radiofrequency ablation for hepatocellular carcinoma: a retrospective comparative study. J Gastroenterol. 2005; 40(11):1054-60.
22. Schramm W, Yang D, Haemmerich D. Contribution of direct heating, thermal conduction and perfusion during radiofrequency and microwave ablation. Conf Proc IEEE Eng Med Biol Soc. 2006;1:5013-6.
23. Yang D, Converse MC, Mahvi DM, et al. Measurement and analysis of tissue temperature during microwave liver ablation. IEEE Trans Biomed Eng. 2007;54(1):150-5.
24. Skinner MG, Iizuka MN, Kolios MC, et al. A theoretical comparison of energy sources—microwave, ultrasound and laser—for interstitial thermal therapy. Phys Med Biol. 1998; 43(12):3535-47.
25. Bhardwaj N, Strickland AD, Ahmad F, et al. A comparative histological evaluation of the ablations produced by microwave, cryotherapy and radiofrequency in the liver. Pathology. 2009;41(2):168-72.
26. Yu NC, Chang X, Lu DS, et al. Microwave liver ablation: influence of hepatic vein size on heat-sink effect in a porcine model. J Vasc Interv Radiol. 2008;19(7):1087-92.
27. Awad MM, Devgan L, Kamel IR, et al. Microwave ablation in a hepatic porcine model: correlation of CT and histopathologic findings. HPB (Oxford). 2007;9(5):357-62.
28. Simon CJ, Dupuy DE, Iannitti DA, et al. Intraoperative triple antenna hepatic microwave ablation. AJR Am J Roentgenol. 2006;187(4):W333-40.
29. Yu NC, Lu DS, Raman SS, et al. Hepatocellular carcinoma: microwave ablation with multiple straight and loop antenna clusters—pilot comparison with pathologic findings. Radiology. 2006;239(1):269-75.
30. Shibata T, Iimuro Y, Yamamoto Y, et al. Small hepatocellular carcinoma: comparison of radio-frequency ablation and percutaneous microwave coagulation therapy. Radiology. 2002; 223(2):331-7.
31. Dong B, Liang P, Yu X, et al. Percutaneous sonographically guided microwave coagulation therapy for hepatocellular carcinoma: results in 234 patients. AJR Am J Roentgenol. 2003;180(6):1547-55.
32. Shiomi H, Naka S, Sato K, et al. Thoracoscopy-assisted magnetic resonance-guided microwave coagulation therapy for hepatic tumors. Am J Surg. 2008;195(6):854-60.
33. Iannitti DA, Martin RC, Simon CJ, et al. Hepatic tumor ablation with clustered microwave antennae: the US phase II trial. HPB (Oxford). 2007;9(2):120-4.
34. Seki S, Sakaguchi H, Iwai S, et al. Five-year survival of patients with hepatocellular carcinoma treated with laparoscopic microwave coagulation therapy. Endoscopy. 2005;37(12): 1220-5.
35. Liang P, Dong B, Yu X, et al. Prognostic factors for survival in patients with hepatocellular carcinoma after percutaneous microwave ablation. Radiology. 2005;235(1):299-307.
36. Xu HX, Lu MD, Xie XY, et al. Prognostic factors for long-term outcome after percutaneous thermal ablation for hepatocellular carcinoma: a survival analysis of 137 consecutive patients. Clin Radiol. 2005;60(9):1018-25.
37. Yin XY, Xie XY, Lu MD, et al. Percutaneous thermal ablation of medium and large hepatocellular carcinoma: long-term outcome and prognostic factors. Cancer. 2009:115(9):1914-23.
38. Seki T, Wakabayashi M, Nakagawa T, et al. Percutaneous microwave coagulation therapy for solitary metastatic liver tumors from colorectal cancer: a pilot clinical study. Am J Gastroenterol. 1999;94(2):322-7.
39. Shibata T, Niinobu T, Ogata N, et al. Microwave coagulation therapy for multiple hepatic metastases from colorectal carcinoma. Cancer. 2000;89(2):276-84.
40. Ogata Y, Uchida S, Hisaka T, et al. Intraoperative thermal ablation therapy for small colorectal metastases to the liver. Hepatogastroenterology. 2008;55(82-83):550-6.
41. Liang P, Wang Y, Yu X, et al. Malignant liver tumors: treatment with percutaneous microwave ablation—complications among cohort of 1136 patients. Radiology. 2009;251(3);933-40.

14 Isolated Hepatic Perfusion with TNF and Melphalan for Patients with Diffuse Hepatic Metastases

Susan B. Kesmodel, H. Richard Alexander Jr

INTRODUCTION

The management of unresectable liver metastases is a significant clinical challenge. In many patients, metastatic disease may be isolated to the liver or the liver may be the predominant site of metastatic disease. Progression of disease in the liver is generally the most significant cause of morbidity and mortality in these patients.

In 2011, it is estimated that over 140,000 people in the United States will be diagnosed with colorectal cancer (CRC).[1] Approximately 20–25% of these patients will have synchronous liver metastases, and an additional 20–30% of the patients will eventually develop hepatic metastases.[2,3] While surgical resection provides the only chance for cure, the majority of the patients will have unresectable disease due to the distribution of hepatic metastases or the presence of extrahepatic disease. Systemic chemotherapy is considered the standard of care for treatment of patients with unresectable CRC liver metastases. Numerous clinical trials have evaluated outcomes in these patients using various chemotherapy regimens combining 5-fluorouracil (5-FU), oxaliplatin, and/or irinotecan with or without targeted biological agents. These studies have demonstrated response rates (RRs) ranging from 35 to 60%, and median survival periods ranging from 15 to 23 months depending on the combination used.[4-10] Second-line therapies are not as efficacious and generally result in RRs of less than 25%, and median survival periods of less than 15 months.[11-15] Therefore, it is clear that alternative therapies for the management of unresectable CRC liver metastases need to be developed.

In addition to CRC, other malignancies such as ocular melanoma and neuroendocrine tumors also have a propensity to metastasize selectively to the liver. In patients with ocular melanoma, the liver is the most common site of metastatic disease. Systemic therapy options for these patients are limited in number and efficacy,[16-19] and although surgical resection, when possible, may improve survival, recurrence rates are high and 5-year survival rates are less than or equal to 20%.[20-22] In the case of neuroendocrine tumors, while prolonged survival may be observed in patients with diffuse liver metastases, significant systemic symptoms may develop due to disease burden and hormone production.[23,24] Therefore, for both malignancies, treatments which target the liver may be of substantial clinical benefit.

Liver-directed treatments—also known as regional therapies—have the advantages of allowing dose intensive therapy to be delivered to the cancer burdened organ while limiting unnecessary systemic toxicities and may have an important role in the management of patients with unresectable liver metastases. Hepatic artery infusion (HAI) or hepatic perfusion have the additional advantage of treating the entire liver at once and target macroscopic as well as microscopic disease.

Isolated hepatic perfusion (IHP) is a technique that has the potential to provide significant benefit in patients who are refractory to other therapies or who have limited treatment options.

DEVELOPMENT OF IHP AND INITIAL CLINICAL RESULTS

The liver-directed therapies that are under development for the treatment of patients with primary and metastatic liver tumors include HAI, IHP, radiofrequency ablation, transarterial embolization (TAE) and selective internal radiation. Several of these therapies including IHP, take advantage of the unique vascular supply of hepatic tumors, which derive their blood flow primarily from the hepatic arterial circulation.[25] This allows for tumors to be targeted for treatment through the hepatic artery while limiting both systemic toxicity and toxicity to the normal liver.

Vascular isolation and regional perfusion of a cancer burdened organ or region of the body was first described by Creech and Krementz in 1958, and was made possible only through the development of extracorporeal oxygenated bypass circuits.[26] Creech and Krementz demonstrated that high dose chemotherapy could be delivered to regional vascular beds while limiting systemic exposure, and anti-tumor effects were also observed. In 1961, Dr Robert Ausman, at the Roswell Park Memorial Institute (now known as the Roswell Park Cancer Institute), published a paper describing the development of a technique for IHP.[27] The technique was first refined in a canine model and was then tested in 5 patients with various hepatic malignancies. Although there was no long-term follow-up and the morbidity was significant, therapeutic effect was likely observed in 2 patients. In 1969, Stehlin et al. demonstrated the synergistic effects of hyperthermia and chemotherapy in regional perfusion, and therefore, the combination of hyperthermia and chemotherapy has become the standard approach.[28]

Because of the significant morbidity and potential mortality associated with IHP, this technique did not gain widespread acceptance over the following three decades. Several small single-institution series were published during this time, but patient selection criteria and perfusion parameters were variable, limiting the utility of these studies.[29-31] In the early 1990s, interest in the field of regional perfusion was renewed following a report by Lienard and Lejeune combining chemotherapy and tumor necrosis factor alpha (TNF) for the treatment of extremity melanoma and sarcoma.[32] This study and the observations of others demonstrated remarkably high RRs with the use of TNF and melphalan against those and other malignancies (Fig. 1). In addition, because of the potential for significant systemic toxicity associated with the use of TNF, there was more focus on standardizing perfusion techniques. Emphasis was placed on ensuring complete vascular isolation, and monitoring systems were developed to assess systemic leaks during perfusion.

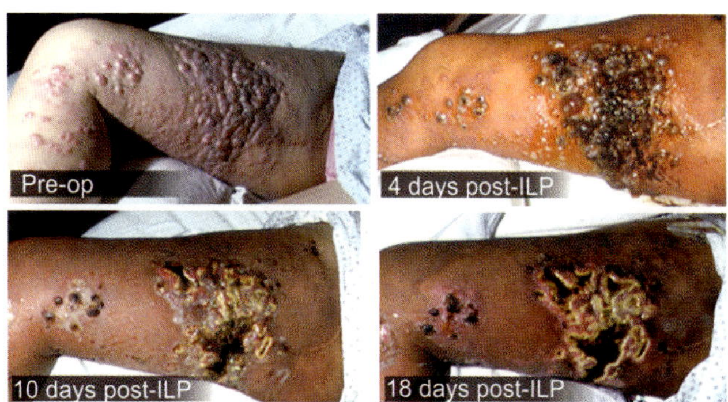

Figure 1 Photographs of a patient showing extensive-in-transit metastases throughout the leg from a primary eccrine gland adenocarcinoma that arose on the heel. Under a single patient compassionate use approval from the FDA, the patient was treated with a 90-minute hyperthermic isolated limb perfusion using tumor necrosis factor and melphalan. The patient experienced rapid Eschar formation and tumor necrosis within days of treatment. Note the sparing of normal skin bridges within the large thigh tumor mass. This was the first observation of this regimen having meaningful clinical efficacy against an adenocarcinoma

During the 1990s, several groups in the United States and Europe developed protocols to evaluate the safety and efficacy of IHP in patients with unresectable liver malignancies.[33-36] One of the most comprehensive studies was a Phase II protocol from the National Cancer Institute (NCI) which evaluated the use of high dose melphalan, TNF and moderate hyperthermia for the management of unresectable malignancies confined to the liver.[33] The maximum tolerated doses (MTD) of melphalan and TNF were established from a previously conducted Phase I study. Complete vascular isolation was confirmed using continuous intraoperative leak monitoring with I-131 human serum albumin. A total of 34 patients were treated, and 33 patients were assessable for response. There was one treatment-related mortality. The majority of the patients (76%) had CRC liver metastases, and 60% had received prior systemic or regional treatment. Grade III or greater hepatic toxicity was observed in 75% of the patients and was reversible in all but one patient. The overall RR was 75% and was maintained in patients with advanced disease or those

Chapter 14

Table 1 Response to IHP based upon number of lesions, diameter of largest tumor, or percent hepatic replacement in 33 evaluable patients

	n	*PR or CR**	*Percentage*
Overall	33	25	75
Number#			
1–4	9	7	78
5–19	13	9	69
20	11	9	81
Diameter largest lesion (cm)			
<5	4	2	50
5–9.9	12	9	75
10	17	14	82
% Hepatic replacement			
< 20	6	5	83
20–49	15	10	66
50	12	10	83

*Partial (PR) or complete (CR) response
#Radiographically imageable lesions
(*Source:* Modified from J. Clin. Oncol. 1998;16:1479)

who had prior treatment (Table 1). This study therefore established IHP as a viable treatment option for patients with unresectable liver metastases, although, it was clear that refinements in the technique and delivery of therapeutic agents needed to be explored.

OPEN TECHNIQUE FOR IHP

Isolated hepatic perfusion using the open approach is a complex surgical procedure. Access to the liver and the porta hepatis is obtained using a subcostal incision. The abdomen is explored to evaluate for peritoneal dissemination or distant lymph node involvement which would be a contraindication to the procedure. Involvement of resectable lymph nodes limited to the porta hepatis is not considered a contraindication to IHP since this has not been shown to adversely affect outcomes.

Hepatic vascular isolation is obtained by first mobilizing the right and left lobes of the liver; taking down the triangular ligaments, and mobilizing the duodenum to expose the inferior vena cava (IVC) below the liver. The right lobe of the liver is then mobilized medially to visualize the entire retrohepatic vena cava to the level of the diaphragm. All venous tributaries from the retroperitoneum to the IVC including the right adrenal vein and phrenic vein are ligated. All collateral vessels to the liver are also ligated. The structures of the porta hepatis, including the proper hepatic artery (PHA), portal vein (PV) and common bile duct, are completely exposed. The

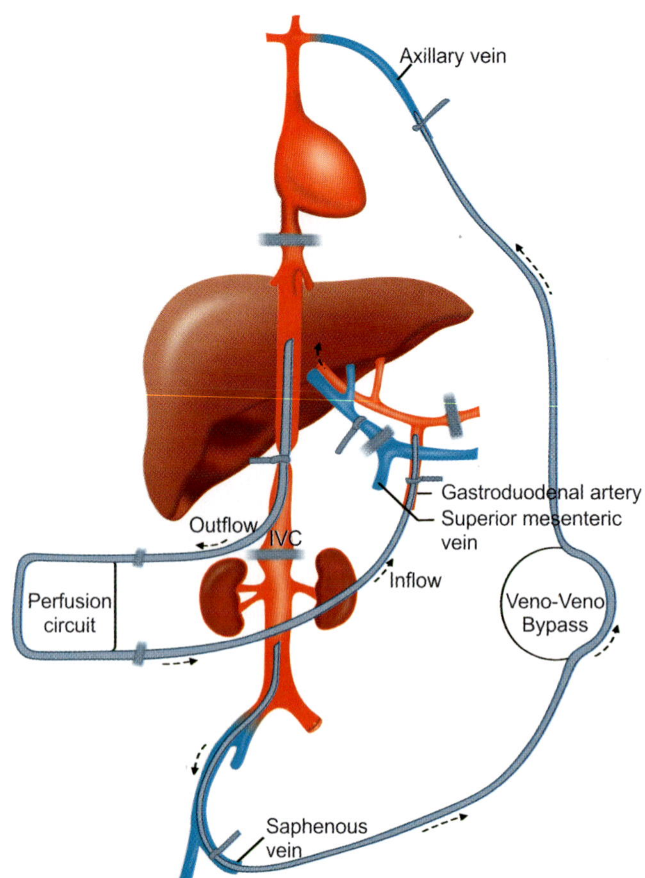

Figure 2 Illustration of the isolated hepatic perfusion circuit. On the patient's right is the extracorporeal perfusion circuit connected to an inflow cannula positioned in the gastroduodenal artery, and an outflow cannula in an isolated segment of the retrohepatic IVC. Note the vascular occlusion clamps on the common hepatic artery and portal vein. A second venovenous bypass circuit is on the patient's left to shunt IVC blood flow back to the heart during perfusion

gastroduodenal artery (GDA) is identified, and serves as the cannulation site for the perfusion. The IHP circuit is depicted in Figure 2.

Systemic anticoagulation using heparin is administered to maintain an activated clotting time of more than 350–400 seconds. A venovenous bypass circuit is then created from the saphenous vein to the axillary vein to maintain systemic venous return. This is necessary since flow in the retrohepatic vena cava will be interrupted with occluding clamps during the perfusion. The saphenous vein is cannulated with a 14–16 Fr catheter with the tip positioned just below the renal veins. A similar 14–18 Fr catheter is placed in the axillary vein and positioned in the central circulation. These two cannulae are then attached to a centrifugal pump and form the venovenous bypass circuit.

To create the perfusion circuit, a vascular clamp is placed across the IVC just above the renal veins.

A venotomy is made in the IVC, and a 20–24 Fr catheter is inserted in the retrohepatic vena cava which serves as the venous outflow for the hepatic perfusion circuit. Alternatively, the retrohepatic venous cannula can be inserted via the femoral vein percutaneously. The PV and common hepatic artery (CHA) are occluded with vascular clamps. The inflow for the perfusion is then created by making an arteriotomy in the GDA while as cannulating this vessel with a 3–4 mm arterial catheter positioned at the orifice of the CHA. Complete isolation of the liver is then achieved by placing a vascular clamp across the suprahepatic vena cava. Temperature probes are placed directly into the liver parenchyma on the right and left side to monitor hyperthermia during the procedure.

The perfusion circuit for the open technique consists of a roller pump, membrane oxygenator and a heat exchanger. The perfusate consists of 700 milliliters (ml) of a balanced salt solution and one unit of packed red blood cells (roughly 300 ml). A unit of packed red blood cells is necessary to ensure adequate oxygen delivery to the hepatic parenchyma during the perfusion. Arterial and venous blood gases are monitored throughout the perfusion to maintain a perfusate pH between 7.2 and 7.3. This is achieved with the addition of sodium bicarbonate to the perfusate. The heat exchanger is utilized to warm the perfusate to maintain hepatic parenchymal temperatures between 38.5°C and 40°C. Flow rates of greater than 400 ml/min should be achieved, and optimal flow rates are 600–800 ml/min (Table 2). Uniform perfusion to both lobes of the liver can be observed by rapid and uniform increase in temperature in both lobes (Fig. 3). During the perfusion, a venous outflow reservoir is monitored for changes in volume. Significant increases or decreases in the reservoir suggest incomplete vascular isolation. If this occurs, all vascular clamps should be evaluated, and any additional collateral vessels to the liver should be identified and ligated. The perfusion continues for 60 minutes and then the liver is flushed with 1500 ml of crystalloid followed by 1500 ml of colloid. The vascular structures are decannulated and repaired, and normal liver perfusion is restored.

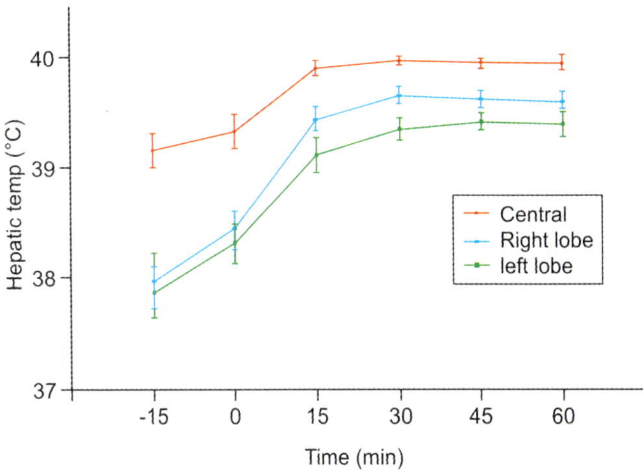

Figure 3 Graph showing the rapid and uniform heating of the hepatic parenchyma during isolated hepatic perfusion

Table 2 Treatment and perfusion parameters used during IHP

Duration	*1 hour*
Hepatic tissue temp	39.5–40°C
TNF[#]	1.0 mg
Melphalan	1.5 mg/kg
Flow rate	600–1,200 ml/min
Arterial line pressure	110–200 mm Hg[*]
Venovenous bypass flow	1.8–2.0 L/min
Perfusate volume	
Perfusate Composition	700 cc crystalloid
	300 cc pRBCs
	2,000 U heparin
	20–40 mEq $NaHCO_3$
Post-perfusion flush	
Hepatic artery	1.5 L crystalloid
	1.5 L colloid
Portal vein	1.0 L crystalloid

[#]Not used currently
[*]Measured pressure in circuit, actual delivered pressure into hepatic artery is lower.

In the past, a leak monitoring system, similar to that utilized for Isolated Limb Perfusion, to confirm complete vascular isolation of the liver was used for IHP. Since complete vascular isolation can be consistently achieved in IHP, this leak monitoring system is no longer used.

ISOLATED HEPATIC PERFUSION FOR CRC LIVER METASTASES

Because of the relatively high frequency of CRC liver metastases and the significant morbidity and mortality that is observed in these patients due to progression of liver disease, the majority of studies that have evaluated IHP have been performed in patients with CRC liver metastases. These studies have utilized multiple types of chemotherapy including mitomycin C,[36] oxaliplatin,[37] and melphalan with or without TNF.[36,38-43]

There are two large series that have been published which have evaluated IHP in patients with unresectable CRC liver metastases.[40,42] Between June 1994 and July 2005, 120 patients with unresectable CRC liver metastases were treated on sequential prospective

Table 3 Results with IHP for patients with CRC liver metastases treated with IHP

Treatment regimen	*# of patients evaluable*	*CR*	*PR*	*Median PFS months*
Overall	114	2	67 59%	7.0
IHP – no HAI	58	0	33 57%	5.8
IHP – HAI	46	2	30 65%	13.0
IHP (TNF alone)	10	0	4	3.0

Overall survival: median—17.4 months

clinical trials at the NCI using IHP with melphalan alone (n = 69), melphalan and TNF (n = 41), or TNF alone (n = 10).[40] The majority of the patients (80%) had been treated with previous chemotherapy prior to IHP. Postoperatively, 46 patients (38%) were treated with HAI using floxuridine. There were five (4%) treatment-related mortalities; response was evaluable in 114 patients. Overall RR was 59% with a median time to hepatic progression of 7.0 months. RRs were similar in patients who received postoperative HAI therapy compared to those who did not; 65% versus 57% respectively. However, patients who received HAI therapy had a longer time to hepatic progression than those patients who did not receive HAI therapy; 13.0 months versus 5.8 months respectively (Table 3). The most common toxicities were transient elevations in serum transaminases and total bilirubin. Median overall survival (OS) was 17.4 months. Factors associated with response were the dose of melphalan and the use of TNF. With respect to OS, only the use of HAI therapy and a preoperative carcinoembryonic antigen level of less than or equal to 30 ng/ml were significant on multivariate analysis (Table 4).

Similar outcomes were reported by van de Velde and colleagues, who treated 105 patients with unresectable CRC liver metastases over a 10-year period between August 1994 and December 2004.[42] In contrast to the NCI study, all patients were treated with a fixed high-dose of melphalan (200 mg), and almost all patients were perfused simultaneously through the hepatic artery and PV. In this series, approximately half of the patients had received prior systemic chemotherapy for the treatment of liver metastases before undergoing IHP. Treatment-related morbidity and mortality were similar to that observed in the NCI study. The median progression-free survival (PFS) was 7.4 months, while the median duration of hepatic response was 11.4 months. The overall RR was 50% (52/105 patients). The median OS was 24.8 months. In patients who responded to IHP, the median OS was 32.7 months compared to 16.2 months in patients who did not respond to IHP. On multivariate analysis, the use of adjuvant chemotherapy was associated with response and PFS while a greater number of hepatic metastases, PV perfusion alone, and postoperative complications were associated with decreased OS.

Using this same group of patients treated with IHP, van Iersel et al. recently reported a case-control study that compared the use of IHP with melphalan to systemic chemotherapy in patients with unresectable CRC liver metastases.[43] The IHP group consisted of 99 patients treated between August 1994 and December 2004. The systemic chemotherapy group consisted of 111 patients who were enrolled in the CApecitabine, IRinotecan, Oxaliplatin (CAIRO) study of the Dutch Colorectal Cancer Group and received either sequential chemotherapy with first-line capecitabine, followed by second-line irinotecan, and then third-line capecitabine and irinotecan or combination chemotherapy with first-line capecitabine and irinotecan followed by second-line capecitabine and oxaliplatin. Patient characteristics in both groups were similar except that the IHP patients were younger. In the IHP group, major postoperative complications were observed in 35% of the patients,

Table 4 Cox proportional hazards models (following backward elimination) showing the relationship between OS and liver PFS in 120 patients with diffuse CRC LM treated with IHP and in 105 patients for whom preoperative CEA was known

Survival (n = 120)	*Parameter estimate*	*P-value*	*Hazard ratio (HR)*	*95% CI for HR*
HAI	0.58	0.0039	1.78	1.20, 2.64
Survival (n = 105)				
HAI	0.54	0.013	1.72	1.12, 2.63
Preoperative CEA	0.83	0.0012	2.29	1.39, 3.78
Liver PFS (n = 120)				
HAI	1.02	< 0.0001	2.79	1.87, 4.16
Liver PFS (n = 105)				
HAI	1.17	< 0.0001	3.22	2.06, 5.03
Preoperative CEA	0.85	0.0006	2.35	1.44, 3.82

Section 4

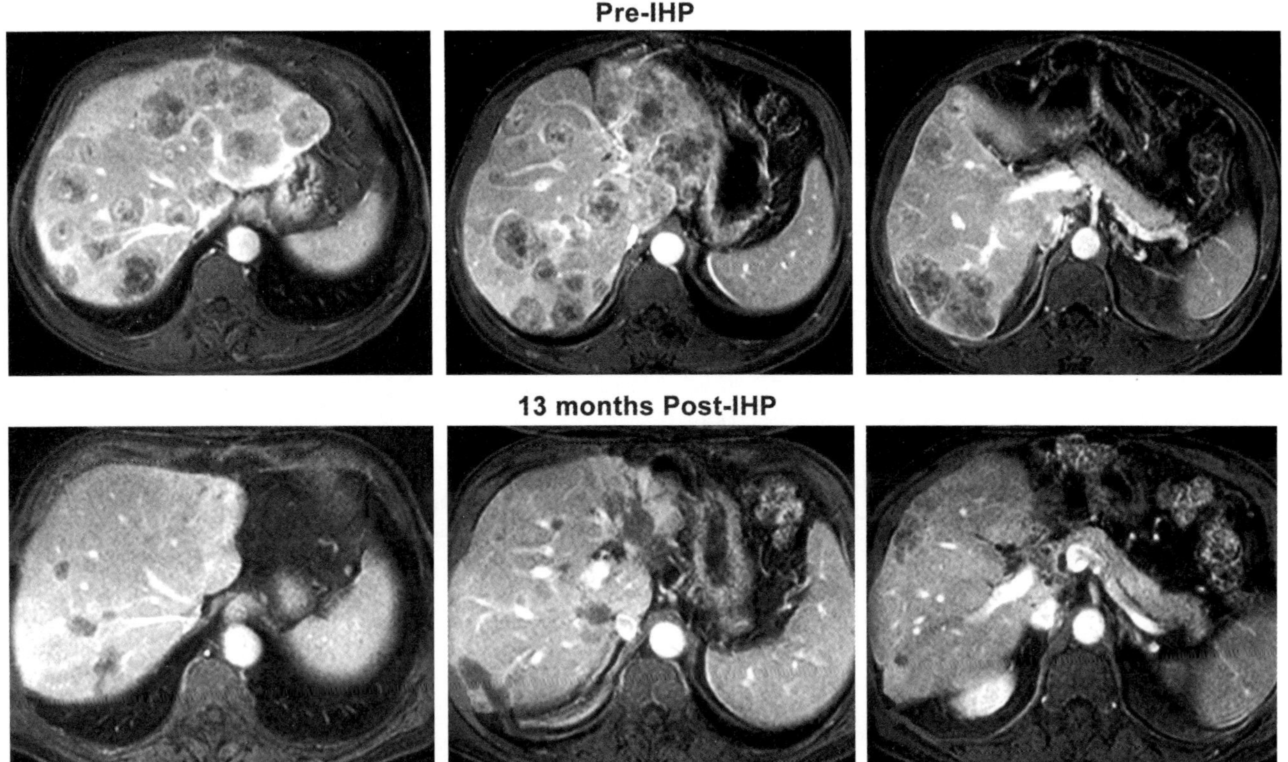

Figure 4 Gadolinium enhanced magnetic resonance imaging study from a patient with extensive hepatic metastases from colorectal cancer who had been previously treated with systemic and regional chemotherapy. The patient had a marked response to a 60-minute isolated hepatic perfusion as reflected in the lower images obtained over one year after treatment

and perioperative mortality was 6%. Sixteen patients received systemic therapy immediately after IHP, and 72 patients received systemic treatment at the time of disease progression. The overall RR for IHP was 47%, and the median time to disease progression was 7.3 months. In the systemic chemotherapy group, grade III/IV toxicity was observed in 52% of the patients, and treatment-related mortality was 2%. The overall RR to first-line therapy was 37%, and the median time to disease progression was 7.9 months. There was no significant difference in OS between the two groups; 25.0 months for those treated with IHP and 21.7 months for patients treated with systemic chemotherapy alone. Those patients who were treated with IHP as first-line therapy (50 patients) had an OS of 28.9 months, which was not significantly different compared to the systemic therapy group (p = 0.24). Only patients who were able to undergo metastasectomy after chemotherapy or IHP (total 15 patients) had a significant improvement in OS. Because IHP demonstrated no significant survival benefit when compared to systemic chemotherapy alone, the authors of this study concluded that systemic therapy remains the standard of care for management of patients with unresectable CRC liver metastases and that IHP should be considered in the context of prospective clinical trials.

Although the role of IHP as first-line therapy for patients with unresectable CRC liver metastases may be limited, there is a potential role for IHP in patients who are refractory to systemic chemotherapy. Alexander et al. published a series specifically focusing on 25 patients with unresectable CRC liver metastases refractory to irinotecan-based therapy who were treated on protocol at the NCI with IHP using melphalan between March 1993 and February 2003.[39] Twenty-two of the patients received irinotecan-based therapy as second-line treatment for CRC liver metastases, while 3 patients received this as first-line therapy. Similar to other IHP studies, the patients had significant tumor burden with a median number of 10 hepatic metastases and a median percent hepatic replacement by tumor of 25% (Fig. 4). The overall RR was 60% (1 complete, 14 partial), and the median duration of response in the liver was 12 months. Systemic progression occurred in 13 patients (54%) at median 5 months. The median OS was 12 months with a 2-year survival of 28%. These results are quite favorable when compared to second-line chemotherapy where RRs are generally less than 25%, and median OS is usually less than 15 months. Therefore, there may be a role for IHP as second-line or third-line therapy in selected patients with unresectable CRC liver metastases who are refractory to systemic chemotherapy.

ISOLATED HEPATIC PERFUSION FOR OCULAR MELANOMA

Ocular melanoma accounts for approximately 3–6% of all cases of melanoma, and 30–60% of the patients with ocular melanoma will develop liver metastases.[44-49] The options for systemic treatment in these patients are limited in number and efficacy,[16-19] and although surgical resection has been attempted in selected patients with modest results,[20-22] most patients have diffuse metastases—many of which are not visible on imaging studies (Fig. 5). Given the limited alternative treatment options, multiple studies have evaluated the use of IHP in these patients.

Similar to IHP for CRC, several protocols were developed at the NCI to evaluate IHP in patients with ocular melanoma liver metastases. Alexander et al. reported a Phase I-II Study of IHP in patients with ocular melanoma and unresectable hepatic metastases.[50] Twenty-two patients were treated between 1994 to 1999 in two Phase I studies using escalating doses of melphalan with or without TNF, and in a Phase II study using melphalan and TNF. Half of the patients received melphalan alone, and the other half were treated with melphalan and TNF. Patients generally had advanced disease with a median number of metastatic nodules at 25 (range, 5 to less than 50); a mean percentage of hepatic replacement at 25% (range, 10–75%) and the mean size of the largest lesion was greater than 7 cm. The overall RR was 62%; 2 complete responses (CR, 10%) and 11 partial responses (PR, 52%). Of those patients treated with melphalan alone, 7 out of 10 (70%) had a response, while 6 out of 11 patients (54%) treated with melphalan and TNF had evidence of a radiographic response. There was one treatment-related mortality (5%). Transient hepatic toxicity was observed in approximately 80% of the patients. More hepatic and systemic side effects were observed in patients who received TNF, although, these were also transient. The median PFS was 9 months in all patients and was significantly longer in patients who received TNF (14 months vs 6 months, $p = 0.04$). The OS was 11 months. These results were very promising given the high RR, and the acceptable morbidity and mortality that were observed.

A follow-up study was published in 2003, and reported outcomes in 29 patients with metastatic ocular melanoma to the liver treated at the NCI using IHP with melphalan alone between 1997 and 2002.[51] This study included 6 patients from the previous report. Similar to the prior study, the overall RR was 62% with 3 CRs (10%) and 15 PRs (52%). The actuarial median hepatic PFS in the 18 patients who demonstrated evidence of a response was 12 months, and the OS in all patients was 12.1 months. There were no treatment-related deaths, and the most common side effect was transient grade III or greater hepatic toxicity which occurred in 65% of the patients. On multivariate analysis, only baseline lactate dehydrogenase (LDH) was identified as a significant independent prognostic factor for survival, suggesting that baseline LDH level may have a role in patient selection (Fig. 6).

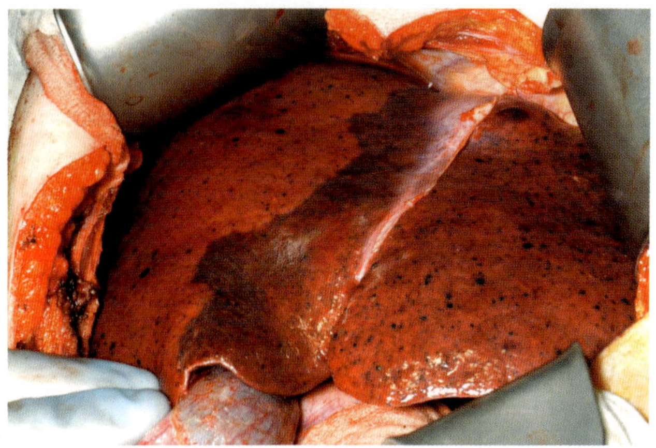

Figure 5 Operative photograph of a patient with diffuse miliary metastases isolated to the liver from a primary ocular melanoma. Note the geographic wave of tumor extending through segment 4. Most of the metastases were not imaged on preoperative magnetic resonance imaging or computed tomography

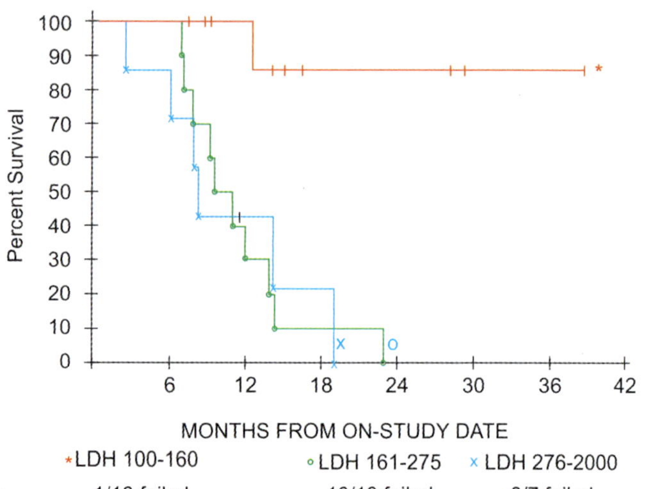

Figure 6 Actuarial overall survival curves of patients following isolated hepatic perfusion for ocular melanoma metastatic to the liver showing the favorable prognosis in those with a normal baseline lactate dehydrogenase (LDH) level

Smaller series in the literature have also achieved results that are comparable to those of the NCI. Noter et al. reported on 8 patients treated with IHP with high dose melphalan (200 mg) for ocular melanoma metastases.[52] The overall RR was 50% (all partial), the median PFS was 6.7 months, and the median OS was 9.9 months. Transient hepatic toxicity was observed in 3 patients, and veno-occlusive disease eventually developed in 2 patients. A follow-up report from the same center which included a total of 19 patients treated with IHP—13 with ocular melanoma metastases—demonstrated an RR of 33% in patients with ocular melanoma metastases; a median time to hepatic progression of 8.2 months, and a median OS of 10 months.[53]

Based on these studies, it appears that in patients with unresectable ocular melanoma liver metastases, RRs of less than 50% can generally be obtained using IHP with melphalan with or without TNF with mortality rates of less than 5% and transient morbidity. These results are better than those obtained with systemic therapy alone and appear to be comparable to those obtained with other regional therapies including TAE and HAI.[54-60] Therefore, the use of IHP in these patients has the potential to provide significant clinical benefit.

ISOLATED HEPATIC PERFUSION FOR NEUROENDOCRINE TUMORS

Approximately 75% of the patients with neuroendocrine tumors will have metastatic disease at presentation, and the most common site for metastasis is the liver.[23,24,61] While surgical resection is effective and can improve 5-year survival rates to greater than 50%, complete surgical resection is usually difficult since patients often present with multifocal or bilateral disease.[23,24,62-64] Even with diffuse liver metastases, 5-year survival rates of approximately 30% have been observed without treatment.[24] However, patients may develop debilitating local and systemic symptoms related to tumor burden and hormone production. In addition, liver-directed therapies have the potential to improve long-term outcomes by controlling progression of disease. Therefore, treatment of hepatic metastases has become an important component in the overall management of these patients.

The only report in the literature which documents the use of IHP to treat neuroendocrine hepatic metastases in a substantial number of patients is a study from the NCI.[65] This report details treatment and outcomes in 13 patients with neuroendocrine liver metastases treated with IHP on various protocols between 1993 and 2003. Ten patients were treated with melphalan alone; 2 patients received a combination of melphalan and TNF, and 1 patient was treated with TNF alone. Reversible grade III/IV hepatic toxicity was observed in 62% of the patients, which is consistent with toxicity observed in other IHP studies. There was one treatment-related mortality. Overall RR was 50%, and the median actuarial survival was 48 months. Given the effectiveness of surgical resection and other liver-directed therapies[23,66-70] in the management of patients with neuroendocrine liver metastases, it is likely that IHP will only play a significant role in the management of patients with quite advanced disease. It is possible, however, that with the continued development and evaluation of percutaneous IHP techniques, IHP will become a more important treatment modality for these patients in the future.

PERCUTANEOUS HEPATIC PERFUSION

Isolated hepatic perfusion using the open technique has the potential for significant morbidity, and a major drawback of the technique is that it cannot be repeated. Given the excellent RRs that are observed after a single perfusion, it is possible that multiple perfusions may provide more durable responses and improve OS. Therefore, over the last two decades, a technique for percutaneous hepatic perfusion (PHP) has been developed to potentially decrease the morbidity of hepatic perfusion and to allow for sequential treatments (Fig. 7).

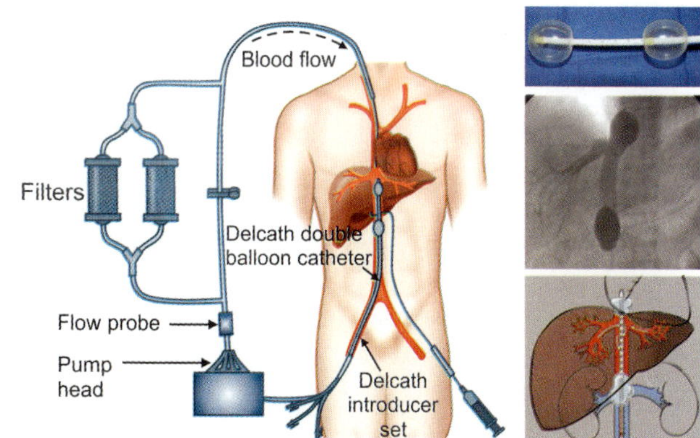

Figure 7 Diagram of the Delcath® Catheter System. Melphalan is administered directly into the hepatic artery through an infusion catheter placed percutaneously via the femoral artery. Hepatic venous outflow is isolated via a double balloon catheter in the retrohepatic IVC (shown top right). Blood is drawn out of the retrohepatic IVC through multiple fenestrations located along the length of the catheter between the cranial and caudal balloons. The blood is then pumped through a pair of activated charcoal filters prior to returning to the systemic circulation via an internal jugular vein catheter.
Fluoroscopic image of the isolated retrohepatic IVC segment obtained by retrograde injection of contrast through the intra-balloon fenestrations; to confirm the absence of systemic leak is shown in the middle right

Chapter 14

Patients undergoing PHP are treated under general anesthesia. The technique utilizes a double-balloon catheter system (produced by Delcath Systems, New York, NY) which is positioned percutaneously in the retrohepatic vena cava under fluoroscopic guidance. The double-balloon catheter has a unique construction with a large central lumen, three accessory lumina, and fenestrations throughout its length that allows for collection of hepatic venous outflow (Fig. 7). The two balloons on either end of the catheter are positioned inferior and superior to the hepatic veins and are inflated under fluoroscopy independently. The venous outflow from the liver is filtered through an extracorporeal filtration system and is then returned to the systemic circulation through a catheter in the internal jugular vein. The arterial catheter is placed percutaneously from the femoral artery and is positioned in the PHA under fluoroscopic guidance. Accessory arteries may also be embolized to ensure that the chemotherapy infusion is truly isolated to the liver. Once vascular isolation is confirmed, chemotherapy is administered as a continuous infusion over 30 minutes. The filtration circuit is then continued for an additional 30 minutes after the perfusion to ensure that all the chemotherapy is removed. Anticoagulation is required during the perfusion and is reversed using protamine and fresh frozen plasma at the end of the perfusion. Temporary use of vasopressors is necessary after balloon inflation to maintain hemodynamic stability.

Initial experience and results using PHP were first reported in the early 1990s.[71-73] Ravikumar et al. reported a series of 58 PHP that were performed in 21 patients using escalating doses of 5-FU or doxorubicin. In this study, the extraction efficiency of the filter ranged from 64–91%.[73] The most common grade III/IV toxicities were transient hypotension at the time of IVC occlusion and myelosuppression. There were no mortalities. Curley et al. reported similar outcomes using PHP with escalating doses of doxorubicin in 10 patients with hepatocellular carcinoma.[72] Both of these studies demonstrated that the technique was feasible; however, the clinical efficacy of the procedure was not evaluated.

In 2005, Pingpank et al. reported a Phase I study of PHP using melphalan in patients with unresectable hepatic malignancies.[74] A total of 74 procedures were performed in 28 patients. Twelve patients were treated at an initial melphalan dose of 2.0 mg/kg, which was then escalated to an MTD of 3.5 mg/kg over subsequent cohorts of 3 patients. The majority of the patients—21 in number (75%)—had received previous treatment for liver metastases. The patients who had not received previous treatment all had metastatic ocular melanoma. The most common grade III/IV toxicities were myelosuppression; mainly neutropenia and thrombocytopenia which were observed at all dose levels. Grade III/IV hepatic toxicity occurred after less than 20% of the treatments and was transient. The filtration efficiency ranged from 58.2 to 94.7% with a mean of 77%. The overall RR in 27 assessable patients was 30% (CR = 2, PR = 6). In patients with metastatic ocular melanoma, the overall RR was 50% (CR = 2, PR = 3). This study established the MTD of melphalan at

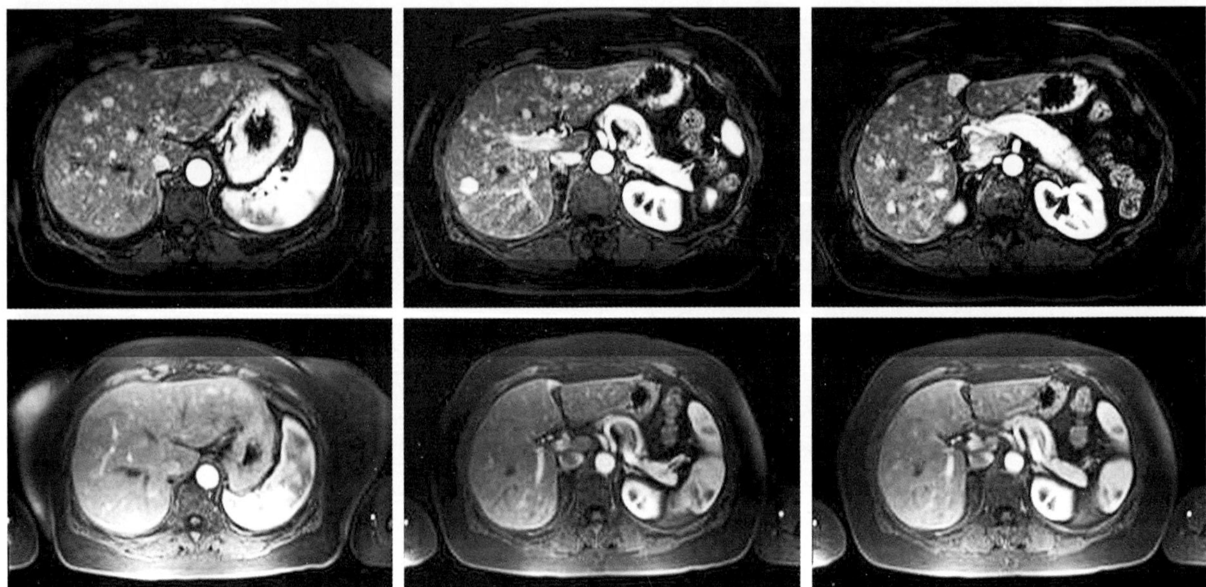

Figure 8 Gadolinium enhanced magnetic resonance images of a patient with diffuse liver metastases from ocular melanoma (top panels) and corresponding images taken 20 months after three PHP treatments

3.0 mg/kg; demonstrated that PHP could be performed with manageable toxicities and also, demonstrated anti-tumor effects for multiple histologies. Marked responses may be obtained after PHP as shown in Figure 8 from a patient with ocular melanoma liver metastases. A multicenter random assignment trial comparing PHP to best alternative care in patients with diffuse metastatic melanoma primarily isolated to the liver has recently been completed and demonstrated a significantly longer hepatic PFS in those treated with PHP.

CONCLUSION

Isolated hepatic perfusion is a liver-directed therapy that may be utilized to treat patients with unresectable liver metastases. Numerous studies in patients with various tumor histologies have generally demonstrated RRs of greater than 50% with transient morbidity and acceptable mortality. While systemic therapy remains the standard of care for the treatment of patients with unresectable CRC liver metastases, there may be a role for IHP in patients who are refractory to systemic therapy given the excellent RRs and OS that have been observed in these patients treated with IHP. For patients with unresectable ocular melanoma liver metastases, the role for IHP may be more significant because of the lack of efficacy and availability of other treatment options. The ability to perform PHPs may increase the role of hepatic perfusion for the treatment of multiple tumor histologies since this procedure allows for sequential treatments to be delivered with lower morbidity. The management of unresectable liver metastases is a significant clinical problem that requires the combined efforts of multiple providers to develop an integrated approach for each patient. Continued evaluation of hepatic perfusion in these patients is necessary so that the role of hepatic perfusion in this integrated approach can be more clearly defined.

REFERENCES

1. American Cancer Society. Colorectal Cancer Facts & Figures 2011-2013. Atlanta: American Cancer Society, 2011. Ref Type: Electronic Citation.
2. Leporrier J, Maurel J, Chiche L, et al. A population-based study of the incidence, management and prognosis of hepatic metastases from colorectal cancer. Br J Surg. 2006;93(4):465-74.
3. Scheele J, Stangl R, Altendorf-Hofmann A. Hepatic metastases from colorectal carcinoma: impact of surgical resection on the natural history. Br J Surg. 1990;77(11):1241-6.
4. Fuchs CS, Marshall J, Mitchell E, et al. Randomized, controlled trial of irinotecan plus infusional, bolus, or oral fluoropyrimidines in first-line treatment of metastatic colorectal cancer: results from the BICC-C study. J Clin Oncol. 2007;25(30):4779-86.
5. Goldberg RM, Sargent DJ, Morton RF, et al. A randomized controlled trial of fluorouracil plus leucovorin, irinotecan, and oxaliplatin combinations in patients with previously untreated metastatic colorectal cancer. J Clin Oncol. 2004;22(1):23-30.
6. Hurwitz H, Fehrenbacher L, Novotny W, et al. Bevacizumab plus irinotecan, fluorouracil, and leucovorin for metastatic colorectal cancer. N Engl J Med. 2004;350(23):2335-42.
7. Saltz LB, Clarke S, Díaz-Rubio E, et al. Bevacizumab in combination with oxaliplatin-based chemotherapy as first-line therapy in metastatic colorectal cancer: a randomized phase III study. J Clin Oncol. 2008;26(12):2013-9.
8. Tournigand C, Andre T, Achille E, et al. FOLFIRI followed by FOLFOX6 or the reverse sequence in advanced colorectal cancer: a randomized GERCOR study. J Clin Oncol. 2004; 22(2):229-37.
9. Tournigand C, Cervantes A, Figer A, et al. OPTIMOX1: a randomized study of FOLFOX4 or FOLFOX7 with oxaliplatin in a stop-and-Go fashion in advanced colorectal cancer—a GERCOR study. J Clin Oncol. 2006;24(3):394-400.
10. Van Cutsem E, Köhne CH, Hitre E, et al. Cetuximab and chemotherapy as initial treatment for metastatic colorectal cancer. N Engl J Med. 2009;360(14):1408-17.
11. Bidard FC, Tournigand C, André T, et al. Efficacy of FOLFIRI-3 (irinotecan D1,D3 combined with LV5-FU) or other irinotecan-based regimens in oxaliplatin-pretreated metastatic colorectal cancer in the GERCOR OPTIMOX1 study. Ann Oncol. 2009;20(6):1042-7.
12. Giantonio BJ, Catalano PJ, Meropol NJ, et al. Bevacizumab in combination with oxaliplatin, fluorouracil, and leucovorin (FOLFOX4) for previously treated metastatic colorectal cancer: results from the Eastern Cooperative Oncology Group Study E3200. J Clin Oncol. 2007;25(12):1539-44.
13. Peeters M, Price TJ, Cervantes A, et al. Randomized phase III study of panitumumab with fluorouracil, leucovorin, and irinotecan (FOLFIRI) compared with FOLFIRI alone as second-line treatment in patients with metastatic colorectal cancer. J Clin Oncol. 2010;28(31):4706-13.
14. Rothenberg ML, Cox JV, Butts C, et al. Capecitabine plus oxaliplatin (XELOX) versus 5-fluorouracil/folinic acid plus oxaliplatin (FOLFOX-4) as second-line therapy in metastatic colorectal cancer: a randomized phase III noninferiority study. Ann Oncol. 2008;19(10):1720-6.
15. Van Cutsem E, Bajetta E, Valle J, et al. Randomized, placebo-controlled, phase III study of oxaliplatin, fluorouracil, and leucovorin with or without PTK787/ZK 222584 in patients with previously treated metastatic colorectal adenocarcinoma. J Clin Oncol. 2011;29(15):2004-10.
16. Albert DM, Ryan LM, Borden EC. Metastatic ocular and cutaneous melanoma: a comparison of patient characteristics and prognosis. Arch Ophthalmol. 1996;114(1):107-8.
17. Bedikian AY, Legha SS, Mavligit G, et al. Treatment of uveal melanoma metastatic to the liver: a review of the M. D. Anderson Cancer Center experience and prognostic factors. Cancer. 1995;76(9):1665-70.
18. Bedikian AY, Papadopoulos N, Plager C, et al. Phase II evaluation of temozolomide in metastatic choroidal melanoma. Melanoma Res. 2003;13(3):303-6.

19. Pyrhönen S, Hahka-Kemppinen M, Muhonen T, et al. Chemoimmunotherapy with bleomycin, vincristine, lomustine, dacarbazine (BOLD), and human leukocyte interferon for metastatic uveal melanoma. Cancer. 2002;95(11):2366-72.
20. Mariani P, Piperno-Neumann S, Servois V, et al. Surgical management of liver metastases from uveal melanoma: 16 years‘ experience at the Institut Curie. Eur J Surg Oncol. 2009;35(11):1192-7.
21. Pawlik TM, Zorzi D, Abdalla EK, et al. Hepatic resection for metastatic melanoma: distinct patterns of recurrence and prognosis for ocular versus cutaneous disease. Ann Surg Oncol. 2006;13(5):712-20.
22. Rivoire M, Kodjikian L, Baldo S, et al. Treatment of liver metastases from uveal melanoma. Ann Surg Oncol. 2005; 12(6):422-8.
23. Chamberlain RS, Canes D, Brown KT, et al. Hepatic neuroendocrine metastases: does intervention alter outcomes?. J Am Coll Surg. 2000;190(4):432-45.
24. Moertel CG. Karnofsky memorial lecture. An odyssey in the land of small tumors. J Clin Oncol. 1987;5(10):1503-22.
25. Breedis C, Young G. The blood supply of neoplasms of the liver. Am J Pathol. 1954;30(5):969-77.
26. Creech O Jr, Krementz ET, Ryan RF, et al. Chemotherapy of cancer: regional perfusion utilizing an extracorporeal circuit. Ann Surg. 1958;148(4):616-32.
27. Ausman RK. Development of a technic for isolated perfusion of the liver. N Y State J Med. 1961;61:3393-7.
28. Stehlin JS Jr. Hyperthermic perfusion with chemotherapy for cancers of the extremities. Surg Gynecol Obstet. 1969;129(2):305-8.
29. Aigner K, Walther H, Tonn J, et al. First experimental and clinical results of isolated liver perfusion with cytotoxics in metastases from colorectal primary. Recent Results Cancer Res. 1983;86:99-102.
30. Schwemmle K, Link KH, Rieck B. Rationale and indications for perfusion in liver tumors: current data. World J Surg. 1987;11(4):534-40.
31. Skibba JL, Quebbeman EJ. Tumoricidal effects and patient survival after hyperthermic liver perfusion. Arch Surg. 1986;121(11):1266-71.
32. Lienard D, Ewalenko P, Delmotti JJ, et al. High-dose recombinant tumor necrosis factor alpha in combination with interferon gamma and melphalan in isolation perfusion of the limbs for melanoma and sarcoma. J Clin Oncol. 1992;10(1): 52-60.
33. Alexander HR Jr, Bartlett DL, Libutti SK, et al. Isolated hepatic perfusion with tumor necrosis factor and melphalan for unresectable cancers confined to the liver. J Clin Oncol. 1998;16(4):1479-89.
34. Hafström LR, Holmberg SB, Naredi PL, et al. Isolated hyperthermic liver perfusion with chemotherapy for liver malignancy. Surg Oncol. 1994;3(2):103-8.
35. Lindnér P, Fjälling M, Hafström L, et al. Isolated hepatic perfusion with extracorporeal oxygenation using hyperthermia, tumour necrosis factor alpha and melphalan. Eur J Surg Oncol. 1999;25(2):179-85.
36. Marinelli A, Vahrmeijer AL, van de Velde CJ. Phase I/II studies of isolated hepatic perfusion with mitomycin C or melphalan in patients with colorectal cancer hepatic metastases. Recent Results Cancer Res. 1998;147:83-94.
37. Zeh HJ 3rd, Brown CK, Holtzman MP, et al. A phase I study of hyperthermic isolated hepatic perfusion with oxaliplatin in the treatment of unresectable liver metastases from colorectal cancer. Ann Surg Oncol. 2009;16(2):385-94.
38. Alexander HR Jr, Libutti SK, Bartlett DL, et al. Hepatic vascular isolation and perfusion for patients with progressive unresectable liver metastases from colorectal carcinoma refractory to previous systemic and regional chemotherapy. Cancer. 2002;95(4):730-6.
39. Alexander HR Jr, Libutti SK, Pingpank JF, et al. Isolated hepatic perfusion for the treatment of patients with colorectal cancer liver metastases after irinotecan-based therapy. Ann Surg Oncol. 2005;12(2):138-44.
40. Alexander HR Jr, Bartlett DL, Libutti SK, et al. Analysis of factors associated with outcome in patients undergoing isolated hepatic perfusion for unresectable liver metastases from colorectal center. Ann Surg Oncol. 2009;16(7):1852-9.
41. Rothbarth J, Pijl ME, Vahrmeijer AL, et al. Isolated hepatic perfusion with high-dose melphalan for the treatment of colorectal metastasis confined to the liver. Br J Surg. 2003;90(11):1391-7.
42. van Iersel LB, Gelderblom H, Vahrmeijer AL, et al. Isolated hepatic melphalan perfusion of colorectal liver metastases: outcome and prognostic factors in 154 patients. Ann Oncol. 2008;19(6):1127-34.
43. van Iersel LB, Koopman M, van de Velde CJ, et al. Management of isolated nonresectable liver metastases in colorectal cancer patients: a case-control study of isolated hepatic perfusion with melphalan versus systemic chemotherapy. Ann Oncol. 2010;21(8):1662-7.
44. Cohen VM, Carter MJ, Kemeny A, et al. Metastasis-free survival following treatment for uveal melanoma with either stereotactic radiosurgery or enucleation. Acta Ophthalmol Scand. 2003;81(4):383-8.
45. Kujala E, Mäkitie T, Kivelä T. Very long-term prognosis of patients with malignant uveal melanoma. Invest Ophthalmol Vis Sci. 2003;44(11):4651-9.
46. Lorigan JG, Wallace S, Mavligit GM. The prevalence and location of metastases from ocular melanoma: imaging study in 110 patients. AJR Am J Roentgenol. 1991;157(6):1279-81.
47. McLaughlin CC, Wu XC, Jemal A, et al. Incidence of noncutaneous melanomas in the U.S. Cancer. 2005;103(5): 1000-1007.
48. Seregard S, Kock E. Prognostic indicators following enucleation for posterior uveal melanoma. A multivariate analysis of long-term survival with minimized loss to follow-up. Acta Ophthalmol Scand. 1995;73(4):340-4.
49. Singh AD, Topham A. Incidence of uveal melanoma in the United States: 1973-1997. Ophthalmology. 2003;110(5): 956-61.
50. Alexander HR, Libutti SK, Bartlett DL, et al. A Phase I-II study of isolated hepatic perfusion using melphalan with or without tumor necrosis factor for patients with ocular melanoma metastatic to liver. Clin Cancer Res. 2000;6(8):3062-70.
51. Alexander HR Jr, Libutti SK, Pingpank JF, et al. Hyperthermic isolated hepatic perfusion using melphalan for patients with ocular melanoma metastatic to liver. Clin Cancer Res. 2003;9(17):6343-9.

52. Noter SL, Rothbarth J, Pijl ME, et al. Isolated hepatic perfusion with high-dose melphalan for the treatment of uveal melanoma metastases confined to the liver. Melanoma Res. 2004;14(1):67-72.
53. van Iersel LB, Hoekman EJ, Gelderblom H, et al. Isolated hepatic perfusion with 200 mg melphalan for advanced noncolorectal liver metastases. Ann Surg Oncol. 2008;15(7): 1891-8.
54. Fiorentini G, Aliberti C, Del Conte A, et al. Intra-arterial hepatic chemoembolization (TACE) of liver metastases from ocular melanoma with slow-release irinotecan-eluting beads. Early results of a phase II clinical study. In Vivo. 2009; 23(1):131-7.
55. Gupta S, Bedikian AY, Ahrar J, et al. Hepatic artery chemoembolization in patients with ocular melanoma metastatic to the liver: response, survival, and prognostic factors. Am J Clin Oncol. 2010;33(5):474-80.
56. Huppert PE, Fierlbeck G, Pereira P, et al. Transarterial chemoembolization of liver metastases in patients with uveal melanoma. Eur J Radiol. 2010;74(3):e38-44.
57. Leyvraz S, Spataro V, Bauer J, et al. Treatment of ocular melanoma metastatic to the liver by hepatic arterial chemotherapy. J Clin Oncol. 1997;15(7):2589-95.
58. Mavligit GM, Charnsangavej C, Carrasco CH, et al. Regression of ocular melanoma metastatic to the liver after hepatic arterial chemoembolization with cisplatin and polyvinyl sponge. JAMA. 1988;260(7):974-6.
59. Peters S, Voelter V, Zografos L, et al. Intra-arterial hepatic fotemustine for the treatment of liver metastases from uveal melanoma: experience in 101 patients. Ann Oncol. 2006; 17(4):578-83.
60. Sato T, Eschelman DJ, Gonsalves CF, et al. Immunoembolization of malignant liver tumors, including uveal melanoma, using granulocyte-macrophage colony-stimulating factor. J Clin Oncol. 2008;26(33):5436-42.
61. Norheim I, Oberg K, Theodorsson-Norheim E, et al. Malignant carcinoid tumors. An analysis of 103 patients with regard to tumor localization, hormone production, and survival. Ann Surg. 1987;206(2):115-25.
62. Benevento A, Boni L, Frediani L, et al. Result of liver resection as treatment for metastases from noncolorectal cancer. J Surg Oncol. 2000;74(1):24-9.
63. Chen H, Hardacre JM, Uzra A, et al. Isolated liver metastases from neuroendocrine tumors: does resection prolong survival? J Am Coll Surg. 1998;187(1):88-92.
64. Que FG, Nagorney DM, Batts KP, et al. Hepatic resection for metastatic neuroendocrine carcinomas. Am J Surg. 1995;169(1):36-42.
65. Grover AC, Libutti SK, Pingpank JF, et al. Isolated hepatic perfusion for the treatment of patients with advanced liver metastases from pancreatic and gastrointestinal neuroendocrine neoplasms. Surgery. 2004;136(6):1176-82.
66. Cao CQ, Yan TD, Bester L, et al. Radioembolization with yttrium microspheres for neuroendocrine tumour liver metastases. Br J Surg. 2010;97(4):537-43.
67. Gaur SK, Friese JL, Sadow CA, et al. Hepatic arterial chemoembolization using drug-eluting beads in gastrointestinal neuroendocrine tumor metastatic to the liver. Cardiovasc Intervent Radiol. 2011;34(3):566-72.
68. Ho AS, Picus J, Darcy MD, et al. Long-term outcome after chemoembolization and embolization of hepatic metastatic lesions from neuroendocrine tumors. AJR Am J Roentgenol. 2007;188(5):1201-7.
69. Mazzaglia PJ, Berber E, Siperstein AE. Radiofrequency thermal ablation of metastatic neuroendocrine tumors in the liver. Curr Treat Options Oncol. 2007;8(4):322-30.
70. Saxena A, Chua TC, Bester L, et al. Factors predicting response and survival after yttrium-90 radioembolization of unresectable neuroendocrine tumor liver metastases: a critical appraisal of 48 cases. Ann Surg. 2010;251(5):910-6.
71. Beheshti MV, Denny DF Jr, Glickman MG, et al. Percutaneous isolated liver perfusion for treatment of hepatic malignancy: preliminary report. J Vasc Interv Radiol. 1992;3(3):453-8.
72. Curley SA, Newman RA, Dougherty TB, et al. Complete hepatic venous isolation and extracorporeal chemofiltration as treatment for human hepatocellular carcinoma: a phase I study. Ann Surg Oncol. 1994;1(5):389-99.
73. Ravikumar TS, Pizzorno G, Bodden W, et al. Percutaneous hepatic vein isolation and high-dose hepatic arterial infusion chemotherapy for unresectable liver tumors. J Clin Oncol. 1994;12(12):2723-36.
74. Pingpank JF, Libutti SK, Chang R, et al. Phase I study of hepatic arterial melphalan infusion and hepatic venous hemofiltration using percutaneously placed catheters in patients with unresectable hepatic malignancies. J Clin Oncol. 2005;23(15):3465-74.

Index

Page numbers followed by *f* refer to figure and *t* refer to table

E

F

G

H

I

K

L

Index